Premodern Health, Disease, and Disability

Premodern Health, Disease, and Disability is an interdisciplinary series devoted to all topics concerning health from all parts of the globe and including all premodern time periods: Antiquity, the Middle Ages and Early Modern. The series is global, including but not limited to Europe, the Middle East, the Mediterranean, and Asia. We encourage submissions examining medical care, such as health practitioners, hospitals and infirmaries, medicines and herbal remedies, medical theories and texts, care givers and therapies. Other topics pertinent to the scope of the series include research into premodern disability studies such as injury, impairment, chronic illness, pain, and all experiences of bodily and/or mental difference. Studies of diseases and how they were perceived and treated are also of interest. Furthermore, we are looking for works on medicinal plants and gardens; ecclesiastical and legal approaches to medical issues; archaeological and scientific findings concerning premodern health; and any other studies related to health and health care prior to 1800.

Gender, Health, and Healing, 1250-1550

Edited by
Sara Ritchey and
Sharon Strocchia

Amsterdam University Press

Cover illustration: *Saint Elizabeth of Hungary Washing a Leper*, 1480-1500, winged retable, Parish Church of St. Giles, Bardejov, Slovakia
By permission of the Institute for Material Culture, University of Salzburg

Cover design: Coördesign, Leiden
Typesetting: Crius Group, Hulshout

ISBN 978 94 6372 451 7
e-ISBN 978 90 4854 446 2 (pdf)
DOI 10.5117/9789463724517
NUR 684

Printed and bound by CPI Group (UK) Ltd, Croydon, CR0 4YY

Table of Contents

List of Figures and Tables

Figures

Tables

Acknowledgments

The editors wish to express their deepest gratitude to the many scholars and friends who have invested their intellectual energy, organizational talent, and good cheer in the making of this volume. The genesis of this collection was a 2018 workshop hosted by the a.r.t.e.s. Graduate School for the Humanities at the University of Cologne and organized by Eva-Maria Cersovsky and Ursula Gießmann. "Gender(ed) Histories of Health, Healing, and the Body, 1250-1550" aimed to situate questions about gender and medicine within the context of the broader social, cultural, religious, and economic concerns of this period. The workshop convened historians from far-flung countries, distinct disciplines, and all career stages, and thereby provided a generative forum for reflecting on the methodological and theoretical frameworks for producing histories of gender, health, and healing. The diverse sources and toolkits on display throughout the weekend enhanced the workshop's productive conversations and convinced the editors of this volume to continue and share those conversations in print. We are grateful to our organizers, fellow participants, and the University of Cologne for fostering such a long-lasting and fruitful dialogue.

From workshop to publication our efforts have been aided by a generous community of scholars who offered feedback and provided intellectual resources and inspiration that have greatly enriched the volume. We wish to single out in particular Montserrat Cabré, Joan Cadden, Sandra Cavallo, Monica Green, Mary Fissell, Katharine Park, and Linda Voigts. Both of the editors participated in Monica Green's NEH Summer Institute on Health and Disease in the Middle Ages, held at the Wellcome Library in 2009 and 2012, and are deeply grateful for the knowledge and ongoing mentoring she has provided. Our editors at Amsterdam University Press have given these essays an elegant home while ensuring a smooth publication process. Our sincere thanks to Walt Schalick, Wendy Turner, and Christina Lee, who first showed such enthusiasm for the project. Thanks also to Shannon Cunningham and Vicki Blud for guiding us from manuscript to print, and to the press's outside reviewers, Patricia Skinner and Joseph Ziegler, for offering thorough and constructive feedback.

Sara Ritchey would like to thank the history department at the University of Tennessee, which provided travel funding and leave time for research and writing undertaken for this volume. Sara is also incredibly grateful to Sharon Strocchia for envisioning this project from the get-go, for her generous invitation to serve as an editorial partner, and especially for the friendship and solidarity she has shared along the way. Sharon Strocchia would like to thank Emory University for ongoing research support that helped make this project possible. She also wishes to extend heartfelt thanks to Sara Ritchey, whose blazing intellect, boundless creativity, and positive attitude throughout the process made her the ideal teammate.

Abbreviations

dm. (pl. dms.)	dirham (a unit of weight)
KBR	Bibliothèque royale de Belgique (Koninklijke Bibliotheek and Bibliothèque royale)
BML 38	Boston Medical Library MS 38
BNCF	Biblioteca Nazionale Centrale di Firenze
Magl.	Magliabechiana
BNM VII 40	Biblioteca Nazionale Marciana, Latin VII 40

Introduction

Gendering Medieval Health and Healing: New Sources, New Perspectives

Sara Ritchey and Sharon Strocchia

The essays in *Gender, Health, and Healing, 1250-1550* take as their point of departure an integrative, hybrid model of analysis that illuminates the intersections between healthcare and other aspects of medieval and Renaissance culture.[1] Taking this integrative approach widens the lens from the narrow terrain of academic, text-based medicine to include common forms of health maintenance and curative practice such as bathing, prayer, the use of cosmetics and wellness products, and other methods of caring for the body and self. By situating a range of caregiving techniques within the more inclusive framework of 'health and healing', the essays place diverse strains of healthcare such as household medicine and spiritual-liturgical therapeutics on a continuum with academic medicine, and then show how these varied modes of healing interacted with and informed one another. The volume thus decentres theoretical medicine to make room for the lived experience of healthcare in all of its diversity at a formative moment in history. The period under examination here, ranging from the thirteenth to the sixteenth centuries, warrants particular scrutiny because it is commonly identified with the emergence of professional medicine as a distinct body of knowledge and practice.[2] During these centuries, university-trained physicians sought to assert their superior professional competencies, in part by laying claim to theoretical principles that governed the natural world

1 Green, 'Integrative Medicine', calls for an approach that incorporates the history of medicine, health, and body maintenance into other historical subdisciplines such as cultural, social, and political history. The essays here build on that call both by foregrounding healthcare practices and by channeling sources, methods, and insights from these subdisciplines in order to demonstrate the latitude of healthcare knowledge and practice in this period.

2 McVaugh, *Medicine before the Plague*, argues for both the medicalization of European life and the beginnings of professional medicine in the thirteenth and fourteenth centuries.

Ritchey, Sara & Sharon Strocchia (eds), *Gender, Health, and Healing, 1250-1550*. Amsterdam, Amsterdam University Press 2020
DOI: 10.5117/9789463724517_INTRO

and human bodies, and to which their extensive education and institutional affiliation gave them unique access.[3] The operation of gender shaped this process in fundamental ways by coding certain acts and identities as professional and others as informal or unskilled.

One of the most significant ways in which this volume achieves an integrative picture of late medieval and Renaissance healthcare is through the intentional expansion of the sources and methods that traditionally constitute medical history. The essays in this volume plumb a wide array of materials that run the gamut from the religious, domestic, and legal to the literary, homiletic, and visual. By taking a more capacious approach to sources beyond canonical texts, the volume showcases the sheer complexity of everyday caregiving and health maintenance in the late medieval and Renaissance period. Drawing on a broader palette of sources informs our understanding of how varieties of bodywork and caregiving were organized and practised on an aggregate social scale as well as in the more intimate realms of household and community. A number of sources used in this volume have been catalogued or 'coded' as religious, literary, household, and even legal sources that refer to matters of the home or ritual practice, rather than to health and healing. A principal aim of this volume, then, is to untether our sources from the categories that have obscured the complex terrain on which healthcare interactions unfolded in this period.

The volume enlarges the scholarly corpus for studying late medieval and Renaissance healthcare in three main ways: by unearthing completely new material or making it available in English translation for the first time; by mining sources whose medical value has been overlooked because they have been considered primarily as 'religious' or 'legal' in nature; and by rereading more familiar canonical sources from a gendered perspective. Some of the sources analysed here, such as manuscript and printed recipe books, belong to the domain of vernacular household medicine that has sparked tremendous interest in recent years. These troves of practical know-how not only substantiate women's widespread ownership of medical knowledge in late medieval and Renaissance societies, but also highlight the authority wielded by experiential knowledge within the domestic realm and beyond. Other types of sources examined in this volume, such as psalters, courtesy books, and manuals for Islamic market inspectors, have been considered either secondary or even unrelated to health and healing. This body of evidence has long been hiding in plain sight but has not been fully exploited

3 See, for example, the analysis by Cabré and Salmón of the dynamic of power and authority at work in the case of Jacoba Felicie in 'Poder académico *versus* autoridad femenina'.

for its 'medical' content. Still other essays in the volume view from new angles little-known medical treatises, vernacular health regimens, and surgeons' manuals, while several contributions tackle established theoretical discourses from both the Christian and Islamicate worlds. Reading this diverse evidence through a gendered lens opens new insights into such topics as breast care, infertility, balneotherapy, postsurgical care, and the corrosive properties of menstrual blood.

This more encompassing approach to source material yields a picture of medical multiplicity in which many varieties of healers tended to bodily needs within homes and princely courts, on city streets, at religious shrines, as well as in hospitals and religious communities. Consequently, these essays reimagine the lived experience of healthcare beyond the limited sphere of scholastic or theoretical medicine. They place on a mutually informing continuum acts of caring and curing, domestic and institutional settings for caregiving, and spiritual and physical approaches to healthcare. In so doing, the essays in this volume reveal the multiplicity of sites for the construction, storage, and transmission of body knowledge that was largely pragmatic in its orientation.[4] Widening the source base for medical history beyond authoritative discourses produces a richer, more nuanced picture of what people actually did to sustain or recover good health and the ways in which they understood their own bodies.

Excavating new or non-traditional sources requires imaginative thinking and painstaking research, but an even greater challenge is the question of how to conceptualize that evidence. The contributors to this volume deploy a variety of perspectives and interpretive frameworks that yield new angles of vision on late medieval and Renaissance healthcare. Borrowing insights from anthropology, feminist critique, the material turn, and contemporary healthcare practices, they document the plurality of medical knowledge and practice and uncover a range of unseen healers, healing practices, and bodily threats. In the process, the authors give sustained attention to knowledge categories that encompass the miraculous and affective, which traditionally have been regarded as unstable and thus unauthoritative means of understanding the body and physical world. They value knowledge claims and body experiences that were expressed in highly local contexts that never sought universal articulation, and recapture aspects of the orally driven, informal knowledge networks that informed the late medieval and Renaissance economy of health and healing.

4 Park, *Secrets of Women*, 82, notes that the body of knowledge amassed by household practitioners in this period was largely 'orally transmitted, experience-based, concrete and bodily oriented'.

The essays also experiment with innovative methods for reading sources in order to make meaning out of textual silences and other forms of 'non-evidence'. Even accounting for references to professional midwives, official records for the late medieval period demonstrate a genuine scarcity of female medical professionals.[5] In part, this absence stems from the fact that, in order to emerge as a distinct professional class, university-trained physicians simultaneously professed their superior knowledge of the body and belittled the untheorized experiential knowledge associated with female practitioners.[6] Consequently, relying on professional documents that were premised on an effort to subordinate feminine caregiving does little to substantiate the vital roles played by women healers in this period. Rather, as the essays collected here demonstrate, scholars must develop new ways of reading non-evidence and archival silences. The authors in this volume do so by valuing local descriptions of healthcare practices and by working creatively with fragmentary evidence.

The major methodological through-line uniting all of these essays, however, is the use of gender as a fundamental tool of analysis. This approach – which in itself is complex rather than uniform – illuminates both the sheer variety of medical care practised by women as well as the discursive constructions of gendered bodies. Studying discourses, spaces, and practices through a gendered lens makes visible healthcare activities performed within the home and other non-institutional settings that were not recorded in systematic, academic, or even 'official' records such as guild registers. Importantly, foregrounding gender enables the contributors to challenge traditional binaries that ahistorically separate health-related texts and practices; at the same time, it illuminates the epistemic and practical boundaries that have detached care from cure, medicine from religion, and domestic healing from paid labour. These separations have been highly consequential: they both conceal and devalue forms of healthcare labour as well as the body knowledge produced and transmitted outside the traditional settings of university, guild, and academy. Since informal nodes of knowledge and practice often constituted a continuum with academic medical theories, attending to the gendered nature of caregiving helps to elucidate the differently calibrated degrees of skill and knowledge involved in caring for the human body.

5 Green, 'Documenting Medieval Women's Medical Practice'. From the twelfth to fifteenth centuries in France, England, and Italy, the number of female specialists, including midwives, constituted between 1.2 and 1.5 per cent of the total population of professional healers. Similar disparities characterize the records in the Hispanic kingdoms.

6 Solomon, *Literature of Misogyny*; Wear, *Knowledge and Practice*, 62-64.

In adopting gender as a principal analytical lens, the contributors build on the work of several generations of feminist scholars who have probed the ways in which intellectual and institutional structures limit the visibility of female practitioners in late medieval and Renaissance societies. Generally speaking, earlier studies, such as Mélanie Lipinska's *Histoire des femmes médecins* and Eileen Power's 'Some Women Practitioners', examined individual cases of female practitioners, along with barriers to women's medical advancement. More recent works have harnessed the analytical power of gender to interrogate the systemic mechanisms of women's erasure from what we commonly understand to be histories of medicine.[7] Studies by Monica Green and Montserrat Cabré, for instance, have provided an interpretive framework for uncovering the presence of female practitioners in premodern medical regimes – one that is sensitive to mechanisms of knowledge transmission beyond the written text.[8]

One of their key conceptual interventions has been to problematize issues of occupational markers, including the absence of these markers within the semantic domain of 'woman'. The roles of women *as* women – that is, as sisters, mothers, daughters, friends, neighbours, and servants – included daily healthcare tasks that were not differentiated from their expected social roles of mothering, cooking, cleaning, and the performance of other routine chores. Cabré has affirmed the wide range of expert activities conducted by women in medieval households to maintain health and treat sickness.[9] Despite the skills involved, these forms of labour were not considered to be professional or full-time occupations, even when performed outside one's immediate household.[10] The makeshift, often situational nature of that work failed to generate the occupational markers that typically locate healthcare practitioners in medieval and early modern societies.

Moving away from professional titles, feminist scholars instead have portrayed women as 'agents of health' who cared for bodies while also

7 Lipinska, *Histoire des femmes médecins*; Power, 'Some Women Practitioners'; for a later period, see Walsh, *Doctors Wanted.* Other foundational works include Pelling, 'Thoroughly Resented', who first articulated the significance of the household as a locus of care; Duden, *Woman beneath the Skin*; and Klapisch-Zuber, 'Blood Parents and Milk Parents'.

8 Green, 'Books as a Source'. Green has shown that female practitioners were active in early Salernitan medical circles, only to be alienated from authoritative medicine due to impediments in accessing Latin texts. On this process see her *Making Medieval Medicine Masculine*.

9 Cabré, 'Women or Healers?'; Green, 'Bodies, Gender, Health, Disease', 3-6; Horden, 'Household Care and Informal Networks'.

10 The lawsuits filed by female household practitioners in late medieval Valencia document the valuable medical services they offered to their community, as well as the difficulties they encountered in obtaining compensation for them; Blumenthal, 'Domestic Medicine'.

facilitating or coordinating healthcare within households and institutions.[11] This reformulation not only opens the way to understanding the place of household medicine within a complex hierarchy of resort, it also underlines the fact that body knowledge acquired through domestic duties could be repurposed to serve broader public health agendas. In sixteenth-century London, for instance, poor elderly women who had amassed a panoply of nursing skills tended the parish sick as paid 'keepers'; this same group of women advanced public health initiatives in their role as 'searchers' of the dead, whose diagnoses formed the statistical backbone of English bills of mortality.[12] Similarly, married women in Italian and German cities carried out hospital work in medical partnerships organized around domestic models.[13]

Among the most critical interventions on display in this volume is the concept of 'bodywork' developed elsewhere by Mary Fissell.[14] This concept provides a crucial framework for thinking about the many varieties of caregivers that treated suffering bodies, as well as the different types of medical agency they exercised. The notion of bodywork reorients what it means to do the history of medieval and early modern medicine by encompassing a broad, highly variegated array of healers beyond such canonical actors as physicians, surgeons, and guild-licensed apothecaries. Bodywork immediately recognizes the value of healing activities performed by herbalists, empiricists, possessors of relics, shrine guards, wise women, and hospital nurses. It also underscores the practical know-how developed by mothers, sisters, daughters, beguines, birth attendants, and domestic servants who diagnosed ailments, made remedies, and tended ailing bodies without ever being identified by a professional title.

Other scholars have used the tools of gender analysis to uncover the social and cultural significance of 'female' and 'male' bodies, that is, the markers of sex difference and the bodily experience of gender in this period. For example, Joan Cadden has assessed how medical, theological, and philosophical discourses intersected when covering topics such as reproduction, embryology, and sexual pleasure.[15] The gendered understandings of

11 Green coined this term in 'Bodies, Gender, Health, Disease'.

12 Munkhoff, 'Poor Women and Parish Public Health'; Munkhoff, 'Searchers of the Dead'.

13 Stevens Crawshaw, 'Families, Medical Secrets and Public Health'; Kinzelbach, 'Women and Healthcare'.

14 Fissell, 'Introduction', 11. In proposing the concept of 'bodywork' Fissell builds on previous scholarship such as Cavallo's notion of 'artisans of the body', Cabré's notion of modification of body surfaces in 'From a Master to a Laywoman', and Green's term 'technologies of the body' in 'Bodies, Gender, Health, Disease'.

15 Cadden, *Meanings of Sex Difference*.

physiology and anatomy that learned male authors produced were sometimes conflicting, at other times mutually reinforcing, but always multivalent and complex.[16] According to these intellectual traditions, the most basic distinction between the sexes was the uterus, which was defined by its function in menstruation, conception, and the generation of offspring. This singular physiological difference cast the uterus as an 'enigmatic space where both life and knowledge began' and launched a whole genre of texts investigating 'the secrets of women'.[17] Discussions of women's 'secrets' in Latin and vernacular texts often fashioned women's bodies as dangerous and women themselves as untrustworthy; yet they also demonstrate a genuine thirst for practical knowledge of gynecology, obstetrics, contraception, and fertility among non-elite practitioners.

Several essays in this volume advance this discussion by emphasizing the importance of bodily function in medieval explanations of sex difference. Stressing the centrality of the uterus and its function within the humoral system, they show how that very centrality became a means of naturalizing certain characteristics for women, such as nurturing and compassion. Their analyses implicitly challenge the argument regarding the prevalence of a 'one-sex model' proposed by Thomas Laqueur, which has enjoyed tremendous staying power among scholars since its publication in 1990.[18] Relying on Galen's fragmentary discussion of the 'one-sex model' in his *The Uses of Parts*, Laqueur asserted that, until the eighteenth century, Europeans operated with an understanding that there was only one sex, based on inverted morphological similarities between male and female genitals. It was the performance of gender, rather than differentiated sex organs, that determined social hierarchies among male and female. While there certainly were some medieval traditions that recapitulated the one-sex model, late medieval and Renaissance notions of sex difference were hardly monolithic.[19] The authors in this volume provide a more nuanced picture by showing that contemporary explications of sex difference hinged on function far more than on morphology or form.

In foregrounding gender as an analytical tool, this collection intersects with other recent work that seeks to enlarge our understanding of medical culture

16 Although the authors surveyed are primarily male, Cadden does include a discussion of Hildegard of Bingen, 70-87. On gender and sex difference in intellectual traditions, see also Park, *Secrets of Women*, and DeVun, 'Jesus Hermaphrodite'.

17 Park, *Secrets of Women*, 35.

18 Laqueur, *Making Sex*.

19 For criticisms of Laqueur's 'one-sex' thesis, see Cadden, *Meanings of Sex Difference*, 3; Park and Nye, 'Destiny is Anatomy'; and King, *One-Sex Body on Trial*.

in this period. The essays in *Medicine, Religion and Gender in Medieval Culture* (2015) similarly argue that gender allows us to think in expansive ways about what 'counts' as medicine.[20] Both collections feature an array of medieval texts – mystical, legal, literary, hagiographic – that reveal the conceptual interdependence of physical and spiritual health and the many different kinds of practitioners that tended to matters of health. Despite sharing a rich feminist legacy, however, the two collections differ in significant ways. The essays in the 2015 collection focused primarily on language and representation – the points 'where literature and medicine collide' – rather than on knowledge and practice, which take centre stage here. Broadly speaking, they examined medical discourse and metaphorical language as a way to better understand literary production, religious experience, and the causal dimensions of sin. By contrast, the essays in the present volume mine documents of practice such as hospital statutes and monastic inventories, literary and hagiographic texts, and material artefacts in order to produce a more comprehensive picture of medieval and Renaissance healthcare – one that includes its caregiving dimensions. This expanded source palette allows the authors to probe some of the under-represented ways that both practitioners and patients negotiated healthcare resources, as when nurses at the Paris Hôtel-Dieu protested their working conditions or when parturient women sought assistance from relics held by a local abbey. Still another difference between the two volumes is geographic. The present collection extends well beyond the earlier volume's tight focus on English and Anglo-French communities to encompass the Mediterranean and to connect it to parts of northern Europe. Putting northern European healthcare practices in conversation with those circulating throughout the Mediterranean basin emphasizes the transregional, cross-confessional construction of humoral knowledge that made it highly adaptable to local practices and faith traditions.

Indeed, the widened geographic scope on display in this volume reflects increasing contact between multiple cultures, languages, and faith traditions in late medieval and Renaissance societies. In this sense, the volume participates in aspects of the 'global turn' currently transforming the field of medieval and early modern studies. Scholars have increasingly recognized that areas within overlapping contact zones shared common experiences with plague outbreaks, and that their disease environments were increasingly integrated by commercial circuits.[21] These interactions occurred

20 Yoshikawa, ed., *Medicine, Religion and Gender.*

21 For the integration of disease environments across broad geographic regions, see Green, ed., *Pandemic Disease in the Medieval World*, and Varlik, *Plague and Empire.*

on multiple scales. Microhistorical evidence, for instance, demonstrates that medically aware travellers utilized a variety of medical traditions when traversing the maritime highways between the Mediterranean and Indian Ocean.[22] Archaeological evidence, meanwhile, establishes extensive borrowings in the spatial architecture of hygienic practice as witnessed, for example, in the Abbasid *hammams* of Spain and the Maghreb, which were adapted from earlier Umayyad traditions, which themselves had evolved from a previous Byzantine model.[23] On an even broader scale, the acceleration of exchanges between and across the Mediterranean basin, the Atlantic world, and Asian maritime colonies after 1500 cross-pollinated practical knowledge and exposed practitioners to new materia medica. Even within more localized settings, however, vernacular health regimens and 'books of secrets' facilitated the circulation of medical knowledge in both Latin and various vernaculars within the heady mix created by manuscript, print, and orality.[24] Differences in language or confession apparently did not pose insurmountable barriers to exchange; in fact, confessional and linguistic differences may have enlarged the scope of local body knowledge and healthcare practice in some instances.[25]

The essays in *Gender, Health, and Healing* mine this hybridity and exchange by considering the multiple pathways through which knowledge transfers took place in these centuries. Specialists and everyday caretakers conveyed practical and theoretical knowledge about the body through professional texts, vernacular regimens and compilations, oral communications, demonstrations of practice, and observation and exchange of the implements of care. As several of the essays show, the vernacularization

22 Lambourn, *Abraham's Luggage*, 219-39, discusses the medicinal substances carried by a twelfth-century Jewish trader who shuttled between Egypt and the western Indian Ocean, which borrowed from Indic, Islamic, and Jewish medical traditions.

23 Boisseuil, ed., *Le bain: espaces et pratiques*, explores bathing practices among Jewish, Christian, and Muslim communities in the Mediterranean. See Cressier, 'Prendre les eaux', for a discussion of Andalusian *hammams*. As with *mikva'ot* constructed for Jewish women, the sex segregation that characterized bathing practices points to the bath as a potential site of feminine transmission of body knowledge; see Marienberg, 'Le bain des Melunaises'.

24 Cavallo and Storey, *Healthy Living*; Leong and Rankin, 'Introduction: Secrets and Knowledge'; Strocchia, *Forgotten Healers*; and more generally, Fissell, 'Marketplace of Print'. Nicoud, *Les régimes de santé*, provides a comprehensive study of the origins and diffusion of health regimens before the age of print.

25 For example, around 1400 three Muslim midwives, Marién, Seynça, and Xency, were summoned to attend at the childbed of the Christian Queen Leonor, who must have desired the particular form of care these women could provide. On this case, see Narbona-Cárceles, 'Woman at Court'. Green also discusses these women in terms of the professionalization of midwifery in 'Bodies, Gender, Health, Disease', 24-25.

of medical knowledge from the twelfth century onward not only enabled the translation of learned medical concepts into local idioms, it also created new forms of knowledge by adapting and blending local and traditional practices with humoral theories and professional standards. The process of vernacularization thus encouraged the decentralization of medical discourses. English medical literature from the late fourteenth century provides a good case in point. Linda Voigts has shown that the production and circulation of medical and scientific texts in Middle English and Anglo-Latin increased dramatically in this period, with Latin transcriptions often appearing next to English treatises in a single codex.[26] These hybrid texts speak volumes about the heterogeneous nature of their audiences.[27] Several essays in this collection extend our understanding of the process of medical vernacularization into early Renaissance France and Italy, where female householders in cities and courts put learned discourse to practical uses in their quest to sustain healthy households and familial interests. They highlight the fact that vernacularization not only braided different kinds of know-how across linguistic and geographical settings, but also frequently involved first-hand experimentation by practitioners eager to develop effective remedies for everyday ailments.

Often, the acquisition and transfer of body knowledge evaded textual documentation altogether. Scholars such as Pamela Smith and Pamela Long have called attention to the importance of embodied knowledge developed by artisans, makers, and practitioners through repeated, hands-on experience over time.[28] This kind of sensory-based, experiential knowledge of the body and the natural world gained greater legitimacy throughout the later

26 Voigts, 'What's the Word? Bilingualism in Late-Medieval England'. In conjunction with Patricia Deery Kurtz, Voigts compiled a database of over 7,700 scientific and medical manuscript texts in Old and Middle English, which is accessible through the *Voigts-Kurtz Search Program*. More recently, Orlemanski, *Symptomatic Subjects*, has explored how the vernacularization and broad dissemination of medical texts in England created new subjectivities.

27 Solomon, *Fictions of Well-Being*, illustrates a similar process in Iberia, where the medical text came to stand in for the professional practitioner. It is also worth noting that the editors of the three-volume primary source anthology, *Women Writing Latin*, call into question the patriarchal and literary canonicity of Latin in the Middle Ages, arguing that there was a 'complicated relationship' between Latin literacy and the development of European vernaculars. They posit that women as producers of Latin texts can be re-embedded into medieval textual culture by focusing on non-literary and collaborative texts; Churchill et al., eds., *Women Writing Latin*.

28 Recent studies of embodied knowledge include P. Smith et al., eds., *Ways of Making and Knowing*; P. Smith, *Body of the Artisan*; and Long, *Artisan/Practitioners and the Rise of the New Sciences*.

Middle Ages and Renaissance. Although embodied knowledge was one of the most important 'ways of knowing' in premodern societies, it is nevertheless difficult to grasp textually or systematically because it was inherently oral, performative, or even liturgical in nature. Rather than being transmitted through texts, embodied knowledge was acquired and circulated through some combination of verbal instruction, informal learning arrangements, and repeated practice, often under the tutelage of a skilled practitioner. The concept of embodied knowledge is central to understanding how medieval and Renaissance women developed and transferred their understandings of regimen, as well as their knowledge of herbal properties, distilling methods, bathing therapies, and other healing skills.[29]

Building on these notions, the essays in this volume recognize that not all sites of knowledge production, storage, and transmission are textual, even though texts can often communicate certain instantiations. Several authors consider the ways in which material objects, collective work arrangements, and the spatial choreography of caregiving facilitated the circulation of embodied knowledge within everyday settings. In so doing, they enlist commonplace objects such as the bathtub and the prayerbook as medical technologies that speak to local, communal circumstances of knowledge exchange; they also highlight the diverse sites and spatial dimensions of care, ranging from the bedside in sixteenth-century German households to stalls in the Syrian marketplace. These thoughtful examinations simultaneously extend the spatial reach of gendered medical interactions while nuancing the class distinctions at play within them.

Other essays allow us to glimpse aspects of embodied knowledge by focusing on what Peregrine Horden has called 'the non-natural environment'.[30] The non-natural environment refers to the six external factors that influenced bodily health in humoral medicine that spanned both Galenic and Arabic systems. The Islamicate physician Hunyan ibn-Ishaq (d. 873 CE) delineated these factors as air, food and drink, diet and rest, sleeping and waking, evacuation and retention, and the passions of the soul.[31] These principles, whose influence varied over time, may have gained greater traction in medieval life as a result of the health regimens proliferating in the thirteenth and fourteenth centuries. Although the non-naturals threaded through distinct humoral systems, they still needed to be adapted to local

29 Rankin, *Panaceia's Daughters*, 139-59, discusses the keen attention to detail and technique involved in making household remedies, which was considered to be a type of skilled handiwork.

30 Horden, 'Non-Natural Environment'.

31 Maurach, ed., 'Johannicius', 160.

circumstances, especially since the non-natural environment encompassed everyday activities such as prayer, pilgrimage, reading, and bathing.[32] Within the household itself, female householders helped manage the non-naturals on a daily basis. Their roles as guardians of healthy living became especially apparent with the resurgence of a preventive paradigm in Italian urban centres after 1500.[33] Friends, family, and caregivers attended to the non-naturals in other ways by helping the sick re-establish a sense of physical and emotional equilibrium through letters, personal visits, and spiritual consolation.[34] Foregrounding the complexity of healing, the essays in this volume urge a rethinking of the historical trajectories that have placed the epistemological centre of gravity in cure rather than care, in academic texts rather than everyday practice, in stable interpretations of basic health principles rather than local and historical variations.

The chapters of this book are organized thematically into four sections that make visible gendered medical practices and the transmission of gendered medical discourse from different angles. This scheme moves topically from religious healing to knowledge production, from infirmity and care to reproductive matters. At the same time, the essays share numerous points of contact that cut across sections. Running throughout the volume are common concerns with bodywork and vernacular knowledge-making; relationships between gender and bodily function that underpinned understandings of sex difference; and innovative ways of making meaning from 'non-evidence'. The volume concludes with an elegant afterword that draws many of these strands together and reflects on directions for future research.

The essays in Part 1, 'Sources of Religious Healing', harness religious sources, specifically psalters and miracle tales, to illuminate the ways that women used prayer, liturgy, pilgrimage, and saintly intercession as an integral component of healthcare practice. They focus on the broader therapeutic role played by seemingly 'religious' texts and objects such as sermons, miracle stories, records of charity, and theological doctrines, which

32 Recent studies of therapeutic reading include McCann, *Soul-Health*; Solomon, *Fictions of Well-Being*; and Olson, *Literature as Recreation*; on music, see Horden, ed., *Music as Medicine*.

33 Cavallo and Storey, *Healthy Living*; see also Cavallo and Storey, eds., *Conserving Health in Early Modern Culture*.

34 Weisser, *Ill Composed*; Strocchia, *Forgotten Healers*, 67-84. Women's epistolary networks have become rich terrain for exploring the circulation of vernacular medical knowledge in the late medieval and early modern period; see inter alia Whitaker, 'Reading the Paston Letters Medically'; Rankin, *Panaceia's Daughters*.

encompassed important healthcare knowledge and practice.[35] As the essays in this section attest, body knowledge existed in the common tradition of religious communities and cults, and in the patterns of repeated practice embodied in liturgical rhythms.

The opening essay by Sara Ritchey navigates the apparent 'absence' of professional medical treatises in women's religious communities by examining the kinds of books women *did* possess: psalters. Archaeological and archival evidence confirm the caregiving mission of the beguines of St. Christopher in Liège, who maintained historic ties with the hospital of St. Christopher and even founded their own hospital and leprosarium. Ritchey therefore asks how their prayer life may have informed their presence in hospitals and at bedsides. Although psalters have typically been understood as 'religious' or 'liturgical' books, Ritchey shows that the prayers, illuminations, and poetry inscribed within a psalter from St. Christopher's (Liège, Bibliothèque de l'Université MS 431) would have fit comfortably into a non-natural environment oriented toward hospital care. Borrowing methods from anthropology and linguistics, she emphasizes the function of performative language in wielding efficacious bedside care. The psalter, she argues, acted as a technology that structured caregiving interactions between patients and their beguine custodians, while also enabling beguines to maintain their own regimens of self-care. As a result, she opens up a new body of evidence – psalters – for thinking about how religious women would have drawn on their skills in the performance of prayer, liturgy, and regimen, as well as the modulation of the passions in order to serve as occasional healthcare practitioners.

In a similar vein, Iliana Kandzha examines the miracles of the German empress St. Cunigunde, outlining the female clientele of the cult seeking her medical intervention. She approaches cult activity with a wide-angle lens to show how sources that scholars typically have interpreted as reflecting religious life can be harnessed to illuminate gendered patterns of healthcare behaviour. In the first century after Cunigunde's death in 1033, the miracles recorded at the Bavarian shrine of this virgin saint demonstrated no discernible preference toward female petitioners. However, by the fifteenth century in faraway Leuven, manuscript evidence such as relic registers and account books indicates the proliferation of material objects supporting Cunigunde's role in facilitating 'an easy delivery in childbirth'. A devotional manuscript used by the Augustinian canonesses at Bethlehem and a cache

35 On the perils of applying 'religion' as an analytical category to premodern peoples, see J. Smith, 'Religion, Religions, Religious'.

of relics (including the saint's girdle and mantle) kept at Bamberg Cathedral and the Benedictine abbey of Michelsberg signify the development of a cult dedicated to Cunigunde's potent intercession in childbirth. Because these obstetric objects represent a localized healthcare practice and a later efflorescence of miraculous activity, they have not been integrated into scholarship on childbirth rituals or on Cunigunde's saintly activity. Kandzha thus elucidates the ways that the economy of relics served as an important source of healing for parturient women during a time when childbirth had not yet been fully medicalized.

The essays in Part 2, 'Producing and Transmitting Medical Knowledge', turn to little-known or recently discovered texts to examine masculine medical constructions of the female body, on the one hand, and feminine constructions of medical knowledge, on the other. Montserrat Cabré and Fernando Salmón examine two medieval medical commentaries on a Hippocratic aphorism to reveal how physicians yoked madness to lactation problems and thus to mothering. Their careful attention to this medical tradition uncovers an interpretive model for understanding female bodies as physiologically predisposed to manic conditions; in the process, they highlight the flexibility of the humoral system and late medieval imaginings of the female body as fundamentally characterized by the function of menstruation.

The co-authors analyse a series of Latin treatises on transformational 'failures' within women's bodies. First, they discuss the condition known as *fascination*. Two Spanish physicians writing in the late fifteenth and early sixteenth centuries, Diego Álvarez Chanca and Antonio de Cartagena, effectively brought this new disease category into being when they described the harmful effects that the accumulation of venomous menstrual blood could have on a woman's body. Because women's health depended on the function of menstruation, these physicians theorized that when menstrual blood stopped 'flowering' it could become potentially poisonous. Humoral epistemology in this period required that blood had to go *somewhere* in order to maintain balance in the fluid economy of the body; hence, the physicians surmised that women's bodies must have expelled the venomous menstrual vapours through their eyes. The vapours then corrupted the air where they threatened to be absorbed into the pores of weak bodies, like those of children. Sudden, inexplicable illnesses or death thus could be blamed on the fascination caused by elderly women. Turning to the dreaded condition of the 'bloodbreast', Cabré and Salmón also note a central paradox in late medieval understandings of female bodies: how was it possible that the generative maternal body could also be potentially venomous? Their exploration of Latin commentaries on a Hippocratic aphorism regarding 'bloodbreast' demonstrates how late medieval physicians wrestled with this paradox. Bloodbreast referred to menstrual blood that failed to properly transform into breast milk, thus causing toxic vapours to rise into the brain where mania set in. Latin authors such as Taddeo Alderotti and Ugo Benzi reconciled the nutritive maternal body with the insufficient one by positing a late onset of the effects of mania. As Cabré and Salmón show, it was the flexibility of the humoral system that enabled physicians to simultaneously uphold the imagined fatal capacities of the elderly female body, the maniacal body beset by bloodbreast, and the idealized maternal body.

The next essay by Belle Tuten continues elements of this discussion by focusing on female physiology and breast care, but shifts the analysis toward vernacular practice and the hybridization of medical knowledge. Tuten studies a short, fifteenth-century Italian medical treatise devoted to breast care, particularly to painful problems accompanying lactation. This little treatise combined sections from the *Lilium medicine* of Bernard de Gordon with original recipes for treating various breast complaints with home-made plasters and poultices. Tuten situates this text within medieval discourses on breastfeeding, as well as within vernacular concerns about maternal health emerging in Italian Renaissance cities. In the fifteenth century, Italian merchants and humanists alike cultivated deep interests in the family, as evidenced by scores of genealogies, family diaries, and vernacular writings. Although this treatise bears no specific authorship or date, its sharp focus on breast complaints spoke to common problems experienced by affluent new mothers as well as paid wet nurses. Tuten also transcribes one of the treatise's original recipes, which utilized ordinary, inexpensive ingredients confected through relatively simple processes – an excellent example of what has often been called 'kitchen physic'. Female householders could readily manufacture this remedy for themselves, their friends and neighbours, and perhaps even their hired wet nurses. Tuten's detailed attention to this treatise allows us to trace with some degree of precision the ways in which academic medicine and household medical knowledge were combined and disseminated.

Continuing the exploration of vernacular knowledge production, Sheila Barker and Sharon Strocchia examine a recently discovered volume of the encyclopedic recipe collection compiled by the Italian noblewoman Caterina Sforza in the early sixteenth century. They demonstrate how the genre of recipe books reflects the experimental terrain on which Renaissance women could engage in medical and scientific discourse. The vast range of Sforza's recipe collection – much of which was tested empirically – included magical incantations, distilling techniques, veterinary medicine, cosmetics, and household remedies focused on common ailments, reproduction, and female sexuality. What united this miscellany was an overarching principle of utility and pragmatism. Barker and Strocchia argue that these 'secrets' must be read intentionally within the context of a household economy writ large – one that simultaneously served the health needs and the political objectives of a Renaissance court. Besides enlarging Sforza's medical and scientific legacy, this newfound manuscript highlights the authority wielded by experiential knowledge within the domestic realm and beyond. At an unknown date, her recipe collection was methodically censored and its contents expunged of all recipes that trafficked in 'magic'. The authors are aided in the task of reading this 'non-evidence' by the discovery of a partial, separate index that documents the excised recipes. Their reconstruction of now-lost evidence reveals how shifting intellectual regimes reshaped the parameters of licit medicine, science, and religion.

The final essay in this section, by Julia Gruman Martins, shows how medical authors capitalized on early print technologies to disseminate knowledge about the female body to a broad vernacular audience. Martins takes us into a world of household knowledge and control of the body by examining how printers and translators adapted one of the earliest 'books of secrets' – the *Dificio di ricette* (House of secrets), first published in Venice in 1529 – in order to satisfy new readers when translating its contents from Italian to French. This cheaply printed booklet, whose influence extended well into the nineteenth century, included ten recipes that both instructed readers about the workings of the female body and facilitated control over them, especially in matters of reproduction. Martins demonstrates how several strands became intricately intertwined in the process of knowledge-making. Female readers could utilize the recipes, practices, and experimental models put forward to actively regulate their own bodies. With the help of this book, they could manage the periodicity, quality, and quantity of menstruation, assure conception, and answer questions about future children. At the same time, clever translators had to adapt the recipes to differing market conditions such as the availability and cost of key ingredients. Martins argues that the publication of the *Dificio* can be considered a turning point in the broader dissemination of vernacular knowledge about the female body in the multiple ways it took readers' concerns into account.

Part 3, 'Infirmity and Care', tackles the medical significations of feminine caregiving in domestic settings. Eva-Maria Cersovsky's essay derives significant meaning from a short biblical proverb taken from the book of Sirach. This proverb, 'Ubi non est mulier, ingemiscit egens', appears in numerous late medieval texts, ranging from conduct manuals to hospital ordinances and literary tracts. In each case, it reflected the role of women as *women* in the provision of effective caregiving. Sometimes this proverb was used to question or even parody a wife's duty to assist a sick or needy husband, as when Chaucer and Rabelais expressed through it an underlying unease with the power women might yield over weakened husbands and their wealth. At other times, it was cited to naturalize women's association with charity, compassion, and almsgiving; for example, both the thirteenth-century statutes governing the hospital of Spoleto and sixteenth-century Parisian hospital legislation invoked this proverb when appealing to religious women's ideals of compassion and service to the sick poor. Cersovsky also observes, particularly in the *querelle des femmes* literature that debated 'womanly' virtues, an Aristotelian framing of sex difference based in the colder, softer nature of women's bodies – a trait that 'naturally' inclined women to pity. For instance, the sixteenth-century humanist physician and theologian Henricus Cornelius Agrippa conjoined the proverb to an Aristotelian construction of women's bodies as naturally suited to caregiving, citing their breast milk as a physical manifestation of their bodily capacity for healing. Contrary to the *fascinatio* treatises discussed by Cabré and Salmón, Agrippa also praised the salubrious powers of menstrual blood for healing both physical and psychological ailments. Through such constructions, the proverb naturalized women's caregiving capacities so completely as to render their very bodies as sources of healing, transforming customary caregiving roles into thaumaturgic flesh.

Utilizing a combination of visual analysis, thick description, and contemporary theories of caregiving, Cordula Nolte interrogates a wide array of sources in order to query the extent to which domestic care was a gendered field of action in sixteenth-century Germany. By attending closely to furnishings, equipment, objects, and bodily choreography, she illuminates the means by which the spatial, material, and performative dimensions of household care were gendered. Her detailed attention to the spatial arrangements for caregiving and its material instruments – for instance, the placement of beds in relation to the heated centre of the house – shows that even domestic spaces were characterized by various vectors of gendered activity. Echoing the biblical proverb discussed above, Nolte gives medical meaning to the scandalous decision made by Bartholomäus Sastrow, mayor of Stralsund, to marry his wife's caretaker shortly after her death. The newly widowed Sastrow feared dying from a suffocating cough; his perceived survival depended so deeply on the intimate presence of a woman dedicated to his care that he was willing to risk social criticism resulting from a hasty cross-class marriage. Moving nimbly across different scales of analysis, Nolte reconstructs urban networks of care that relied on poor women who worked as travelling nurses or who opened their homes to care for the infirm. In tracing these support networks, she demonstrates that domestic and institutional spheres were linked, even when they were spatially separate. Further, by examining the illustration scheme in a German surgical manual for herniotomy, Nolte reveals an intricate choreography of care in which women acted as key bedside caregivers who learned the intricacies of wound care by observing surgeons and other practitioners. In these sensitive readings, Nolte elicits evidence from silence: that is, from bodily performances that took place at a distance from texts.

Turning from a European Christian context of care to an Ottoman Mediterranean one, Ayman Yasin Atat delves into the pharmaceutical encyclopedia written by the fifteenth-century Ottoman physician, Muhammed ibn Maḥmūd al-Shirwānī, in order to examine the therapeutic uses of the bathtub as a home remedy. In this essay, Atat provides the first English-language translation of al-Shirwānī's thirty-third chapter of the *Rawḍat al-ʿiṭr* (Garden of pharmacy/perfumes) devoted to bathtub remedies. Atat's analysis of both the medical conditions and materia medica described in this chapter of the compendium demonstrates the continuity of bathtub therapeutics among Arabic and Ottoman physicians. Bathtubs provided an ideal form of household medicine for several reasons. They permitted external remedies to achieve a significant amount of contact with the skin surface; users gained additional benefits from exposure to the warm water prescribed in treatment; and the therapy could be applied at home without the patient's need to leave, thereby eliminating the difficulties associated with out-of-home treatments. This latter advantage could be especially important in cases of severe pain. Moreover, the ready availability of ingredients prescribed in al-Shirwānī's remedies, which often included ordinary culinary materials, suggests additional reasons for the longevity of this therapy. As Atat observes, the elaboration of this accessible therapy within a formal medical treatise points to the more authoritative standing commanded by household medicine in the mid-fifteenth-century Islamicate world.

The fourth and final section, '(In)Fertility and Reproduction', turns to the intersection of gender and generation. Catherine Rider investigates medieval discussions of sex difference, focusing in particular on the problem of infertility among both sexes. Although the loss of fertility in the aging female body is a paramount concern today, Rider shows that medieval discussions of infertility factored age more prominently than gender. Examining a wide range of Latin texts authored by university-trained physicians from the late eleventh to the fifteenth centuries, she demonstrates an increasing interest and growing level of detail in discussions of infertility. Borrowing heavily from the influx of Islamicate medical treatises, in particular those of Ibn Sīnā and Ibn al-Jazzār, learned medical writers in Europe argued that old age rendered both men's and women's bodies unfit for reproduction, because age similarly affected the quality of their seed and humoral balance. In discussions of age and fertility, then, physicians considered men's and women's bodies in fairly comparable terms so that gender was only one factor affecting fertility rates. Additionally, Rider shows that *practicas* and other specialized treatises on infertility and reproduction authored by physicians found wider audiences in vernacular translations, testifying to a desire among non-elites for practical knowledge about the body and reproduction.

Finally, Sara Verskin's essay on gender segregation in Islamicate medical practice challenges reigning assumptions through a close reading of assorted medical and legal texts. Historians of the last century have largely recapitulated paradigms of modesty that dictated limitations on male contact with female bodies in medieval Islamicate medical practice. By taking a broad chronological, geographic, and typological view of gynecological interactions, Verskin shows that Muslim women did indeed receive gynecological care from male professional practitioners, while revealing the multiple occasions on which female agents could act as trained medical intermediaries. For example, she notes that treatises on medical ethics included many 'conversational' moments that warn against women learning about contraceptives and abortifacients. These exhortations point to social situations in which medical practitioners presumed that women *might* encounter this information. Elsewhere, Verskin notes that jurists writing law books simply assumed that female nudity was an expected component of medical care. Consequently, they outlined a hierarchy of factors, such as religion, familial relationship, and age, for selecting an appropriate practitioner. Verskin also draws on books of *ḥisba*, or manuals for market inspectors, to show that male phlebotomists treated women by cupping and bleeding; her examination of medical ethics literature demonstrates that male practitioners regularly engaged with women in pulse taking and urinalysis. Still other sources point to medical collaborations between male and female practitioners. Surgical treatises indicated that a skilled woman should carry out intimate procedures, while other medical compendia present various obstetric tasks to be performed by the male physician, midwives, female attendants, or sometimes by the patient herself. By attending to the many interactions occurring in diverse sites of care,

Verskin shows that barriers between the sexes did not render impossible the practice of learned gynecological medicine, despite the prevailing culture of modesty in the medieval Islamicate world.

The volume closes with a brief, insightful afterword by Naama Cohen-Hanegbi, who uses a case history recounted by the sixteenth-century Portuguese physician Amato Lusitano as a way to weave together the twin threads of healing women and women healers running throughout the collection. Drawing on his academic training, this learned physician contributed significantly to the medical debates of his day regarding humoral imbalances in women's bodies. His diagnoses of women's ailments concentrated on the uterus, which functioned to balance the fluid humoral economy. Yet hovering in the background of his case history are unnamed female caregivers (*mulierculae assistentes*) who simultaneously performed the day-to-day tasks of healing and acted as narrative agents. It was these practitioners who orchestrated care, determined some of the next steps in treatment, and funneled critical information about the patient's progress to Lusitano as members of a fruitful medical partnership. Cohen-Hanegbi encourages scholars to pursue subtle clues like these in order to reconstruct the vast, largely hidden extent of women's agency and authority in providing healthcare.

Due to their proximity to institutional power and means of textual transmission, learned physicians and the professional practitioners who were their heirs cast historical trajectories that have shaped the way we think about body knowledge and healthcare practice. The essays in this volume strive to dismantle those trajectories. They peel back the dense layers of representation that over time have come to produce a stable and monolithic image of professional knowledge and power. By interrogating the conditions that allowed those professional competencies to emerge, the essays argue instead that healthcare was a communal enterprise dependent on a continuum of reciprocal knowledge and practice. Underneath, beyond, and on the periphery of the canonical texts and the licensed practitioners who projected a powerful image of their own singularity, the contributors in this volume search for the quiet, informal modes of labour and the unseen knowledge transmissions that made possible the daily struggle to survive. By expanding the sources for the history of late medieval and Renaissance healthcare and reading them in new ways, the essays capture the complexity and range of care practices and transmissions of body knowledge. In doing so, they recentre therapeutic epistemologies that unfolded in everyday acts of caregiving as well as the local contexts in which women held sway.

Works Cited

Printed Works

Blumenthal, Debra. 'Domestic Medicine: Slaves, Servants and Female Medical Expertise in Late Medieval Valencia', *Renaissance Studies*, 28.4 (2014), 515-32.

Boisseuil, Didier, ed. *Le bain: espaces et pratiques*, special issue of *Médiévales* 43 (2002).

Cabré, Montserrat. 'From a Master to a Laywoman: A Feminine Manual of Self Help', *Dynamis*, 20 (2000), 371-93.

—. 'Women or Healers? Household Practices and the Categories of Health Care in Late Medieval Iberia', *Bulletin of the History of Medicine*, 82 (2008), 18-51.

Cabré, Montserrat and Fernando Salmón. 'Poder académico *versus* autoridad femenina: la Facultad de Medicina de París contra Jacoba Félicié (1322)', *Dynamis*, 19 (1999), 55-78.

Cadden, Joan. *Meanings of Sex Difference in the Middle Ages: Medicine, Science, and Culture* (Cambridge: Cambridge University Press, 1993).

Cavallo, Sandra. *Artisans of the Body in Early Modern Italy: Identities, Families and Masculinities* (Manchester: Manchester University Press, 2007).

Cavallo, Sandra and Tessa Storey. *Healthy Living in Late Renaissance Italy* (Oxford: Oxford University Press, 2013).

—, eds. *Conserving Health in Early Modern Culture: Bodies and Environment in Italy and England* (Manchester: Manchester University Press, 2017).

Churchill, Laurie J., Phyllis R. Brown, and Jane E. Jeffrey, eds. *Women Writing Latin: From Roman Antiquity to Early Modern Europe*, 3 vols. (London: Routledge, 2002).

Cressier, Patrice. 'Prendre les eaux en al-Andalus: pratique et fréquentation de la Hamma', *Médiévales*, 43 (2002), 41-54.

DeVun, Leah. 'The Jesus Hermaphrodite: Science and Sex Difference in Premodern Europe', *Journal of the History of Ideas*, 69.2 (2008), 193-218.

Duden, Barbara. *The Woman beneath the Skin: A Doctor's Patients in Eighteenth-Century Germany* (Cambridge, MA: Harvard University Press, 1998).

Fissell, Mary E. 'Introduction: Women, Health, and Healing in Early Modern Europe', *Bulletin of the History of Medicine*, 82.1 (2008), 1-17.

—. 'The Marketplace of Print', in *Medicine and the Market in England and its Colonies, c. 1450-c. 1850*, ed. Mark S.R. Jenner and Patrick Wallis (New York: Palgrave Macmillan, 2007), 108-32.

Green, Monica. 'Bodies, Gender, Health, Disease: Recent Work on Medieval Women's Medicine', *Studies in Medieval and Renaissance History*, ser. 3, 2 (2005), 1-46.

—. 'Books as a Source of Medical Education for Women in the Middle Ages', *Dynamis*, 20 (2000), 331-69.

—. 'Documenting Medieval Women's Medical Practice', in *Practical Medicine from Salerno to the Black Death*, ed. Luis Garcia-Balléster, Roger French, Jon Arrizabalaga, and Andrew Cunningham (Cambridge: Cambridge University Press, 1994), 322-52.

—. 'Gendering the History of Women's Healthcare', *Gender & History*, 20 (2008), 487-518.

—. 'Integrative Medicine: Incorporating Medicine and Health into the Canon of Medieval European History', *History Compass*, 7.4 (2009), 1218-45.

—. *Making Medieval Medicine Masculine: The Rise of Male Authority in Pre-modern Gynaecology* (Oxford: Oxford University Press, 2008).

—, ed. *Pandemic Disease in the Medieval World: Rethinking the Black Death*, special issue of *The Medieval Globe*, 1 (2014).

Horden, Peregrine. 'Household Care and Informal Networks: Comparisons and Continuities from Antiquity to the Present', in *The Locus of Care: Families, Communities, Institutions, and the Provision of Welfare since Antiquity*, ed. Peregrine Horden and Richard Smith (London: Routledge, 1998), 21-67.

—. 'A Non-natural Environment: Medicine without Doctors and the Medieval European Hospital', in *The Medieval Hospital and Medical Practice*, ed. B.S. Bowers (Aldershot: Ashgate, 2007), 133-46.

—, ed. *Music as Medicine: The History of Music Therapy since Antiquity* (Aldershot: Ashgate, 2000).

Horden, Peregrine and Richard Smith, eds. *The Locus of Care: Families, Communities, Institutions, and the Provision of Welfare since Antiquity* (London: Routledge, 1998).

King, Helen. *The One-Sex Body on Trial: The Classical and Early Modern Evidence* (Aldershot: Ashgate, 2013).

Kinzelbach, Annemarie. 'Women and Healthcare in Early Modern German Towns', *Renaissance Studies*, 28.4 (2014), 619-38.

Klapisch-Zuber, Christiane. 'Blood Parents and Milk Parents: Wet Nursing in Florence, 1350-1530', in idem, *Women, Family, and Ritual in Renaissance Italy*, trans. Lydia G. Cochrane (Chicago: University of Chicago Press, 1985), 132-64.

Lambourn, Elizabeth A. *Abraham's Luggage: A Social Life of Things in the Medieval Indian Ocean World* (Cambridge: Cambridge University Press, 2018).

Laqueur, Thomas. *Making Sex: Body and Gender from the Greeks to Freud* (Cambridge, MA: Harvard University Press, 1990).

Leong, Elaine and Alisha Rankin. 'Introduction: Secrets and Knowledge', in *Secrets and Knowledge in Medicine and Science, 1500-1800*, ed. Elaine Leong and Alisha Rankin (Farnham: Ashgate, 2011), 1-20.

Lipinska, Mélanie. *Histoire des femmes médecins depuis l'antiquité jusqu'a nos jours* (Paris: Libriarie G. Jacques & Co., 1900).

Long, Pamela O. *Artisan/Practitioners and the Rise of the New Sciences, 1400-1600* (Corvallis, OR: Oregon State University Press, 2011).

McCann, Daniel. *Soul-Health: Therapeutic Reading in Later Medieval England* (Cardiff: University of Wales Press, 2018).

McVaugh, Michael R. *Medicine before the Plague: Practitioners and their Patients in the Crown of Aragon, 1285-1345* (Cambridge: Cambridge University Press, 1993, repr. 2002).

Marienberg, Evyatar. 'Le bain des Melunaises: les juifs médiévaux et l'eau froide des bains rituels', *Médiévales*, 43 (2002), 91-101.

Maurach, Gregor, ed. 'Johannicius: Isagogue ad Techni Galieni', *Sudhoffs Archiv*, 62 (1978), 148-74.

Munkhoff, Richelle. 'Poor Women and Parish Public Health in Sixteenth-Century London', *Renaissance Studies*, 28.4 (2014), 579-96.

—. 'Searchers of the Dead: Authority, Marginality, and the Interpretation of Plague in England, 1574-1665', *Gender & History*, 11 (1999), 1-29.

Narbona-Cárceles, María. 'Woman at Court: A Prosopographic Study of the Court of Carlos III of Navarre (1387-1425)', *Medieval Prosopography*, 22.1 (2001), 31-64.

Nicoud, Marilyn. *Les régimes de santé au Moyen Âge: naissance et diffusion d'une écriture médicale (XIIIe-XVe siècle)*, 2 vols. (Rome: École française de Rome, 2007).

Olson, Glending. *Literature as Recreation in the Later Middle Ages* (Ithaca, NY: Cornell University Press, 1982).

Orlemanski, Julie. *Symptomatic Subjects: Bodies, Medicine, and Causation in the Literature of Late Medieval England* (Philadelphia: University of Pennsylvania Press, 2019).

Park, Katharine. *Secrets of Women: Gender, Generation, and the Origins of Human Dissection* (New York: Zone Books, 2006).

Park, Katharine and Robert Nye. '"Destiny is Anatomy": Essay Review of Thomas Laqueur's *Making Sex*', *New Republic* (18 February 1991), 53-57.

Pelling, Margaret. '"Thoroughly Resented?" Older Women and their Medical Role in Early Modern London', in *Women, Science and Medicine, 1500-1700: Mothers and Sisters of the Royal Society*, ed. Lynette Hunter and Sarah Hutton (Stroud: Sutton, 1997), 63-88.

Power, Eileen. 'Some Women Practitioners of Medicine in the Middle Ages', *Proceedings of the Royal Society of Medicine*, 15 (1922), 20-23.

Rankin, Alisha. *Panaceia's Daughters: Noblewomen as Healers in Early Modern Germany* (Chicago: University of Chicago Press, 2013).

Smith, J.Z. 'Religion, Religions, Religious', in *Critical Terms for Religious Studies*, ed. Mark C. Taylor (Chicago: University of Chicago Press, 1998), 269-84.

Smith, Pamela H. *The Body of the Artisan: Art and Experience in the Scientific Revolution* (Chicago: University of Chicago Press, 2004).

Smith, Pamela H., Amy R.W. Meyers, and Harold J. Cook, eds. *Ways of Making and Knowing: The Material Culture of Empirical Knowledge* (Ann Arbor: University of Michigan Press, 2014).

Solomon, Michael. *Fictions of Well-Being: Sickly Readers and Vernacular Medical Writing in Late Medieval and Early Modern Spain* (Philadelphia: University of Pennsylvania Press, 2010).

—. *The Literature of Misogyny in Medieval Spain* (Cambridge: Cambridge University Press, 1997).

Stevens Crawshaw, Jane. 'Families, Medical Secrets and Public Health in Early Modern Venice', *Renaissance Studies*, 28.4 (2014), 597-618.

Strocchia, Sharon T. *Forgotten Healers: Women and the Pursuit of Health in Late Renaissance Italy* (Cambridge, MA: Harvard University Press, 2019).

Varlik, Nükhet. *Plague and Empire in the Early Modern Mediterranean World: The Ottoman Experience, 1347-1600* (Cambridge: Cambridge University Press, 2015).

Voigts, Linda Ehrsam. 'What's the Word? Bilingualism in Late-Medieval England', *Speculum*, 71(1996), 813-26.

Voigts-Kurtz Search Program, University of Missouri, Kansas City, https://cctr1.umkc.edu/cgi-bin/search (accessed 18 October 2019).

Walsh, Mary Roth. *'Doctors Wanted, No Women Need Apply': Sexual Barriers in the Medical Profession, 1835-1975* (New Haven: Yale University Press, 1977).

Wear, Andrew. *Knowledge and Practice in English Medicine, 1550-1680* (Cambridge: Cambridge University Press, 2000).

Weisser, Olivia. *Ill Composed: Sickness, Gender, and Belief in Early Modern England* (New Haven: Yale University Press, 2015).

Whitaker, Elaine E. 'Reading the Paston Letters Medically', *English Language Notes*, 31 (1993), 19-27.

Yoshikawa, Naoë Kukita, ed. *Medicine, Religion and Gender in Medieval Culture* (Cambridge: D.S. Brewer, 2015).

About the Authors

Sara Ritchey is Associate Professor of History at the University of Tennessee, Knoxville. She is the author of *Holy Matter: Changing Perceptions of the Material World in Late Medieval Christianity* (2014) and a forthcoming book on late medieval religious women's therapeutic knowledge and healthcare practices (2021).

Sharon Strocchia is Professor of History at Emory University in Atlanta. A social and cultural historian of Renaissance Italy, she has published widely on women, religion, and health-related topics. Her most recent book is *Forgotten Healers: Women and the Pursuit of Health in Late Renaissance Italy* (2019).

Part 1

Sources of Religious Healing

1 Caring by the Hours

The Psalter as a Gendered Healthcare Technology

*Sara Ritchey**

Abstract

This essay explores a psalter, Liège, Bibliothèque de l'Université MS 431, as a tool for the construction and transmission of women's therapeutic knowledge. It places the psalter in its institutional context at the beguinage of St. Christopher's, which maintained relationships with hospitals and a leprosarium in Liège. Given its context in feminine circuits of care, the essay argues that several features of this psalter, supported by comparative evidence from other contemporaneous psalters from the region, indicate the ways that beguines incorporated prayer and liturgical performance into their practice of daily caregiving.

Keywords: liturgy, poetry, performance, passions of the soul, beguines, Liège

When young Ida of Nivelles fled her home to escape an unwanted marriage, she slipped out of a window, taking only her psalter, and found refuge among the local beguines living next to the hospital of St. Sépulchre. While living there, Ida often participated in the nursing care that beguines in the region provided. She gathered clothing, footwear, food, and 'other necessary edibles' ('caetera esui necessaria') from residents of Nivelles to distribute to the poor and sick in the hospitals of St. Sépulchre and St. Nicholas. While occupied in these endeavours, a patient at St. Nicholas called Ida over to her bed in order to test her motivation for this constant caretaking. She asked Ida to beg in the streets on her behalf to determine whether she aided the sick

* I am grateful for the valuable feedback on this essay provided by members of the Johns Hopkins University History of Medicine Colloquium in October of 2018.

Ritchey, Sara & Sharon Strocchia (eds), *Gender, Health, and Healing, 1250-1550*. Amsterdam, Amsterdam University Press 2020
DOI: 10.5117/9789463724517_CH01

'purely for God's sake' or for 'flattery and show?'[1] Ida quickly responded to this entreaty, insisting that she did not wish the sick woman to remain indigent ('sustineas indigentiam'). As a result, the hospital patient was convinced of Ida's genuine desire to serve the sick and dying.

As this story indicates, the thirteenth-century *Life* of Ida of Nivelles renders in pious terms her labour to provide nursing services. Tales of Ida's caregiving contributed to her reputation as a 'ready handmaid of Christ' ('statim ancilla Christi'). This hagiographic process suggests how the health agency of religious women ('mulieres religiosae') was encoded in other social norms. Ida's identity as an efficacious bedside healer was conveyed through her gendered connotation as a compassionate handmaid. Her therapeutic actions therefore were not recorded as medical knowledge or practice, but as examples of her intense religiosity, as hagiographic portraits in the *Life* of a 'holy virgin'.[2]

The case of Ida spotlights the kinds of historical trajectories through which these healthcare services have resisted translation as 'medical' sources and thus as 'medical' history. In fact, Ida's caregiving activities were hardly unique in the thirteenth-century southern Low Countries. Hundreds of women living as beguines, anchoresses, Cistercian nuns, and Augustinian canonesses served as nurses, herbalists, midwives, and wonder-workers; they assisted patients using charms, blessings, relics, meditations, and prayers, in addition to more naturalistic healing methods such as herbs, stones, purgatives, phlebotomy, and the maintenance of regimen. Their labour was increasingly necessary during the mid- to late thirteenth century, as immigrants from the countryside flooded into the cities and towns of the southern Low Countries in search of work in the burgeoning textile industries. Beguines, in particular, found low-wage employment as hospital staff and domestic caregivers who nursed the sick and elderly, cleaned, and cared for small children and the dying.

Beguines were among the most active urban communities to develop caregiving institutions devoted to assisting the poor, sick, and indigent in this rapidly urbanizing region. These women were so closely associated with bodily caregiving that some sources use the terms 'beguine hospital'

1 *Vita B. Idae de Nivella*, 203: 'Et ut pure intuitu Dei non adulatorie infirmis succurrere videretur'.

2 Indeed, her casting as a 'holy virgin' would have *enabled* her service to the sick. Ida's status as virgin distinguished her in bodily terms not only as not threatening to the social fabric, but also as spiritually efficacious. Her therapies worked in large part *because of* her reputation as a holy virgin, because her patients expected a certain kind of efficacy from her.

and 'beguine convent' as synonyms.[3] As Walter Simons has shown, the beguinages of Klapdorp in Antwerp, St. Anne in Arras, St. Aubert in Bruges, Ter Arken in Brussels, Wetz in Douai, Poortakker in Ghent, Wierinck in Louvain, le Taye in Mons, and Baerdonc in Ypres were all created as beguine hospitals.[4] Beguines working as hospital nurses founded the court beguinages of Borgloon, Ghent, Lille, Mechelen, Tongeren, and Valenciennes; and at the beguinages of Antwerp, Assenede, Cambrai, Diksmuide, 's-Hertogenbosch, Maubeuge, and Mons, the infirmary was the original building, the founding purpose of the institution being care for sick and elderly women.[5] That so much of their activity and mission was dedicated to healthcare raises vital questions about how these communities of women constructed and transmitted body knowledge. What were the guiding principles of their practice? Where did they receive their training? Where are their records of medical knowledge? These questions address the issue of elusive sources. Even Walter Simons, who has uncovered such vast archival evidence for the healthcare institutions founded and staffed by beguines, went on to note that, although these women *must* have received training, 'such expertise has unfortunately remained undocumented'.[6]

This essay argues that, in fact, we *do* have ample sources for women's healthcare knowledge and practice in this period. These sources come not in the form of coherent academic treatises, but in 'fragile traces' detectable in liturgy, poetry, recipes, meditations, sacred objects, and the everyday behaviours that constituted their world.[7] Here, I examine a source genre that, when understood within late medieval women's circuits of care, can yield fresh insights into women's therapeutic practice and epistemology. Remembering that Ida fled to the beguinage with only one possession, her psalter, I turn to the evidence offered by this type of book. I show that psalters often contain fragmentary traces of practices long forgotten as therapeutic and typically considered now only in terms of religion, devotion, or liturgy.[8] An analysis of Liège, Bibliothèque de l'Université MS 431 demonstrates how psalters structured therapeutic interactions and accrued therapeutic significance in caregiving contexts. After a brief introduction to the psalters from this region, I turn to the caregiving contexts in which they

3 Simons, *Cities of Ladies*, 77.

4 Ibid., 77.

5 Ibid., 76.

6 Ibid., 77-78.

7 The idea of 'fragile traces' here comes from Hunt, 'Acoustic Register'; on the variety of everyday practices that constitute such traces, see Collins, *Black Feminist Thought*, 251-52.

8 Taylor, 'Remapping Genre'.

would have been used. Beguines like Ida of Nivelles consulted these psalters in both private and communal settings in beguinages and in hospitals. After discussing the beguines of St. Christopher in Liège, with whom MS 431 was institutionally connected, I examine three caregiving situations in which the psalter may have been used: at the bedsides of the sick, the parturient, and the dying.

The Psalter as Techne

Psalters, books of hours, and other liturgical and devotional materials provide a veritable archive of women's healthcare practices and feminine therapeutic epistemologies. These books and objects could travel with women from homes, to mass, to funerals, and to other locations in the public sphere.[9] In other words, the prayers they uttered were a form of social action in which meaning depended on a collective setting; the significance and performative action of a prayer's text could change depending on the context in which it was delivered.[10] Psalters were liturgical books used in the Divine Office, the daily round of prayers expected of the secular and regular clergy. Psalters established a set of psalms for each *cursus* of the liturgy so that all 150 psalms were recited within a week.[11] These liturgical books underwent a continual process of evolution during the Middle Ages, but by the twelfth century one could expect the typical psalter to contain a calendar, litany, canticles, collects, and the Office of the Dead, in addition to the Latin text of the psalms.[12] By the mid-thirteenth century, a market for similar prayerbooks developed among the laity, who wished to perform the Hours of the Virgin, a sequence of prayers to the mother of Jesus Christ. These books were known as books of hours because the prayers within them were to be recited throughout the course of the day. They did not contain the full run of psalms but, in addition to the Hours of the Virgin, they often included the Calendar, Gospel lessons, the Hours of the Cross and of the Holy Spirit, the prayers *Obsecro te* and *O intemerata*, the Penitential Psalms and Litany, the Office of the Dead, and Suffrages.[13]

9 Reinburg, *French Books of Hours*, 6.

10 Rappaport, *Ritual and Religion*, 388-95; Tambiah, *Culture, Thought, and Social Action*, pt. 1, 1-166.

11 The distribution could vary according to monastic order or cathedral use. On the development of the psalter throughout the Middle Ages, see Leroquais, *Les psautiers*.

12 Palazzo, *History of Liturgical Books*, 130-32.

13 Wieck, *Painted Prayers*, 9-10.

The art historian Judith Oliver has identified a corpus of 41 Mosan psalters from the thirteenth and early fourteenth centuries, many of which were owned and used by beguines in the region.[14] The term 'Mosan' derives from their provenance in cities and towns like Huy, Mons, and Liège, which dot the Meuse valley in the southern Low Countries. Although programmatic in the sense of their liturgical ordering, the Mosan psalters in this corpus were also highly improvisational, often eliciting the inscription of personal prayers, useful recipes, the names of loved ones or of efficacious saints, and other incidental scribbles. Many of them may be more properly described as psalter-hours, falling somewhere in between a psalter and a book of hours. This highly elastic quality of women's psalters in the region, their inclusion of a varied array of prayers as forms of speech and guides for action, opens a window onto bodily practice in feminine space, such as beguinages and their affiliated hospitals.[15] In beguine caregiving spaces, I argue, the psalter was a therapeutic tool that informed women's healthcare practice.

The corpus of Mosan psalters bear distinctive textual and stylistic attributes. They sometimes feature a variety of additional prayers, vernacular poems, illumination cycles, health rules, mass devotions, liturgical offices, and diagrams known as *computi*, which were used to determine the date of Easter. The health rules, in particular, are only found in this corpus of psalters. Another unique feature of the corpus are the twenty vernacular poems on the life of Christ and the Virgin Mary that appear scattered throughout fourteen of the psalters, each accompanied by full-page miniatures.[16] Although appearing in random combinations, together the poems narrate an abbreviated biblical history beginning with the toxic sin of Adam then focusing on sin's alleviation in the salient events of Christian cosmic history, from the Annunciation to the life and death of Christ. These complex texts and images point to an 'unstable realm' between writing and orality, the realm in which beguines shared medical knowledge and enacted medical practices.[17] The poems participated in a broader culture of performance in which beguine prayer was understood to encourage salubrious effects. An examination of these psalters from the social standpoint of beguines' roles in caregiving institutions reveals fragments of their therapeutic logic and practice. That knowledge and practice was thoroughly oral, performative, and embodied, which is precisely why it has remained undetected until now.

14 Oliver, *Gothic Manuscript Illumination*, 112-19.
15 Metcalf, *Where are YOU/SPIRITS*.
16 Meyer, 'Le psautier'; Sinclair, 'Les manuscrits'.
17 Green, 'Books as a Source', 360.

The Psalter *in Situ*

Liège Bibliothèque de l'Université MS 431 was a psalter-hours produced *c.*1285-90 in Liège. That the psalter's prayers use feminine words such as *ancelle* and do not align with any particular monastic liturgy suggests that the book was made for a beguine. This book, as Oliver has proposed, likely belonged to the liégeois community of St. Christopher.[18] St. Christopher appears atop a gilded tower on the opening folium of the psalter itself (at fol. 12, across from the *Beatus* page). Across from him, nestled in the historiated Q, is the figure of St. Lambert depicted in the throes of martyrdom. Celebrated as the first martyr and patron saint of the city of Liège, Lambert was also the namesake of the mythological founder of the beguines, Lambert le Bègue (d. 1177), who was said to have preached at St. Christopher's and to have been buried there.[19] Indeed, Lambert le Bègue encouraged the pious of Liège to engage in spiritually salubrious forms of theater, such as a vernacular translation of the *Life* and Passion of St. Agnes that he prepared for virgins ('virginibus') or his versified vernacular rendition of the Acts of the Apostles that included well-placed 'exhortations' ('multis loco congruo insertis exhortationes').[20] Lambert explained that he made translations of these biblical narratives for the devout to enact on feast days, supplementing their routine performances, such as 'singing of psalms, hymns, and religious chants'.[21] The vernacularity and versification of these texts points to their social enactments; they would have been read aloud in gatherings, and parts were likely committed to memory for performance apart from the text. The appearance of narrative vernacular poems in a psalter used at St. Christopher's suggests a similar terrain of performed use; in the hospital, as I will show, such a performance would take on therapeutic dimensions.

The beguinage of St. Christopher was one of the oldest and largest in the Low Countries. It grew from a loose federation of privately funded beguine houses and convents in various parts of the parish. The beguinage developed a complicated relationship with the hospital of St. Christopher, which had been in existence in the city from the later twelfth century, staffed by a master following the rule of St. Augustine.[22] A document of

18 Oliver, *Gothic Manuscript Illumination*, 261.

19 On the mythological foundation see Simons, *Cities of Ladies*, 30-34. In the hagiographic *Life* of Odilia, a widow of Liège who lived among the beguines in the thirteenth century, Lambert is referred to as *Lamberto de Sancto Christophoro*; *Vitae B. Odiliae Viduae Leodiensis*, 206-10.

20 Fayen, 'L'Antigraphum Petri'.

21 Ibid., 352: 'in psalmis, in ymnis et canticis spiritualibus expendebant'.

22 De Spiegeler, *Les hôpitaux*, 61-63.

June 1224, issued by Conrad of Urach, the former abbot of Villers who became cardinal and papal legate, sheds light on the early relationship between the women who frequented the hospital and the various men who served as its administrators. Conrad sought to settle a dispute between the monks of nearby St. Laurent and the brothers of the hospital of St. Christopher over the right to elect the priest of St. Christopher.[23] Conrad referred in his judgment to the 'sorores' living near the hospital, ordering that the women should pay an annual rent. These sisters were most likely the first beguines of St. Christopher.[24] In 1241, the hospital received statutes written by Robert of Thourotte, bishop of Liège, stipulating that the women who would live there would occupy a separate space or 'domos mulierem'.[25] The beguines who served St. Christopher's already lived in separate convents and private homes near the hospital, so the statutes likely refer to canonesses who the bishop envisioned living there at some time in the future.[26]

The exact nature of the relationship between the beguines of St. Christopher and the hospital is murky due in part to the informal and ad hoc services they provided in return for participation in the liturgy and sacraments observed at the hospital. A similar relationship among the beguines and the hospital of nearby Tongres is suggestive of the kinds of reciprocal ties maintained between beguines and formal hospital staff. In 1245, Thibaud, a canon of St. Denis and citizen of Tongres, authorized the beguines of Tongres to attend services at the hospital of St. Jacques. They paid the low annual fee of 3 liégeois *oboles* and agreed to split with the hospital the income they received from their work providing assistance in funeral services and from their prayers for the dead.[27] In return, the chaplain of the hospital also acted as rector to the beguines. The beguines of Tongres were thus informally associated with the hospital of St. Jacques, sharing a rector, income, labour, urban space, and prayer, until they established their own beguinage and infirmary in 1257.

The beguines of St. Christopher who made use of MS 431 likely shared comparable proximity and responsibilities with the hospital staff. They

23 Daris, *Extraits*, 152-53.

24 Simons, *Cities of Ladies*, 283; McDonnell, *Beguines and Beghards*, 44.

25 Borgnet and Bormans, *Ly myreur*, 249-52. The document uses the future tense, referring to women who would move there. It is difficult to determine who these *sorores* would be. It seems to indicate that the women who would have taken vows at the hospital would become canonesses. In other cases, such as at the hospital of Notre Dame at Lille, early records use the language of *sorores*, although beguines clearly come to occupy those roles after foundation.

26 De Spiegeler, *Les hôpitaux*, 76-81.

27 Schoolmeesters, *Les regestes de Robert de Thourotte*, 119: 'tres obulos monete Leodiensis'.

may have had a similar relationship to the patients of St. Christopher as Ida of Nivelles had forged with those of the hospitals of St. Sépulchre and St. Nicholas. In those settings, beguines performed caregiving services, ensured that patients' basic material needs were met, provided prayers for them, and performed burial rites. In 1241, the number of beguines living near St. Christopher and participating in liturgical services in its chapel had swelled beyond the hospital's capacity, prompting them to obtain an indulgence for the purpose of constructing a larger church.[28] And by 1267, the beguines had established their own independent hospital, known as the Hôpital Tirebourse, located across the Rue St. Gilles from the hospital of St. Christopher.[29] A 2005 archaeological excavation of the new beguine hospital showed that it remained connected by a series of pathways to the hospital of St. Christopher and to the beguinage, forming a social network dedicated to active charity.[30] As the beguines of St. Christopher executed their daily caregiving tasks, a psalter like Liège MS 431 would have informed their work.

Versified Bedside Comfort

Used at the bedsides of the sick and indigent at the hospital of Tirebourse and the hospital of St. Christopher, Liège MS 431 provided comfort, encouraged salubrious affections, and reassured patients of the Christian significance of their suffering, which would be rewarded with everlasting life. The psalter opens with a single mass prayer, a prayer for the remission of sins that would have been uttered in preparation for receiving the sacrament of Eucharist. The words of the prayer are dialogic, in conversation with the addressee, who is Christ. 'I greet you' ('Je toi salue'), it offers, welcoming the 'bread of angels' that is set upon the altar, the medicinal food that will be ingested after this preparatory prayer and gesture. Again, it repeats, 'I greet you', this time addressing the blood of Christ, the 'chalice of salvation' ('le calisce de salut'). The repetition of *salut* in varied forms throughout the

28 McDonnell, *Beguines and Beghards*, 236.

29 De Spiegeler shows that the process of integration of the hospital was intermittent, only completed in 1473. Next to the hospital the beguinage also established a leprosarium sometime before 1304, called the Leproserie de Florichamps. See Pissart, 'Tirebourse et Florichamps'.

30 Mora-Dieu, 'L'Ancien hôpital Tirebourse'. The excavation showed that little roads connected the hospital to the abbey of St. Laurent and to the hospital of St. Christopher. It also revealed that the patient ward was surrounded by small chapels, presumably in part to keep patients within view of the consecrated host.

prayer unequivocally conjures the term's signification as both health and salvation, as simultaneous, codependent meanings. The intention of *salut* was socially embedded, gathering meaning from the context in which it was uttered, that is, a community dedicated to caregiving. Indeed, it demands, 'deliver me of all of my sins and all of my sicknesses' ('delivres moi de tots mes iniquiteis et des tos mals'), yoking sickness to sin and foregrounding sin's remission as an avenue to health. The words of the prayer strike with illocutionary force, initiating a transformation in the delivery of sin, the alleviation of sickness.[31]

The mass prayer was a form of bodily preparation in anticipation of ingesting the Eucharistic host, the consecrated bread that was theologically identified with the body of Christ. In requesting a purgation of sin, it primed the practitioner's body to house the body of Christ. Although composed as a direct address in the first person singular, in the context of St. Christopher's it was a collective prayer performed by beguines for the sake of the whole community. The book's user and her audience thus together inhabited the 'I' that performed the work of the prayer, unleashing through utterance the processes designed to take effect. In this way, the beguine and her whole surrounding community were incorporated into the rite.[32] Together, their orally delivered prayers issued a collective plea for regeneration, sustenance, and *salus*. That process of regeneration is made clear in the prayer's figuring of an indulgence: 'facet indulgence de tos mes pechies'. The prayer acknowledges the collective enterprise of salvation, offering devotion and praise in exchange for salvation, both in this life and after death.[33] It thus publicizes the notion that participation in the mass continued a form of regeneration of the world, that health was a collective endeavour. This responsibility for communal salvation is echoed in the hospital statutes, which required patients and canons to make regular confession. In other words, through prayer, each member of the hospital, patient and staff, was integrated into a total therapeutic environment.

The total therapeutic environment, or what Peregrine Horden has called 'the non-natural environment', was essential to practical applications of medieval medical theory.[34] In medical theory, the 'non-naturals' referred to the six factors exterior to the body that affected the body's internal humoral

31 Austin, *How to Do Things with Words*, 148-52.

32 Headley, 'Afterword', 231.

33 Bibliothèque de l'Universitè de Liège MS 431, fol. 1v: 'por ta sancta mort rachatas le monde'.

34 On the 'total therapeutic environment', see Horden, 'Religion and Medicine', 139. On his theorization of the 'non-natural environment', see Horden, 'Non-Natural Environment'.

balance and thus, its health. These six factors were: ambient air, food and drink, exercise and rest, sleep and wakefulness, excretion and retention, and the passions of the soul.[35] In practice, beguines and other practitioners tended to the non-natural environment of the hospital by laundering linens, accompanying patients on walks, providing their meals, ensuring their comfort, maintaining hygienic conditions, and praying for them. These tasks, which were required to preserve the health-giving properties of any setting – whether a home, hospital, or abbey – were coded as 'women's work'.[36] As Eva-Maria Cersovsky's essay in this volume demonstrates, an array of late medieval and Renaissance discourses intersected in naturalizing these daily caretaking labours as feminine.[37] It should come as no surprise, then, that the first *regimen* dedicated to elucidating methods of maintaining the six non-naturals was composed in the vernacular for a woman, Beatrice of Savoie, the Countess of Provence.[38] This *régime du corps*, written by Aldobrandino of Siena in 1256, enjoyed wide circulation in women's communities, particularly in northern France and the southern Low Countries.[39] In other words, there was a general cultural expectation that women would oversee regimen and other aspects of the non-natural environment.

Among the six non-naturals, it was the last, the 'passions of the soul', that allowed a range of activities – listening to music and poetry, observing affective performances – to function as therapeutic. The passions of the

35 Maurach, ed., 'Johannicius', 151. Hunayn's work was translated from Arabic into Latin by Constantine the African as the *Isagogue* of Johannitius. It would enter European medical training in this Latinized version.

36 Cabré, 'Women or Healers?'

37 Cersovsky, '*Ubi non est mulier*'.

38 Nicoud has shown that, around the early fourteenth century, the organization of *regimina* began to change across all examples of the genre, from a chapter-by-chapter discussion of treatment according to body parts and afflictions to a schema following the maintenance of each of the six factors in the non-natural environment; Nicoud, *Les régimes de santé*, 153-84. Aldobrandino of Siena's was the first regimen to register this organizational change.

39 The treatise was distributed widely in Flemish, Catalan, and Italian, as well as French; Jacquart and Nicoud, 'Les régimes de santé'. It was also adapted into a full-length treatise on the connection between the health of the body and the soul, which appeared in the fourteenth-century Low Countries. The *Lyen du corps a l'ame et de l'ame au corps* can be found in three extant manuscripts, the earliest of which is Brussels, Bibliothèque royale de Belgique (KBR, Koninklijke Bibliotheek and Bibliothèque royale), MS 11130-32 (xiv, southern Netherlands); the other two are Valenciennes, Bibliothèque municipale, MS 329, and Rome, Biblioteca Apostolica, MS Pal. Lat. 1990. See Féry-Hue, 'Le régime du corps'. Regimental advice sometimes circulated with psalters; see, for example, British Library, MS Sloane 1611, which includes a regimen, psalms, marginal recipes on lactation and childbirth, and a *Life* of Margaret of Antioch, which was frequently used in labour and delivery.

soul were defined as the 'incidental states of the soul [that] have an effect on the body, such as those which bring the natural heat from the interior of the body to the surface of the skin'.[40] The material or bodily bearing of the passions meant that, by altering their internal affects, a person might transform their physical composition. Certain emotions, such as delight or hope, were considered as salubrious and even potentially curative; whereas others, like grief and anger, were deleterious to one's health. Cheerfulness was a particularly healthful passion because it drew the body's internal heat outward and purified the blood.

When performed in the context of the beguine hospital, the poems in Liège MS 431 could facilitate healing by modifying the passions of patients' souls. In this capacity, the poems functioned less as texts for passive reading than as scripts for performance. Their form – rhymed couplets – facilitated the healing process. The experience of poetry and music had the potential to induce a kind of humoral harmony. The poems might have enacted what the Parisian master, John of Garland, described as the work of lyric poetry: to 'embrace the harmony and concord of the humours'.[41] A person's pulse revealed their internal humoral harmony or disharmony, 'elucidat[ing] the passions of the soul'.[42] Ibn Sīnā (Avicenna) elaborated a musical index for describing the movement of the pulse, which included its metre, rhythm, harmony, measure, and accent.[43] The ideal pulse exhibited a slow metre and infrequent rhythm, a pattern that reflected the gradual outward movement of blood induced by a cheerful affect.

But cheerfulness was a challenging passion to maintain in the thirteenth-century European hospital ward, a space where few could reasonably expect to make full recovery. Hospital patients more often experienced the threatening passion of melancholy, which channelled the body's heat and *spiritus* inward, causing lethargy and even physical disability.[44] The antidote to *tristitia* was moderate cheerfulness, delight, and tranquility.[45] Music and lyric poetry were considered some of the most efficient tools for conjuring

40 Maurach, ed., 'Johannicius', 160: 'Sunt quaedam accidentia animae quae faciunt intra corpus, sicut ea, quae commovent calorem ab interiori parte ad superficiem cutis'.

41 John of Garland, *Parisiana poetria*, 7: 'in humanam, que constat in proportione et Concordia humorum'.

42 The phrase comes from the thirteenth-century anonymous *Summa pulsuum* or *Epitome on Pulses*; the treatise can be found in Grant, *Sourcebook in Medieval Science*, 745-48.

43 Avicenna, *Liber canonis*, bk. 1, fen 2. On the role of music in medieval healing practices, see the essays in Horden, ed., *Music as Medicine*.

44 For example, see Avicenna, *Liber canonis*, bk. 3, fen 11.

45 Bartholomew of Salerno, *Practica magistri*, 4: 353. On *tristitia* see also Arnald of Villanova, *Opera medica omnia*, vol. 10.1.

these salubrious affects. Aldobrandino of Siena, for example, prescribed as a means of thwarting melancholy the practice of purgation, a certain Galenic remedy, and the arousal of cheer induced by musicality.[46] Used as a method of affective arousal, the performance of the psalter's poems at the bedsides of the sick was a caregiving practice, one that created an experience of joy and harmony that carried therapeutic benefits for both body and soul.

The contents of the poems address the ultimate salvation and comfort achieved in both body and soul by contemplation of Christ and Mary and participation in the mass and liturgy. When readers of MS 431 encountered the poetic demand that Mary 'enflame the heart of your servant by heat', it is quite possible that they drew on knowledge of the cold complexions of women and the salubrious role of certain affects in thirteenth-century health regimens.[47] This poem, copied on folio 9r, praises Mary as the flower of the tree of Jesse who bore the salvific fruit of Jesus Christ. Accompanied by a full-page miniature with images of the tree of Jesse, the Annunciation, the Visitation, as well as martyr figures including Peter, Paul, and John the Baptist, the poem worked in multiple mediums as text, image, and lived performance. It describes, and also imparts, the kind of experiential knowledge available through the collective performance of chanting, listening, and witnessing the words of the poem itself. Enacted at bedsides, the poem made present Mary and Christ by inspiring ardour ('ardor'), love ('amur'), and the 'spirit of knowledge' ('l'ispirs de science'). For example, it calls on spiritual *consilii* to guide 'my being and my thoughts my existence and my words'.[48] The poem enfolds its users, practitioner and patient together, into a knowledge-making process. 'Make me feel' wisdom's *consilia*, it commands, 'enclose in me' this knowledge.[49] The poem thus describes a process of embodying knowledge, receiving spiritual and scriptural wisdom within the bodily self of practitioner and patient. The performance of this poem can be seen as an enactment of ritual in Roy Rappaport's sense of the term as producing an embodied truth, in this case bonding practitioner and patient in a truth about salvation history.[50] This poem not only provided a

46 As methods of altering insalubrious passions, he cites purgation, a medicine called *lecticia Galieni* (Galen's electuary), and cheerfulness and joy. The manuscript tradition features a musician decorating the capital 'I' in the regime's chapter on the accidents of the soul, suggesting musicality as a means of generating salubrious passions. See, for example, British Library, MS Sloane 2435, fol. 10v, where a fiddler plays music to a person suffering from melancholy.

47 MS Liège 431, fol. 9r: 'Le cuer de ton ancelle enspren de la chalur'.

48 Ibid.: 'Mon ester et mon penser, mon vivre et mon parler'.

49 Ibid.: 'ferme en moi'.

50 Rappaport, *Ritual and Religion*, 119-23.

script for the verbal assent to the wisdom of Mary as the mother of Christ, it also positioned its performers and auditors collectively as those who had 'tasted the fruit' of Mary's womb. That is, they had ingested the medicinal host and had been substantially altered as a result.

Birthing by the Book

The poems of Bibliothèque de l'Universitè de Liège MS 431 suggest that one of the foremost therapeutic roles among beguines was their presence in acts of witnessing during critical moments of transition in the life cycle. Beguines lent their presence and prayers to births, serving as marshals in greeting new life; they also provided care and consolation at the bedsides of the dying, ushering them into a new spiritual state. They were custodians of these rites of passage, rendering natural and biological events into cultural and religious drama. By incorporating these poems and prayers into the process of dying and of giving birth, beguines assigned spiritual meaning to those experiences, making them more manageable by ritualizing them.

For example, the poem *Avez de nostre saignor* (fols. 222r-223v) demonstrates how, through repetition, poetry could unfold into formulaic speech, like medical charms that were delivered over bodies with the expectation of cure.[51] The poem's string of Aves creates an incantatory, almost hypnotic chain of pleas. They are addressed to Christ, who appears as a source of healing grace. With each Ave, the performer insisted upon a transformation, on the efficacy of the poem's work. 'Receive the prayers of your servants', it commands, 'Grant us your company.'[52] Through these words, Christ was made imaginatively present in caregiving acts. He was made physically and experientially present as well, as the poem instructs its audience that the divine grace of healing is found in the Eucharist: 'hail, glorious bread of life' ('Ave, glorious pains de vie'). 'If anyone shall drink of it through you', referring to the grace unleashed in the bread and wine, '[they] will live to all days without end'.[53]

The uniquely truncated form of 'Avez de nostre saignor' suggests some possibilities for its therapeutic use in beguine hospitals and other caregiving sites. Although the poem's base text totals 200 lines, in MS 431 it terminates

51 Here I refer in particular to the musicality presupposed in charms as *carmen* (song). On birthing charms, see Olsan and Jones, 'Performative Rituals'.

52 Liège MS 431, fol. 222v: 'rechoiz proieres de tes sers'; fol. 223r: 'otroie nos ta compaignie'; trans. Ricketts, 481.

53 Liège MS 431, fol. 222v: 'ki par toi en beverat, a toz jors sain fin viverat'; trans. Ricketts, 481.

at line 88.[54] While it is possible that the lines missing from the poem in MS 431 were originally included in a quire that was lost or removed in subsequent bindings, another possibility, based on comparative evidence, is that the women who used MS 431 possessed an embodied familiarity with the poem. In this scenario, the poem's abbreviation points to an oral context of performance that took place beyond the text of the codex. The oral-aural experience of the poetic Aves supports a degree of adaptability, allowing its users to modify the performance of the poem for specific needs or purposes.

This kind of abbreviation for adaptability was common among birthing charms and amulets used by birth attendants from the thirteenth through fifteenth centuries. Don Skemer, for instance, has collected examples of manuscripts that altered formulaic orders in order to cater them to the needs of childbirth. For example, a southern French 'birthing kit' features abridged saints' *Lives* such as that of Margaret of Antioch, Gospel readings, a charm for epilepsy, a crucifixion scene (among other images, principally of saints), and a list of divine names with an indulgence protecting against death, including death in childbirth.[55] The abbreviated forms of well-known texts enabled the users of this manuscript to make choices about appropriate reading performances and to elaborate on and improvise those performances as necessary. As Marianne Elsakkers has shown in her examination of manuscript versions of the peperit charm, words, lines, and phrases of well-known texts could be repeated cyclically throughout the course of labour. In the case of the peperit charm, birth assistants could synchronize their utterances with the rhythm of the parturient's contractions, and they could improvise by expanding or shortening the litany of holy mothers invoked in the charm, depending on the timing needs of the birth process.[56] In a predominantly oral society, poetry and ritual, including medical ritual, were embedded in a culture of performance that operated at a distance from texts.[57] As Iliana Kandzha shows in the following chapter, the relics of locally revered saints also participated in these performative birth rituals; touching or gazing upon a relic while in labour could be combined with the audition of prayers and chants, as well as the recitation of the saint's miracles and *Life*.[58]

54 The base text of this poem is Brussels, KBR, MS IV-36. There are a total of eight manuscripts that include the poem; all are thirteenth-century Mosan psalters. On the distribution of the poems and their relationship to one another, see Ricketts, 'Critical Edition'.

55 Skemer, *Binding Words*, 242. The birthing kit is in a private collection in southern France.

56 Elsakkers, 'In Pain You Shall Bear Children', 205.

57 Symes, *Common Stage*, 2.

58 Kandzha, 'Female Saints as Agents of Female Healing'.

The same process of tailoring the performance of the Aves, or even the psalms themselves, to the situational needs of the parturient was available to the users of MS 431. The beguines could intone the entirety of the Aves in order to foster a meditative state by modulating notes and words according to the pace of labour. Illustrations in MS 431 suggest that they may have served as a kind of apotropaic or meditative purpose, providing positive images onto which a labouring mother could latch, identifying herself and her birth process with the saintly and successful births that preceded hers. For example, at the Antiphon, 'Corde et voce', which opened the Hours of the Nativity of the Virgin, the manuscript offers a depiction of Anne's birth of the Virgin Mary, who is accompanied by a birth attendant or midwife (Figure 1.1). The attendant swaddles the baby and hands him to Joachim. Above this image, we see that the attendant has bathed the baby, and on the facing page, she prepares a meal to continue caring for the mother in bed.[59]

This illustration of Mary's birth, accompanied by the Hours of her Nativity, may have served as a multimedial means of calming the parturient, who gazed upon it while beguines tended to her needs and chanted psalms, Aves, and other salubrious orations. As the parturient focused on the image, she would have placed hope in the outcomes of the birthing process, guaranteed by prayers for Mary's intercession.

The illustrations of Mary's birth may have also functioned as a kind of graphic instruction for beguines learning about obstetric care. We know that beguines were acting as midwives, even if they did not bear this formal occupational label, because statutes from the beguinages in cities like Herentals, Dendermonde, and Mechelen sought to outlaw this activity.[60] Additionally, Thomas of Cantimpré, who developed close relationships with beguines and other *mulieres religiosae* in the region, included in his encyclopedia recipes for childbirth so that priests could provide instruction to midwives in their parishes.[61] Although Thomas lamented that few knowledgeable midwives were available, he also recommended in Book 1

59 For an account of midwives in practice, see the court case of the Jewish midwife, Floreta d'Ays, which is analysed, transcribed and translated in Green and Smail, 'Trial of Floreta d'Ays (1403)'. The case shows that, in the French Mediterranean, midwifery was still a specialization regarded as necessary for certain difficult labours. The beguines of thirteenth- and fourteenth-century Liège would not likely have held occupational markers as midwives and might more appropriately be called 'birth attendants' in their role as practitioners of parturient care.

60 Simons, *Cities of Ladies*, 78.

61 The passage is difficult to interpret. On the one hand, Green has convincingly argued that the priest who could not find a knowledgeable midwife could use these recipes. On the other, since Thomas expected priests to gather midwives, it is also possible that these recipes were used by priests to instruct midwives; Green, *Making Women's Medicine Masculine*, 145-50.

Figure 1.1 Hours of Nativity of the Virgin, at Matins showing birth of the Virgin with midwife handing baby to Joachim and midwife bathing the baby

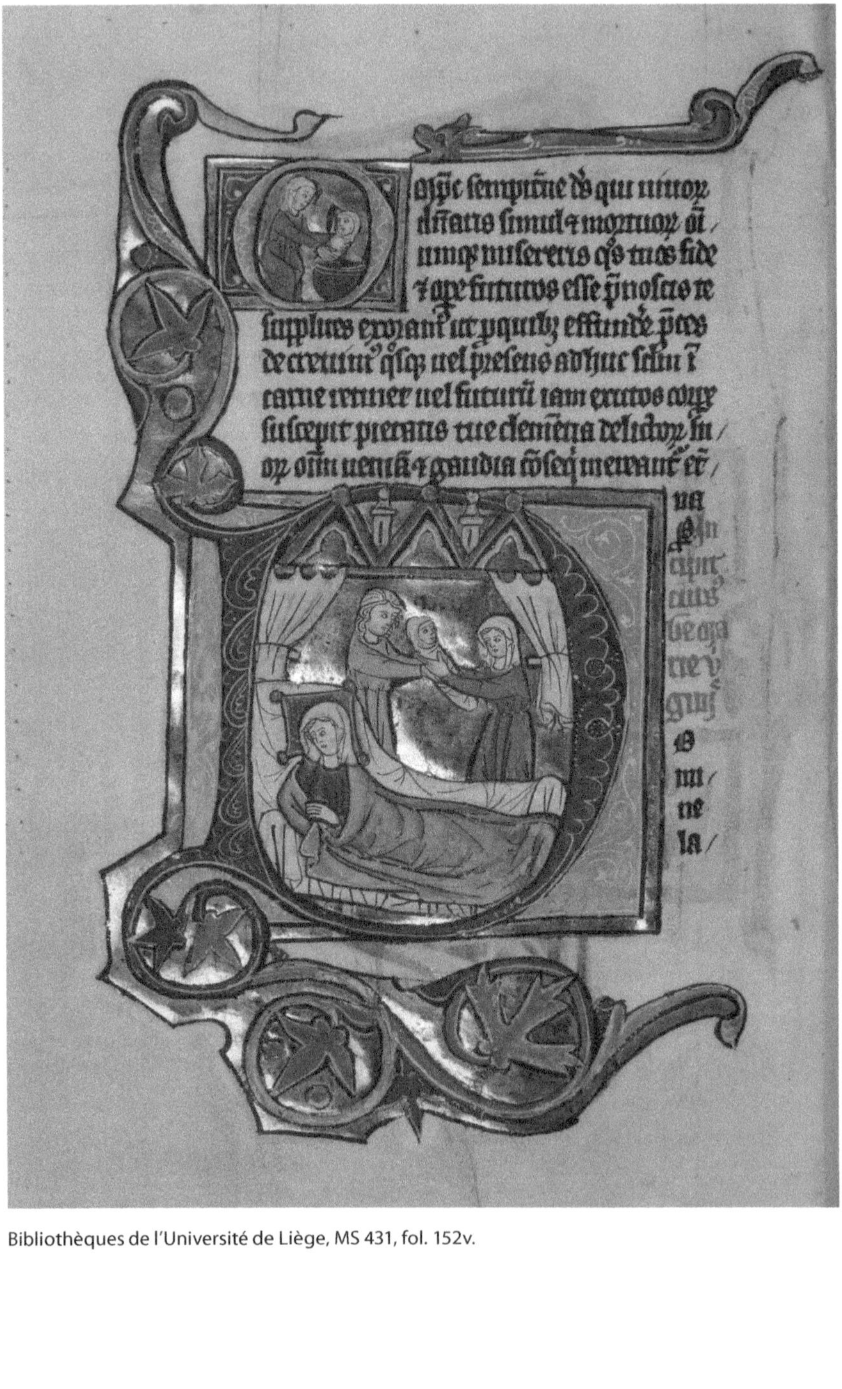

Bibliothèques de l'Université de Liège, MS 431, fol. 152v.

of *On the Nature of Things* (*Liber de natura rerum*) that his readers might 'convene some of the more discreet midwives and instruct them in private, and through them some of the others might more easily be instructed'.[62] This passage emphasizes the oral transmission of knowledge among midwives and other birth attendants who might have conveyed verbally certain authoritative recipes and procedures, and then elaborated on them with examples drawn from their own experience. The women who used MS 431, then, likely possessed an embodied knowledge of basic obstetric procedure, which they communicated orally, through performance.

Death Care

On the other end of the life cycle, beguines participated in care of the dying and performed several of the rituals surrounding death. Wills, testaments, and statutes indicated that beguines of the Low Countries and northern France were known regionally as specialists in care of the dead.[63] Laypeople often called upon these women, either singly or in groups ranging from four to twenty, to be present at their dying moments, to prepare bodies for burial, conduct wakes, sing psalms, and escort bodies to the grave.[64] The Rule for the beguinage in Bruges, for example, prohibits beguines from acting playfully when caring for the bodies of the dead in their charge during wakes.[65] At St. Elizabeth's in Ghent, beguines provided prayers and intercessions at funerals, in addition to holding vigils, fasting, and chanting psalms.[66]

The care provided by beguines to the dying was not intended to prolong life, but to afford comfort, and to assuage fear, assuring them of a good death and the chance at everlasting life in heaven. Hagiographic portraits bolster this picture of the beguines' provision of end-of-life services. For example, Jacques of Vitry commented on Marie of Oignies's constant aid to the mother of a monk, whom she accompanied at bedside until the woman's eventual death.[67] In another instance, Jacques reported on

62 Thomas of Cantimpré, *Liber de natura rerum*, bk. 1.76

63 Deregnaucourt, 'Le dernier voyage', 81-88; see also Schmitt, *Mort d'une hérésie*.

64 Simons, *Cities of Ladies*, 78-79.

65 Ziegler, *Sculpture of Compassion*, 91.

66 *Cartulaire du béguinage de Sainte-Elisabeth à Gand*, 75: 'devotis orationibus et suffragiis visitabant, ac quelibet pro alia mortua devota suffragia abstinentie, vigiliarum, psalmorum et orationum'.

67 *Vita Mariae Oigniacensis*, 572-81, at 2.6.3 (50).

Marie's assistance at the sick bed of the dying John of Dinant; after his death, she always bowed in acknowledgment when passing his gravesite in Oignies.[68] Thomas of Cantimpré similarly asserted that the saintly beguine Christina 'assisted the dying most willingly and gladly exhorted them to a confession of their sins'.[69] He later described her at bedside, eliciting such a confession from the dying Count of Loon, Louis II.[70] In his bedchamber, Count Louis prostrated himself at Christina's feet in a final act of confession before dying.

MS Liège 431 offers a material example of the complex of prayer, imagery, and performance the dying might expect when they called upon beguines from the region. A beguine might offer to help the dying make a purgative act of confession, as in the example of Christina of St. Trond or the opening prayer in MS 431. A priest would have been called in for the administration of final sacraments but, as Richard Trexler has noted, the remainder of the 'transition' for the dying would be punctuated by the presence of chanting, praying women.[71] For example, the poem *Uns faisseles de myrre est mes amis a moi* ('A bundle of myrrh is my beloved to me') (fol. 11r) is rendered as a form of narrative passion meditation, describing the sufferings of Christ that the orant, as proxy for the community, wished to 'experience' ('sentir').[72] The experience the poem ultimately offered, however, was not one of suffering, but of collective identification with the fruits of Christ's suffering, that is, with health and salvation. The poem only offers the briefest allusion to the 'sharp beatings' ('aigres batures') that Christ endured. The remainder of the thirty-line poem is empty of narrative content from the passion. Rather, it conjures repeatedly the delightful smells ('bone odor'), the honor of suffering ('l'onor'), and the happiness of contemplation ('bieneurteit') of Christ's salvific act. The process of contemplating ('comprendre') Christ's crucifixion was designed not to produce suffering, but to generate a sweetness ('doce') and delight for the person willing to focus on the meditation ('qui metroit son penser'). The poem was tailored for those facing certain death. It positioned the performer 'at the end of my life' ('el fin de mon eet') uttering a confession and greeting the moment when 'life will be everlasting and health enduring'

68 Ibid., 2.6.3 (53).

69 Thomas of Cantimpré, *Vita beatae Christinae mirabilis*, 637-60, at 1.27: 'Libentissime ac benignissime morientibus assistebat, exhortans ad peccatorum confessionem'; trans. Newman and King in *Collected Saints' Lives*, 148-49.

70 Thomas of Cantimpré, *Vita beatae Christinae mirabilis*, 1.44.

71 Trexler, *Public Life*, 360-61.

72 The poems are edited and translated in Ricketts, 'Critical Edition'. My transcription is based directly on MS 431; I have used my own translations here, relying on Ricketts for cross reference.

('la vie serat et la santeis durable') and they will experience 'eternal joy' ('joie aront permanable').

To assist with this pleasure-inducing process of contemplating Christ's suffering, the poem includes a full-page miniature that must have had particular resonance for the sick, indigent, and elderly (Figure 1.2). The image of Christ appears in action sequences of mercy and compassion. In four inner medallions he can be seen washing the feet of the poor, feeding his friends in the last supper, praying at Gethsemane, and finally facing his own crucifixion, an act that the poem describes as bringing healthful salvation to the whole world ('le monde at salveit'). The roundels on the periphery of Christ's caregiving acts amplify these salubrious gestures, carrying them forward in time by displaying Christ's future followers, including saints of the church, replicating his caregiving actions. For example, two martyrs endure torture, Dominic feeds the hungry, Martin gives his precious coat to a street beggar, and the Frankish Queen Clotilde curries favour with an imprisoned Leonard who interceded on her behalf for safe delivery.[73]

These images illustrate and vivify the poem, grounding its significations in a Christian concept of *salus* that mingled health and salvation. Like the martyrs who endured suffering for a spiritual purpose, the poem implored its audience to transform their self-understanding, to reinterpret the meaning of their pain and infirmity. The 'source of pain' ('dolur traitier'), it insisted, could be redirected through poetic meditation to become a salubrious process. Contemplation of Christ's myrrh, which was associated with death and mourning in biblical tradition, enabled the practitioner to 'easily carry the burden of tribulation' ('je puisse porter legierement le fais de tribulation'). To those who experienced the painful burdens of the 'flesh and the world' ('le chars et li mons'), it counselled contemplation and confession ('la confession'). The poem thus reassigned meaning to bodily pain and tribulation. It enabled the dying to reimagine their pain from the perspective of Christ's analogous suffering. In this way it gave salvific significance to their suffering and dying. Ingesting the bitter myrrh of Christ's death through the poetic process would ultimately, 'guard my soul at the end of my life' ('garir en puist mi arme el fin de mon eet'). A poem like this one places the beguines of St. Christopher at the bedside of the dying, assisting them in the final process of achieving 'a good death', that is, of dying comfortably while having made the sacrament of confession that ensured 'health everlasting'. Their poetic performances brought consolatory power.

73 On the illustrations, see Brassine, *Le psautier liégeois*.

Figure 1.2 Full-page miniature featuring Christ washing feet, Last Supper, Gethsemene, Crucifixion; exterior roundels depict saints Dominic, Leonard, Martin, Bartholomew, Denis, and Lawrence

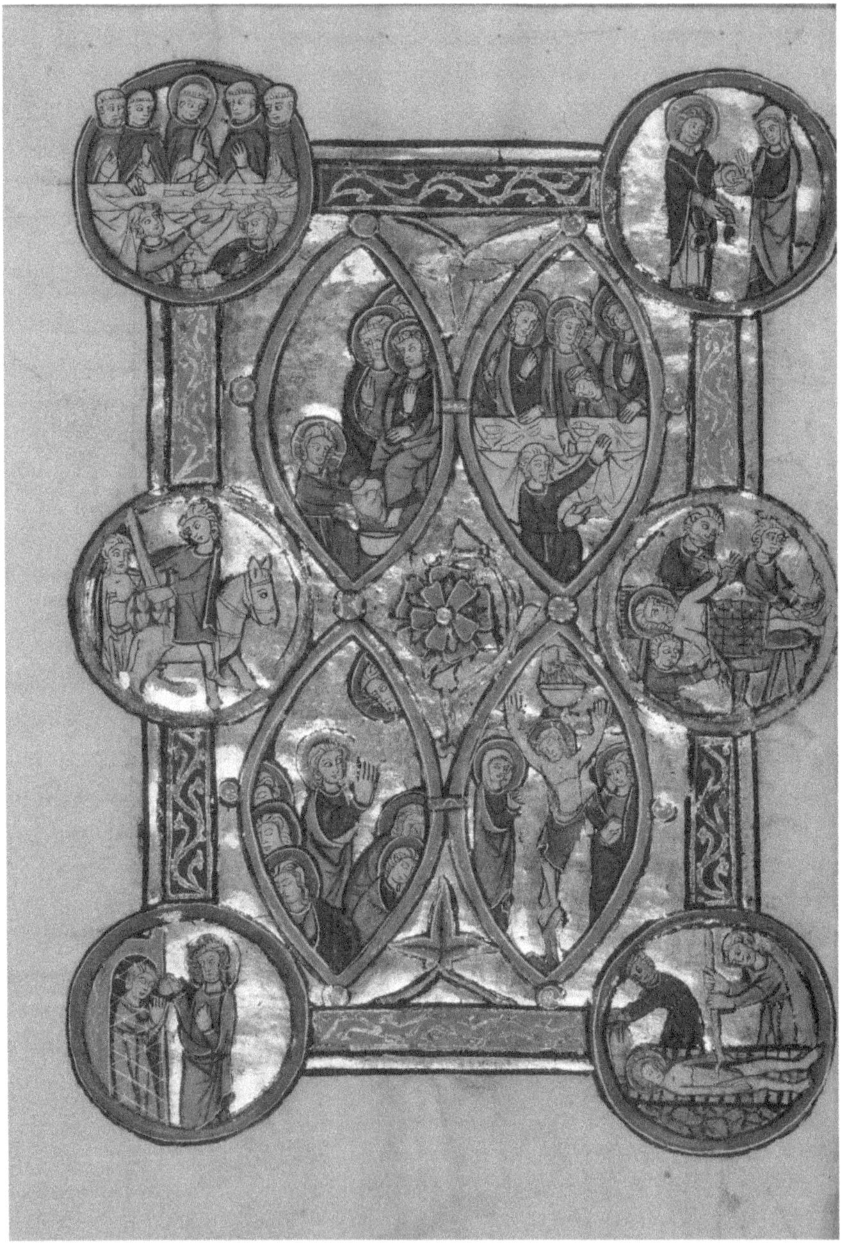

Bibliothèques de l'Université de Liège, MS 431, fol. 10v.

Feminine Therapeutic Epistemologies

MS Liège 431 provides a glimpse into a therapeutic world in which beguines drew on oral, performed, and embodied knowledge when caring for the sick, parturient, and dying. Poetic injunctions to Christ as the source of health and eternal life ('la vie serat et la santeis durable') have heretofore been regarded as the stuff of devotion and liturgy, examples of the affective excesses of thirteenth-century liégeois 'female spirituality'. But the sacramental medicine described in MS 431 was hardly mere metaphor. Informed by the institutional context of hospitals and leprosaria where Mosan beguines often worked, it is necessary to read the psalter's poetry and performance as a means of communicating knowledge and structuring relationships of care in these communities. Beguine psalters show that their therapeutic knowledge was not premised on universal claims in the way that scholastic physicians positioned their own medical theories. Rather, beguine care was adaptable to the needs of individual bodies and their frailties, both spiritual and material. It was improvisational, suited to the specific birthing needs, sins, or the dying wishes of their patients.

The historical legacies of the marginalization and silencing of the production of feminine knowledge about the body, health, and dying well mean that women's therapeutic epistemology is not available on a coherent plane for analytic investigation, a perfect object for the scholar's gaze.[74] Rather, it is enmeshed in disparate scenes, uncanny stories, and fragments of text, image, and object that coalesced into therapeutic microcommunities, that is, into small gatherings around sickbeds, tombs, relics, and prayerbooks from which stories of healing were generated. It is in these local circumstances of knowledge production that we can begin to recuperate silenced voices in lost healing practices, lost texts, and lost intimate moments surrounding sickness and death. These practices, texts, and performances did not seek to lay claim to grand, universal principles or to reduce the human body to a solitary, predictable, impenetrable entity.[75] A source like Liège MS 431 offers access to an everyday world of body knowledge and therapeutic practice in thirteenth-century western Europe and allows us to reframe what really 'counts' as a medical source, a medical practitioner, and a bodily threat.[76]

74 Stewart, *Ordinary Affects*.

75 Gomez, *Experiential Caribbean*, 3.

76 On what 'counts' as medicine, see Langwick, *Bodies, Politics, and African Healing*.

Works Cited

Manuscripts

Brussels, KBR, MS IV-36.
Brussels, KBR, MS 11130-32.
Liège, Bibliothèque de l'Université, MS 431.
London, British Library, MS Sloane 1611.
London, British Library, MS Sloane 2435.
Rome, Biblioteca Apostolica, MS Pal. Lat. 1990.
Valenciennes, Bibliothèque municipale, MS 329.

Printed Works

Aldobrandino of Siena. *La régime du corps de maître Aldebrandin de Sienne: texte français du XIIIe siècle, publié pour la première fois d'après les manuscrits de la Bibliothèque nationale et de la Bibliothèque de l'Arsenal*, ed. Louis Landouzy and Roger Pepin (Geneva: Slatkine, 1978).

Arnald of Villanova. *Arnaldi de Villanova Opera medica omnia*, ed. Luis Garcia-Ballester and Michael R. McVaugh (Barcelona: Ediciones Universitat Barcelona, 1996).

Austin, J.L. *How to Do Things with Words* (Oxford: Oxford University Press, 1962).

Avicenna. *Liber canonis, De medicinis cordialibus, et Cantica* (Venice: Iuntas, 1555).

Bartholomew of Salerno. *Practica magistri Bartholomei Salernitani*, in *Collectio Salernitana*, ed. Salvatore De Renzi (Naples: Filiatre-Sebezio, 1859, repr. 2001), 321-406.

Borgnet, Adolphe and Stanislas Bormans. *Ly myreur des histors ou chronique et geste de Jean des Preis dit d'Outremeuse* (Brussels: Publications de la Commission royale d'Histoire, 1864-87).

Brassine, Joseph. *Le psautier liégeois du XIIIe siècle* (Brussels: Vromant, 1923).

Cabré, Montserrat. 'Women or Healers? Household Practices and the Categories of Health Care in Late Medieval Iberia', *Bulletin of the History of Medicine*, 82 (2008), 18-51.

Cartulaire du béguinage de Sainte-Elisabeth à Gand, ed. Jean Bethune (Bruges: Zuttere, 1883).

Cartularium van het Begijnhof van Dendermonde, ed. Jan Broeckaert (Dendermonde: August De Schepper-Philips, 1902).

Cersovsky, Eva-Maria. '*Ubi non est mulier, ingemiscit egens*? Gendered Perceptions of Care from the Thirteenth to Sixteenth Centuries', in *Gender, Health, and Healing, 1250-1550*, ed. Sara Ritchey and Sharon Strocchia (Amsterdam: Amsterdam University Press, 2020), 191-214.

Collins, Patricia Hill. *Black Feminist Thought: Knowledge, Consciousness, and the Politics of Empowerment* (New York: Routledge, 2002).
Daris, Joseph. 'Extraits du cartulaire de Saint-Laurent', *Bulletin de la Société d'Art et d'Histoire du Diocèse de Liège*, 2 (1882), 321-85.
Deregnaucourt, Jean-Pierre. 'Le dernier voyage: l'ambulation funèbre à Douai aux 14e et 15e siècles', in *La sociabilité urbaine en Europe du Nord-Ouest du XIVe au XVIIIe siècles* (Douai: Imprimerie Lefebvre-Lévêque, 1983).
De Spiegeler, Pierre. *Les hôpitaux et l'assistance à Liège (Xe-XVe siècles): aspects institutionnels et sociaux* (Paris: Belles Lettres, 1987).
Elsakkers, Marianne. 'In Pain You Shall Bear Children (Gen 3:16): Medieval Prayers for a Safe Delivery', in *Women and Miracle Stories: A Multidisciplinary Exploration*, ed. Anne-Marie Korte (Leiden: Brill, 2001), 179-207.
Fayen, Arnold. 'L'Antigraphum Petri et les lettres concernant Lambert le Bègue, conservées dans le manuscrit de Glasgow', *Bulletin de la Commission royale d'histoire*, 68 (1899), 255-356.
Féry-Hue, Françoise. 'Le Régime du corps d'Aldebrandin de Sienne: complément a la tradition manuscrite', *Scriptorium*, 58.1 (2004), 99-108.
Gomez, Pablo. *The Experiential Caribbean: Creating Knowledge and Healing in the Early Modern Atlantic* (Chapel Hill: University of North Carolina, 2017).
Grant, Edward. *A Sourcebook in Medieval Science* (Cambridge, MA: Harvard University Press, 1974).
Green, Monica. 'Books as a Source of Medical Education for Women in the Middle Ages', *Dynamis*, 20 (2000), 331-69.
—. *Making Women's Medicine Masculine: The Rise of Male Authority in Pre-modern Gynaecology* (Oxford: Oxford University Press, 2008).
Green, Monica and Daniel Smail. 'The Trial of Floreta d'Ays (1403): Jews, Christians, and Obstetrics in Later Medieval Marseilles', *Journal of Medieval History*, 34 (2008), 185-211.
Headley, Stephen. 'Afterword: The Mirror in the Mosque', in *Inside and Outside the Mosque: Islamic Prayer across the Indian Ocean*, ed. David Parkin and Stephen Headley (Surrey: Curzon, 2000), 213-39.
Horden, Peregrine. 'A Non-natural Environment: Medicine without Doctors and the Medieval European Hospital', in *The Medieval Hospital and Medical Practice*, ed. Barbara Bowers (Aldershot: Ashgate, 2007), 133-46.
—. 'Religion and Medicine: Music in Medieval Hospitals', in *Religion and Medicine in the Middle Ages*, ed. Peter Biller and Joseph Ziegler (York: York Medieval Press, 2001), 135-54.
—, ed. *Music as Medicine: The History of Music Therapy since Antiquity* (New York: Routledge, 2000).

Hunt, Nancy Rose. 'An Acoustic Register, Tenacious Images, and Congolese Scenes of Rape and Repetition', *Cultural Anthropology*, 23.2 (2008), 220-53.

Jacquart, Danielle and Marilyn Nicoud. 'Les régimes de santé au XIIIe siècle', in *Comprendre le XIIIe siècle*, ed. Pierre Guichard and Danièle Alexandre-Bidon (Lyon: Presses universitaires de Lyon, 1995), 201-14.

Jacques de Vitry. *Vita Mariae Oigniacensis*, in *Acta sanctorum*, ed. D. Papebroek, June, pt. 5 (Paris: Palme, 1867), 542-72.

John of Garland. *The Parisiana Poetria of John of Garland*, ed. and trans. Traugott Lawler (New Haven: Yale University Press, 1974).

Kandzha, Iliana. 'Female Saints as Agents of Female Healing: Gendered Practices and Patronage in the Cult of St. Cunigunde', in *Gender, Health, and Healing, 1250-1550*, ed. Sara Ritchey and Sharon Strocchia (Amsterdam: Amsterdam University Press, 2020), 67-90.

Langwick, Stacey. *Bodies, Politics, and African Healing: The Matter of Maladies in Tanzania* (Bloomington, IN: University of Indiana Press, 2011).

Leroquais, Victor. *Les Psautiers: manuscrits latins du bibliothèques publiques de France* (Paris: Protat Frères, 1940).

McDonnell, Ernest. *Beguines and Beghards in Medieval Culture with Special Emphasis on the Belgian Scene* (Rutgers, NJ: Rutgers University Press, 1954).

Maurach, Gregor. 'Johannicius: Isagogue ad Techni Galieni', *Sudhoffs Archiv*, 62 (1978), 148-74.

Metcalf, Peter. *Where are YOU/SPIRITS: Style and Theme in Berawan Prayer* (Washington, DC: Smithsonian Institution Press, 1989).

Meyer, Paul. 'Le Psautier Lambert le Bègue', *Romania*, 29 (1900), 536-40.

Mora-Dieu, Guillaume. 'L'Ancien hôpital Tirebourse, à Liège: resultats de l'èvaluation Archaeologique', *La Lettre du Patrimoine*, 8 (October-December 2005), 132-34.

Nicoud, Marilyn. *Les régimes de santé au Moyen Âge* (Rome: École Française de Rome, 2007).

Oliver, Judith. *Gothic Manuscript Illumination in the Diocese of Liège, 1250-1350* (Leuven: Peeters, 1988).

Olsan, Lea and Peter Murray Jones. 'Performative Rituals for Conception and Childbirth in England, 900-1500', *Bulletin of the History of Medicine*, 89.3 (2005), 406-33.

Palazzo, Eric. *A History of Liturgical Books from the Beginning to the Thirteenth Century*, trans. Madeleine Beaumont (Collegeville, MN: Liturgical Press, 1998).

Pissart, Madeleine. 'Tirebourse et Florichamps', *Annuaire d'histoire Liégeoise*, 4 (1950), 285-99.

Rappaport, Roy. *Ritual and Religion in the Making of Humanity* (Cambridge: Cambridge University Press, 1999).

Reinburg, Virginia. *French Books of Hours: Making an Archive of Prayer, 1400-1600* (Cambridge: Cambridge University Press, 2012).

Ricketts, Peter T., trans. 'Critical Edition of the Poems of the Mosan Psalters', in *The Feast of Corpus Christi*, ed. Barbara Walters, Vincent Corrigan, and Peter T. Ricketts (University Park, PA: Pennsylvania State University Press, 2006), 445-531.

Schmitt, Jean-Claude. *Mort d'une hérésie: l'église et les clercs face aux béguines et aux béghards du Rhin supérieur du XIVe au XVe siècle* (Paris: Mouton, 1978).

Schoolmeesters, Émile. *Les regestes de Robert de Thourotte: prince-évêque de Liège* (Liège: Cormaux, 1906).

Simons, Walter. *Cities of Ladies: Beguine Communities in the Medieval Low Countries, 1200-1565* (Philadelphia: University of Pennsylvania Press, 2001).

Sinclair, Keith. 'Les manuscrits du Psautier de Lambert le Bègue', *Romania*, 86 (1965), 22-47.

Skemer, Don. *Binding Words: Textual Amulets in the Middle Ages* (University Park, PA: Pennsylvania State University Press, 2006).

Stewart, Kathleen. *Ordinary Affects* (Durham, NC: Duke University Press, 2011).

Symes, Carol. *A Common Stage: Theater and Public Life in Medieval Arras* (Ithaca, NY: Cornell University Press, 2007).

Tambiah, Stanley. *Culture, Thought, and Social Action: An Anthropological Perspective* (Cambridge, MA: Harvard University Press, 1985).

Taylor, Diana. 'Remapping Genre through Performance: From "American" to "Hemispheric" Studies', *PMLA* 122.5 (2007), 1416-30.

Thomas of Cantimpré. *Liber de natura rerum* (Berlin: De Gruyter, 1973).

—. 'The Life of Christina the Astonishing', in *Thomas of Cantimpré: The Collected Saints' Lives*, ed. Barbara Newman and Margot King (Turnhout: Brepols, 2008), 127-57.

—. *Vita beatae Christinae mirabilis*, in *Acta sanctorum*, ed. Joannes Pinnius, July, pt. 5 (Antwerp: Jacobus de Moulin, 1727), 637-60.

Trexler, Richard. *Public Life in Renaissance Florence* (Ithaca, NY: Cornell University Press, 1980).

Vita B. Idae de Nivella, in *Quinque prudentes virgines*, ed. Chrysostomo Henriquez (Antwerp: Cnobbaert, 1630), 199-297.

Vitae B. Odiliae Viduae Leodiensis, in *Analecta Bollandiana*, 13 (1894), 197-287.

Wieck, Roger. *Painted Prayers: The Book of Hours in Medieval and Renaissance Art* (New York: George Braziller, 1997).

Ziegler, Johanna. *The Sculpture of Compassion: The Pieta and the Beguines in the Southern Low Countries, 1300-1600* (Brussels: Institut Historique Belge du Rome, 1992).

About the Author

Sara Ritchey is Associate Professor of History at the University of Tennessee, Knoxville. She is the author of *Holy Matter: Changing Perceptions of the Material World in Late Medieval Christianity* (2014) and a forthcoming book on late medieval religious women's therapeutic knowledge and healthcare practices (2021).

2 Female Saints as Agents of Female Healing

Gendered Practices and Patronage in the Cult of St. Cunigunde

Iliana Kandzha

Abstract

This essay studies the mechanics informing the construction of a single healing cult, that of the virgin saint Empress Cunigunde (*c.*980-1033) and its gender aspects. The shrine of St. Cunigunde in Bamberg was well known as a healing space after her canonization in 1200, although the first miracle collection does not reveal any medical specialization of the cult. Using previously neglected late medieval narrative and archival material, the essay shows that Cunigunde was a popular female patron whose assistance was sought by women, especially during childbirth. This case of female medical patronage is analysed alongside similar practices in the cults of other saints and is regarded as one of the resources for female convalescence in the medical market of that time.

Keywords: miraculous healing, healing relics, Bamberg, holy virgins, female health

One of the most common medical practices available in the Middle Ages was miraculous healing performed through the intercession of saints.[1] Cults of saints created and successfully maintained a powerful economy of miraculous aid throughout the medieval period and beyond.[2] This economy rested on

1 For more on miraculous healing see Ward, *Miracles and the Medieval Mind*; Park, 'Medicine and Society'; Metzler, *Disability in Medieval Europe*, 126-85.

2 The groundbreaking analyses of medieval miracles in the regions of modern-day England and France by Finucane and Sigal reveal that around 90 per cent of the miracles from the analysed

Ritchey, Sara & Sharon Strocchia (eds), *Gender, Health, and Healing, 1250-1550*. Amsterdam, Amsterdam University Press 2020
DOI: 10.5117/9789463724517_CH02

a profound belief in the efficacy of saints' powers, accessed by a devotee through an invocation or contact with a relic, which attracted immense financial and human resources to veneration sites. While some cults achieved a European-wide reputation, most saints exercised their powers within local communities and were invoked to remedy specific maladies.[3] This medical specialization among saints, most evident in the late Middle Ages, was ridiculed by contemporaries, as when Erasmus of Rotterdam parodied, 'Each saint has his distinct office allotted to him, and is accordingly addressed to upon the respective occasions: as one for the tooth-ache, a second to grant an easy delivery in child-birth, a third to help persons [find] lost goods, another to protect seamen in a long voyage, a fifth to guard the farmer's cows and sheep, and so on; for to rehearse all instances would be extremely tedious'.[4] As Erasmus's comments suggest, miraculous interventions functioned as an important resource for healing and relief, including relief in matters of gynecology and obstetrics.[5] However, the role of saints and of God's therapy has not yet been fully incorporated into our understanding of medieval medical practice.[6] This essay seeks to enhance our understanding of the social dynamics and cultural circumstances that led to distinctive allocations of saints' 'offices', and in particular, to account for their development from the perspective of the social history of medicine and gender history.

The case of the cult of St. Cunigunde, the virgin German empress (*c.*980-1033, can. 1200), demonstrates how the constitution of a cult could shift over time as medical significations accrued to a certain saint. Cunigunde was venerated in the diocese of Bamberg in southern Germany and in several other locations. By the end of the fifteenth century, St. Cunigunde had acquired fame for granting 'an easy delivery in childbirth', a capacity included in the list of saints' offices that Erasmus found so tedious. Previous studies of her healing cult have been based almost exclusively on the

corpora concerned healing. These results suggest a distinctive role for the cults of saints in medieval understandings of healthcare. See Finucane, *Miracles and Pilgrims*; Sigal, *L'Homme et le miracle*. On modern practices of religious healing see Duffin, *Medical Miracles*.

3 Vauchez, *Sainthood in the Later Middle Ages*, 145-246, discusses popular and local sainthood.

4 Erasmus, *In Praise of Folly*, 68-69. On the specializations of saints see the classic study by Kræmer, *Les maladies*. Bartlett provides an excellent survey of contemporary scepticism towards the veneration of saints in *Why Can the Dead Do Such Great Things?*, 587-608.

5 Evidence for miraculous healings facilitating pregnancy is discussed by Krüger, 'Elisabeth von Thüringen und Maria Magdalena'; Cormack, 'Better Off Dead'; Powell, 'Miracle of Childbirth'; Morse, 'Thys Moche More Ys Oure Lady Mary Longe'.

6 Green has suggested that scholars should investigate 'how much religious belief served as a supplement to or substitution for other forms of health intervention'; Green, 'Recent Work on Medieval Women's Medicine', 22.

socio-statistical analysis of her miracle collection, created around 1200, quantitatively describing her miracles and their recipients.[7] In this essay, I consider previously overlooked textual traditions and various readings of Cunigunde's hagiographies as well as evidence concerning her relics. I do so in order, first, to outline her cult as one that provided assistance for parturient mothers; second, to contextualize Cunigunde's female patronage alongside other available medical practices and similar developments in the European religious landscape; and, finally, to consider why the cult of Cunigunde, first represented as welcoming all genders and harbouring all ills, acquired a specialized function in the fifteenth century as a local healing resource for pregnant women.

Understanding the Miracle Collection of St. Cunigunde

Cunigunde was one of the first female saints to be officially canonized by the Catholic Church. The canonization bull, issued by Innocent III on 3 April 1200, brought an almost decade-long canonization investigation to conclusion, propagated by the bishop of Bamberg with support from other episcopal authorities and clergy from the region.[8] The inclusion of Cunigunde in the *communio sanctorum* added to the glory of the city of Bamberg, where the cult of her spouse Emperor Henry II (973-1024, can. 1146) had already been well-established since the middle of the twelfth century.[9] Henry and Cunigunde were believed to have lived in a chaste marriage and were known for their donations to the church. These virtues, along with a number of miracles that their hagiographies and visual arts portray as having occurred during their lives, made them subjects of intense veneration. Their shrines became a popular destination for pilgrims from the Bamberg diocese and neighbouring regions, as evidenced in their miracle collections and reflected in the broad distribution of their relics and cult-related objects.[10] Cunigunde can be considered the first contemporary female saint of this German region, preceded only by two German queens

7 Harmening, 'Fränkische Mirakelbücher'; Wenz-Haubfleisch, 'Der Kult der hl. Kunigunde'.
8 Petersohn, 'Die Litterae Papst Innozenz III'.
9 The foundational study on the cults of Henry and Cunigunde in eleventh- to thirteenth-century Bamberg is Klauser, *Der Heinrichs- und Kunigundenkult*. More recent literature on the cult of Cunigunde, her canonization proceedings, and imagery includes Petersohn, 'Die Litterae Papst Innozenz III'; Guth, 'Kaiserin Kunigunde'; Meyer, 'Die konstruierte Heilige'; Dick et al., *Kunigunde, consors regni*; Schneidmüller, 'Heinrich II. und Kunigunde'.
10 Linke, *Beitrag zur Kulttopographie*.

– Mathilda and Adelheid – whose brief veneration was a prominent part of propaganda efforts of the ruling Ottonian dynasty in the tenth century.[11] Thus, it would be tempting to assume that Cunigunde's cult compensated for the lack of local contemporary female saints and promoted a sacred 'medical marketplace', possibly targeted at women.[12]

On 1 August 1199, the feast of St. Peter ad Vincula (also known as Petri Kettenfeier), a mentally impaired man was healed at the tomb of Empress Cunigunde in the Bamberg Cathedral.[13] The fame of a new healing cult spread rapidly and, as Cunigunde's miracle collection narrates, around a hundred people were healed from various diseases or given help at the tomb of Cunigunde between August 1199 and March 1200. Presumably, miracles that occurred at Cunigunde's shrine in the cathedral were first written down in 1200 to support her canonization process. Pope Innocent III advocated for a record of post-mortem miracles as necessary justification for canonization, thus the collection of miracles acquired the function of a legal document. While a chaste lifestyle and pious deeds were praiseworthy virtues, it was post-mortem miracles that served as a clear sign of holiness.[14] Since that time, the date of Cunigunde's first miracle was liturgically celebrated throughout the Bamberg diocese. Every year, the flock was reminded of their patron saint's miracle-working powers.[15]

Several scholars of Christian miracles have conceptualized the miraculous and religious healings evident in the many other miracle books similar to

11 The cults of the sainted queens Mathilde (d. 968) and Adelheid (931-999) were orchestrated by the ruling dynasty to enhance its prestige; hence, these cults did not flourish for too long even in places of their active veneration. See Corbet, *Les Saints ottoniens*, and Gilsdorf, *Queenship and Sanctity*. Even though Cunigunde and Henry II belonged to the same dynasty, it would be erroneous to describe the Ottonians as *beata stirps*, as discussed by Corbet.

12 Goetz has revealed a strong correlation between the gender of a saint and the gender of his or her clientele. Even though many early medieval cults were described as *utrisque sexus*, highlighting the saint's efficaciousness for both men and women, large-scale quantitative analysis has shown that women tended to seek intercession and healing from female saints. See Goetz, 'Heiligenkult und Geschlecht'. The present article further investigates this assumption that female saints acted as agents of female healing.

13 'Vita et miracula S. Cunegundis', 825 (1). There are two existing editions of the *vita* and the miracle collection of St. Cunigunde in the *Acta sanctorum* and *Monumenta germaniae historica*, both of which are incomplete. For the current study, the following manuscripts were analysed, containing the two earliest redactions of the miracle collection of St. Cunigunde: Bamberg, Staatsbibliothek, R.B. Msc. 120; and Leipzig, Universitätsbibliothek, Rep. II 64. For convenience, references will be given to the *Monumenta germaniae historica* edition where possible.

14 Vauchez, *Sainthood in the Later Middle Ages*, 425-77.

15 On the commemoration *propter primum miraculum eius* and Cunigunde's liturgy in Bamberg, see Klauser, *Der Heinrichs- und Kunigundenkult*, 154-56, and Farrenkopf, *Breviarium Eberhardi cantoris*, 159.

that of Cunigunde. In his pioneering studies, Roger Finucane explained the therapeutic effects of contact with a shrine or a relic by drawing on the psychosomatic origins of physical or mental impairments, which in turn were relieved through a psychological effect.[16] Scholars operating within the linguistic turn have shown that miracles are narrative constructions, a means of exercising power and controlling access to the sacred, which leaves unanswered the question of belief and occurrence.[17] Even though some medieval intellectuals and lay people already expressed a fair amount of scepticism towards miracles, these narratives, taken at least partially at face value, stimulated the belief in a specific saint and in God's thaumaturgy, which were seen as a reward for one's devotion and donations. The case of Cunigunde – whose miraculous activities were recorded in the miracle collection, reflected upon in the canonization bull, translated into the vernacular, and commemorated in liturgy – indicates that these miracles were actualized and demanded in different circumstances. Prospective patients, believers, and readers thus understood them both as real events and as powerful narratives. However, narrated miracles also contained the 'many, sometimes conflicting voices' of those who influenced the appearance of a miracle collection and those who received it in the form of a written or oral narrative.[18] Hence, a proper understanding of the miraculous event requires not only a thorough analysis of the healing cures, but also of their textual history, probable audience, and the various media through which these narratives were publicized.

Quantifying the Miraculous in the Early Cult of St. Cunigunde

The miracles of Cunigunde, as recorded in their two earliest redactions now in the libraries in Bamberg and Leipzig, reflect the first phase of the cult taking shape around the canonization in 1200.[19] Viewed through the prism of her miracle collection, it is clear that Cunigunde had a reputation as a healing saint

16 Finucane argued that patients in a cult understood emotionally triggered alleviation of pain as healing; Finucane, *Rescue of the Innocents*, 1-16.

17 On these and other attempts to conceptualize medieval religious belief, see the introduction to Korte, *Women and Miracle Stories*, and Justice, 'Did the Middle Ages Believe in their Miracles?'

18 Goodich, *Miracles and Wonders*, 4.

19 The redactions are preserved in Bamberg, Staatsbibliothek, R.B. Msc. 120, fols. 37v-46r, and Leipzig, Universitätsbibliothek, Rep. II 64, fols. 39v-55r. For the beginnings of the cult of St. Cunigunde and her miracle collections, see Klauser, *Der Heinrichs- und Kunigundenkult*, 96-100, and Wenz-Haubfleisch, 'Der Kult der hl. Kunigunde'.

in thirteenth-century upper Franconia. Among the 153 people who sought her assistance, 144 of them had health problems or disabilities.[20] Here I define a healing miracle as a claim that those with physical or mental impairments and other illnesses were restored to full health. This process is usually described in the sources by the general formula *sanatus/a est* or more disease-specific wordings, such as *illuminatus/a est*.[21] The list of illnesses tackled by Cunigunde and often explicitly named in the Latin text of her collection included paralysis, blindness, deafness and muteness, mental illness, and wounds.[22]

The narrative patterns of these healing miracles are repeated throughout the collection. They contain information about how the devotee became familiar with the cult, the devotee's place of origin, malady, and often his or her age and gender. Finally, each miracle story declared that full health was obtained, sometimes describing the means of coming into contact with the shrine. For example, in one case, the dust ('pulvis') from Cunigunde's tomb was applied to the body of a supplicant.[23] The length and density of details provided varied from a few lines to a full column in the codex, although even a short miracle story exemplified the way in which a healing was recorded; for example, 'A certain young woman from the town of Nuremberg, with the soles of her feet crooked inwards and her knees constricted, obtained health.'[24]

The miracle collection of Cunigunde was analysed extensively by Annegret Wenz-Haubfleish.[25] Her quantitative analysis provided insights into Cunigunde's clientele: their social status, gender, age, and place of origin. She also classified the diseases against which Cunigunde was understood to be effective. While only two miracle stories claimed that Cunigunde resurrected a drowned child, and one reported that she performed exorcism, her most numerous cures (over 70 per cent) involved sensorimotor disabilities, including physical and mental impairments such as paralysis, blindness, or insanity.[26] These sensorimotor disorders are also widespread in other miracle

20 These numbers are taken from Wenz-Haubfleisch, 'Der Kult der hl. Kunigunde', in which she analysed the profile of the devotees of Cunigunde based on her miracle collection. The number of *miraculée* at Cunigunde's tomb and the exact percentage of impairments cured can vary due to different readings of the two redactions as well as different methods of quantification.

21 On the vocabulary describing diseases and healings in miracle accounts see Wenz-Haubfleisch, *Miracula post mortem*, 136-38.

22 Wenz-Haubfleisch, 'Der Kult der hl. Kunigunde', 174.

23 'Vita et miracula S. Cunegundis', 825, 827 (20, 76).

24 Ibid., 825 (14): 'Quedam puella de burgo qui dicitur Nurenberc plante pedis sursum recurve et geniculi contracti sanationem optinuit'.

25 Wenz-Haubfleisch, 'Der Kult der hl. Kunigunde'.

26 Ibid., 174.

collections: for example, a huge corpus of twelfth-century miracle books (recording over 3,500 individual miracles) from one region of France revealed similar, if not identical, healing patterns to those of the cult of Cunigunde.[27]

This prevalence of a specific group of sensorimotor problems among various healing cults could be an intentional replication of New Testament miracles, which were seen as a typological ideal for narrators of saints' miracles and expected by the audience.[28] At the same time, curing a sensorimotor illness was immediately noticeable and made it easy to provide testimony in a pre-canonization interrogation. This immediacy is also performative: its spectacle makes a miracle an influential tool for the conversion of onlookers.[29] Lastly, as Irina Metzler has noted, most of these illnesses fall under the category of incurable sicknesses from the standpoint of medieval medicine. Blindness, deafness, and partial or full physical impairments are best described as disabilities for which religious healing seemed the only possible remedy.[30] In this way, medical practice and religious healing constituted complementary resources.

As for the gender division of Cunigunde's devotees, slightly less than half of the pilgrims recorded as visiting the tomb were women.[31] Yet, in this miracle collection, Cunigunde is never mentioned as a helper in any exclusively gendered experiences, such as pregnancy, child care, or issues related to infertility.[32] All the cures of female pilgrims fall into the same pattern sketched above. From these data, Wenz-Haubfleish concluded that the cult of Cunigunde was not gender-oriented at its inception at the turn of the thirteenth century, nor were female pilgrims specifically attracted by the image of a virgin empress.

However, it is also worth taking into account the fact that women were much more restricted in their ability to travel long distances than men and therefore were less present in miracle collections. Vauchez explained

27 The numbers from Sigal's *L'Homme et le miracle* are presented in Bartlett, *Why Can the Dead Do Such Great Things?*, 342-43.

28 Kee, *Medicine, Miracle and Magic in New Testament Times*; Goodich, *Miracles and Wonders*, 4-7.

29 The miracle collection of Cunigunde contains an example of a 'performative' miracle. After a wealthy imperial officer was healed by the saint, he immediately revealed it to bystanders; numerous bells started to ring to call people's attention to the event and to praise the saint; 'Vita et miracula S. Cunegundis', 827 (69). Goodich assumed the main function of a miracle from the papal standpoint to be conversion; Goodich, 'Vision, Dream and Canonization Policy'.

30 Metzler, *Disability in Medieval Europe*, 140.

31 According to Wenz-Haubfleisch, 43 per cent of devotees (56 women out of 130 pilgrims whose gender is stated) were female; Wenz-Haubfleisch, 'Der Kult der hl. Kunigunde', 170-72.

32 In a few cases involving drowned and lost children, petitioners included not only their mothers but both parents as well as onlookers.

the generally low number of childbirth miracles (between 1.2 and 3.3 per cent) found in medieval collections by noting that parturient women could not travel to a distant cult or spend a night at the tomb, as was common practice.[33] Similar conclusions can be reached from the analysis of the cult of St. Elizabeth of Hungary, based on her canonization protocols and miracle collection. While hosting a slightly larger percentage of female *miraculées* (48 per cent) than Cunigunde, the cult of St. Elizabeth did not seem to specialize in female healings either, at least as seen through the prism of her miracle collection.[34] However, these patterns stand in striking contrast to the active patronage of St. Elizabeth, whose intercession was sought by expectant and parturient women of different social standing.[35] Some of Elizabeth's relics were well-known for their soothing powers during pregnancy and childbirth. These considerations and the comparison with St. Elizabeth raise questions about whether the gender-specialization of a cult should be analysed primarily through a miracle collection, as has been the practice so far.

In fact, the main purpose of the miracle collection of Cunigunde, composed around 1200 during her canonization procedure, was to present her as a universally acceptable and applicable saint. Indeed, the compilers of this and other miracle collections hoped their audiences, especially those in power who could legitimize the prospective cult, would believe in a roughly even gender distribution among *miraculés* and in the powers of the shrine, especially regarding those conditions that could not be cured by physicians. The recurring narrative of a sick person turning to a saint after vainly seeking relief from mundane doctors falls under this agenda.[36] When meticulously calculating the types of impairments and their correlation with the gender of a cured person, we become trapped in an illusion of the general efficacy of the healing cult – an illusion carefully constructed by the compilers of its miracle collection. Hence, the cult of Cunigunde might not have been depicted in her first collection of miracles as targeting a female

33 Vauchez, *Sainthood in the Later Middle Ages*, 466-77. By contrast, in her analysis of the cult of St. Thomas Becket, Powell suggests that pregnant women actually did come to shrines to seek relief, although their stories were deliberately not recounted. Only with a change in the status of lay testimony did stories of successful childbirths enter miracle collections; Powell, 'Miracle of Childbirth'.

34 Jansen, *Medizinische Kasuistik*, esp. 99-100.

35 Krüger, 'Elisabeth von Thüringen und Maria Magdalena'.

36 This narrative of failed earthly medicine is also present in Cunigunde's miracles. 'Vita et miracula S. Cunegundis', 825 (9): 'Item in diocesi nostra nobilis femina, de castello, quod Wischenuelt [Wikenfeld] nuncupatur, immoderatum dolorem sustinens, quia nullo medicorum remedio curari poterat. Se celesti medico commendans, pristinae sanitati restituitur'. See also Metzler, *Disability in Medieval Europe*, 141-46.

audience simply because it would have satisfied neither the requirements of the papal curia nor the ambitions of the diocese of Bamberg.

St. Cunigunde as a Female Healer

Incorporating additional sources into our analysis and considering the developments of St. Cunigunde's cult over time serves as a 'corrective method' when assessing the image portrayed in her initial miracle collection. Previous research on Cunigunde's healing cult in Bamberg has not taken later textual transmissions of the miracle collection into account, and thus has failed to recognize her prominence as a patron for female supplicants.[37] Archival documents and catalogues of relics provide additional evidence concerning the social and gendered constitution of the cult and its visitors. These sources substantiate important changes in the healing economy of St. Cunigunde's cult in Bamberg in later centuries.

A hitherto overlooked addition to Cunigunde's miracles from a late fifteenth-century Belgian codex provides insight into gendered practices involving her relics and presents the saint as a promoter of female healing. This codex contains a collection of saints' lives – including those of St. Henry and St. Cunigunde – written down in 1480 for a female convent in Bethlehem near Leuven.[38] This codex, although originating at a distance from the Bamberg region, apparently contains the first explicit mention of a specific devotion to Cunigunde among pregnant women in Bamberg.

The passage reports on the tunic ('tunica') of St. Cunigunde, which the queen herself made after the death of her husband. This object, kept in Bamberg, especially attracted pregnant women. The codex describes its miraculous healing powers as follows:

> And this [tunic] is said to be of such capacity that to any pregnant woman and those in difficulties of childbearing, who confidently invoke the patronage of the same Virgin and respectfully touches or puts on [the tunic], in an instant it easily brings good health in the labour; and, moreover, it most perfectly releases and protects from the dangers of this sort. And

37 For example, Klauser's study only mentioned the fact that St. Cunigunde was favoured by her female following, referring in this assumption more to the local twentieth-century oral tradition than to medieval sources. See Klauser, *Der Heinrichs- und Kunigundenkult*, 114.

38 Brussels, KBR, MS 3391-99, fols. 172r-180v. Excerpts from this codex are also given in 'De S. Cunigunde Imperatrice', in *Acta sanctorum martii* 1, 279. Since some sentences are not included or rephrased in the printed version, I provide additional citations based on the manuscript.

> then a practice is established in that community that pregnant women, soon approaching the time of delivery, according to the custom, go to the church. After the confession of sins, they protect themselves with the sacred body, and at last approaching the sacred relics of the virgin, they touch or dress in the aforesaid tunic with all respect and devotion.[39]

This passage provides persuasive testimony of Cunigunde being regarded as a healing saint among the women of Bamberg. Moreover, she heals and brings relief to the specifically gendered experience of childbearing. The popularity of this practice cannot be estimated based on this passage alone. However, the compiler of the collection regarded it as worth recounting, while the other almost one hundred miracles from the initial redaction (with two exceptions) were left out.[40]

The same passage also stated that 'the tunic, surely because of devotion to the Virgin adorned with marvellous gems and embellished with innumerable pearls, is not denied to anybody; and in fact is presented upon demand to any women in need'.[41] One might imagine that some of the rich embellishments on the tunic were the gifts of thankful devotees, who wished to express gratitude for the miraculous powers of the virgin saint. The text does not state whether any fee for access to these relics was charged, though archival evidence reveals that a payment of 1 gulden was usually required to see the relics of St. Henry and Cunigunde kept in the cathedral.[42] All in all, this text clearly indicates that the women of Bamberg recognized the healing capacities of Cunigunde and, importantly, had a 'custom' of using them.

39 Brussels, KBR, MS 3391-99, fol. 179v: 'Quae tantae fertur esse virtutis, ut cuilibet mulieri praegnanti, et in partus difficultate virginis eiusdem patrocinium confidenter imploranti, reverenter applicita vel induta, confestim conferat leniter pariendi prosperitatem, et ab huiusmodi periculo perfectissime liberet atque tueatur. Unde habet consuetudo illius civitati, quod mulieres praegnantes, instante iam partus sui tempore, sicuti moris est, ecclesiam adeuntes; post peccatorum confessionem, sacro se corpore se muniant, et demum ad virginis sacrae reliquias accedentes, praedictam tunicam cum omni devotione devotioneque contingant vel induant'. The duplication of the word 'devotione' in the last phrase can be credited to a scribal mistake, thus suggesting that the passage was copied from another source; in a printed edition of the legends of Henry and Cunigunde that appeared in Brussels, which contained the above passage, the phrase reads as 'reverentia devotioneque'. See *Legendae sanctorum Henrici imperatoris et Kunigundis imperatricis*, fol. 45r-v.

40 The manuscript recounts only the first two miracles from the 'standard' collection of Cunigunde's miracles (namely, the miracle that happened *ad vincula petri* and about a lame man from St. Aegidius).

41 Brussels, KBR, MS 3391-99, fol. 179v: 'Quae nimirum tunica ob reverentiam virginis gemmis micantibus adornata et perlis innumeris constipata nemini negatur, sed absque ulla personarum acceptione cunctis indigentibus exhibetur postulata'.

42 Baumgärtel-Fleischmann, 'Die Kaisermäntel im Bamberger Domschatz', 110-11.

As previously stated, a miracle is not only an occasion for healing, it is also a story, transmitted orally, textually, or visually, and often shaped for each specific use. Hence Cunigunde's relics were useful not only for actual devotees in Bamberg, but also for readers of these narratives. Still, we must ask under what circumstances readers in Leuven would know the story of Cunigunde's tunic and her skill in assisting with labour. Who were these readers? And why was a German healing cult for pregnant women of any interest in a completely different religious landscape?

The codex containing examples of parturient women using Cunigunde's relics was created for a convent of Augustinian nuns in Bethlehem, near Leuven, in 1480. This hagiographic collection contains the *Lives* of saints, with additional accounts of their miracles and translations, and could be used as exempla and devotional readings for nuns. The process of selecting and arranging the readings in the codex reshaped their meaning in a way that reflected the identity of community members from the vantage point of their position in Brabant as well as their femininity. Thus, several local saints are included in the hagiographic collection with additional information provided about their relics located in the vicinity of the convent.[43] More than half of the hagiographies belong to female saints. They include not only late antique virgin martyrs, whose cults were widely recognized, but also Merovingian, Carolingian, and more recent female saints, such as St. Elizabeth or St. Cunigunde herself. The lives, martyrdoms, and miracles of twenty-four saintly women (as opposed to only fourteen male saints) provided both edifying reading material and powerful examples of the reconciliation of femininity and a holy lifestyle, as desired by the Augustinian nuns.[44] Hence it is not surprising that the compiler of the collection included the *Life* of Cunigunde with reports of her exclusively female patronage.[45] This miraculous power, appealing to female experiences, could have strengthened bonds between the female community and the saint.

43 For example, the collection recounts the *vitae* of St. Ragenufle and St. Ermeline, early medieval Brabantine saints who were known for their refusal to live a married life and their subsequent hermitage. The legends of a seventh-century 'holy family' from Mons – St. Waltrude, her husband Madelgaire, and their children – are also included.

44 The difference in numbers between male and female saints included in this hagiographic collection is especially striking when considering the overall majority of male saints. According to Schulenburg, only 15 per cent of the medieval *communio sanctorum* were women. See Schulenburg, *Forgetful of their Sex*, 12.

45 It is hard to establish whether the author recorded an orally transmitted story or copied it from a now-lost textual tradition. Similar versions of Henry and Cunigunde's lives are found in another Belgian codex from the Groenendaal priory: Brussels, KBR, MS 219-221, fols. 108v-114r. Even though their cult was not actively venerated there, the personae of Henry and Cunigunde were known in the Flemish region, as demonstrated by their hagiographies being printed as a

Additional evidence of gendered healthcare practices in Cunigunde's late medieval cult can be found in the vernacular translation of the *Lives* and miracles of Henry and Cunigunde drafted by Nonnosus Stettfelder (d. 1529) and published in Bamberg in 1511. On the last page of the book, Nonnosus tried to imagine what Cunigunde looked like.[46] To estimate Cunigunde's height and waist span, Nonnosus used her belt ('gürtel'), a precious relic from the Michelsberg monastery in Bamberg, which was kept there together with her mantle ('mantel'). He also mentioned that these relics facilitated easy childbearing for women who wore the belt and dressed in the mantle.[47] Additionally, he related that one could view these and other relics of Cunigunde – such as her tunic ('rock'), kept in the cathedral treasury – once every seven years during the *Heiltumsweisung*, a festive demonstration of relics.[48]

Both texts – the Belgian codex and the vernacular translation of the saints' legends – describe the same procedure of making physical contact with Cunigunde's relics, and testify to their healing effect upon pregnant women. Nevertheless, the relics discussed were different and apparently were housed in different sites as well. Although the Belgian narrative does not explicitly state where the tunic was kept and where those healings occurred, the catalogues of relics and their treatment by Nonnosus Stettfelder suggest that the tunic in question was housed in the cathedral.[49] At the same time Nonnosus, who worked as a secretary to abbot Andreas Lang at Michelsberg and apparently was knowledgeable about the content of the monastic treasury, stated that the belt and the mantle were kept at the monastery. These objects were also believed to heal women in need, or at least were deliberately described as having such powers. It appears that two distinct ecclesiastical communities in Bamberg – not only the cathedral but also the Benedictine monastery – preserved healing relics of Cunigunde and profited from the pilgrimage of parturient women. In this way, the monastic space could function as a site for healing encounters

single collection in Brussels by the Brethren of the Common Life. See the *Legendae sanctorum Henrici imperatoris et Kunigundis imperatricis*.

46 Nonnosus Stettfelder, *Dye Legend und Leben*, fol. 70r.

47 Ibid., fol. 70r: 'Zu trost schwangern weybern den solche gürtel umb gegurt und mantel angelegt wirt da von sy dan in geperung sunderliche leicterung entpfahen'.

48 Ibid., fol. 70r: 'Solche gürtel und mantel mit sampt yrem rock der in den dumbstiefft zu Bamberg fur heiltumb behaltten wirt werden auch in sybenjaren mit anderm heilgumb dosebst gewyesen'. For more about the tradition of exhibiting relics in general and with respect to Bamberg, see Kühne, *Ostensio reliquiarum*, 275-92, and Cárdenas, *Die Textur des Bildes*.

49 Baumgärtel-Fleischmann, 'Die Kaisermäntel im Bamberger Domschatz'.

particularly suited for women in need, much as Sara Ritchey notes with regard to beguinages elsewhere in this volume.[50]

Renate Baumgärtel-Fleischmann has conducted research on the garments attributed to St. Henry and St. Cunigunde, in which she suggests that, of the six garments kept in the cathedral treasury, the one known as the tunic of St. Cunigunde was the one credited with healing capacities.[51] In 1452, it was even given to the wife of Albert III of Brandenburg to ease the delivery of her child.[52] Moreover, by looking at fifteenth-century account books, Baumgärtel-Fleischmann has discovered evidence of this tunic undergoing constant repair. This might testify to its frequent use, especially considering reports that pregnant women actually donned the tunic.[53] This evidence supports the Belgian account: namely, that the tunic of Cunigunde kept in the Bamberg Cathedral was a source of healing for women. Additionally, both Nonnosus Stettfelder and the anonymous author of the Belgian codex emphasized that Cunigunde either wore or crafted the belt and the garments with her own hands. This was regarded as a proof for devotees that these objects were authentic contact relics that preserved the healing power of the saint herself. However, the Queen could not possibly have worn at least two of them: the belt and the mantle were originally liturgical objects (a stole and an altar cover) from the eleventh century, which by the fourteenth century had acquired a connection to Cunigunde.[54] All these objects, together with other textiles allegedly belonging to the holy royal couple, were indeed preserved intact in Bamberg and were listed in the multiple late medieval books of relics prepared for the *Heiltumsweisung* (Figure 2.1).

The above-mentioned sources testify to the different objects used among parturient women: the tunic housed in the cathedral and the mantle and belt preserved in the monastery. Apparently, women in late medieval Bamberg could have resorted to multiple healing options when they had problems related to childbirth, all of which were connected to the image of St. Cunigunde. This vibrant scene of female miraculous medicine could potentially have created competition for the attention of pilgrims between the two ecclesiastical communities of Bamberg Cathedral and the Michelsberg monastery.[55]

50 Ritchey, 'Caring by the Hours'.

51 Baumgärtel-Fleischmann, 'Die Kaisermäntel im Bamberger Domschatz', 97-100.

52 Ibid., 98, n. 27. The mentioned document: Bamberg, Stadtarchiv, Rep. B7, no. 61, fol. 199r.

53 Baumgärtel-Fleischmann, 'Die Kaisermäntel im Bamberger Domschatz', 98, n. 28.

54 Baumgärtel-Fleischmann, 'Die Kaisermäntel im Bamberger Domschatz'.

55 Competition for pilgrims between the cults of Henry and Cunigunde, whose main shrine was in the cathedral, and of St. Bishop Otto of Bamberg, whose shrine was in Michelsberg, has

Figure 2.1 Fragment from the catalogue of relics of Bamberg Cathedral showing one of the mantels of Cunigunde and her tunic with the belt

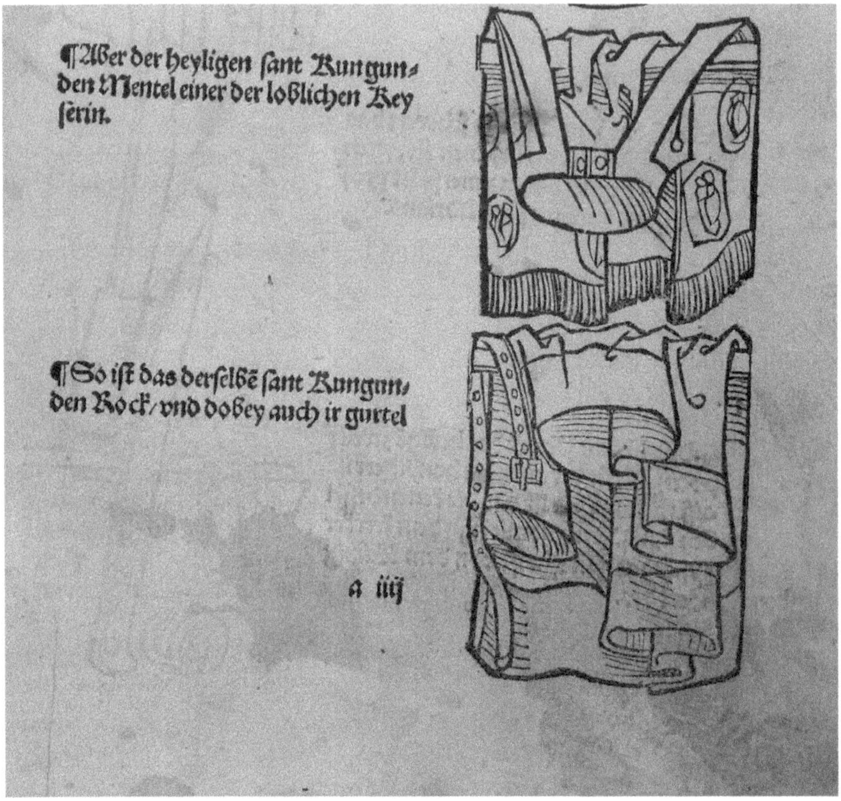

¶Aber der heyligen sant Kungun-
den Mentel einer der loblichen Key-
serin.

¶So ist das derselbē sant Kungun-
den Rock/ vnd dobey auch ir gurtel

a iiij

From *Die weysung vnnd auszruffung des Hochwirdigen heylthumbs zu Bamberg* (Bamberg: Johann Pfeil, 1509), fol. 4r. Bamberg, Staatsbibliothek, R.B. Msc. 3. License: CC-BY-SA 4.0.

Saints' Relics as Obstetric Tools

Reading a wide variety of sources on the cult of Cunigunde reveals that the cult became one of the resources for relief and healing available to women in their specific, gendered health experiences. However, it is still unclear when and why a virgin, childless queen appealed to a female audience in Bamberg, and

already been noted by Wenz-Haubfleisch, *Miracula post mortem*, 216-20. I tentatively suggest (in the event that both sources, Nonnosus Stettfelder and the Leuven narrative, were correct in their description of the relics) that, at the peak of its popularity in the fifteenth century, the cult of Cunigunde may have been another source of discord between the two neighbouring ecclesiastical institutions.

what processes in the late medieval understanding of her cult led to Cunigunde becoming an agent of healing for women. It is clear that by the end of the fifteenth century her tunic, mantle, and belt were already used as obstetric tools, although the connection may have originated earlier at the end of the fourteenth century, when these relics became explicitly linked to the image of Cunigunde. Indeed, one of the factors that may have attracted female pilgrims to seek Cunigunde's help during pregnancy could have been the accessibility and preservation of her relics in the form of intact pieces suitable for wearing and other practices. Moreover, those relics (the belt and two garments) resembled those of other saints already petitioned for similar purposes.

Contact relics, similar to those of Cunigunde, were known in abundance in cults of both male and female saints. Belts, girdles, and tunics became popular objects of devotion because they retained an intimate connection to saints' bodies. Binding a sick person with a holy girdle implored assistance from that saint and stimulated hope of recovery.[56] Some of these objects also were used to facilitate delivery and ensure the health of a child.[57] Often they were placed over the body of a pregnant woman, as was the case with Cunigunde's relics; sometimes a charm or a prayer was sewn into the girdle.[58] If an expectant mother could afford it, a prestigious saint's girdle was used, since its miraculous powers were believed to secure the mother a painless delivery and the infant good health.

The practice of putting a belt on the body of a parturient woman originated from older customs of 'measuring, binding and loosing' surrounding childbirth.[59] Some of these girdles and belts were crafted to a purported measurement (usually height) of Christ, the Virgin Mary, or other saints. The ritual of 'measuring to a saint' is attested as a widespread healing practice in the late Middle Ages, used not only by parturient women, but also applied, for example, to sick children.[60] The popularity of such a healing practice might explain the interest of Nonnosus Stettfelder in the stature of Cunigunde and

56 Morse explains the birth-girdle ritual in more detail in 'Thys Moche More Ys Oure Lady Mary Longe'.

57 For more about these and other examples, see Schulenburg, *Forgetful of their Sex*, 228-33; Bartlett, *Why Can the Dead Do Such Great Things?*, 246-47, 354.

58 Skemer, 'Amulet Rolls and Female Devotion in the Late Middle Ages'; Morse, 'Thys Moche More Ys Oure Lady Mary Longe'.

59 These customs included putting her husband's belt around the body of a pregnant woman in order to evoke principles of 'sympathetic medicine'. Another common practice was to attach a charm for a safe delivery, such as the *peperit* charm, to a belt. See Elsakkers, 'In Pain You Shall Bear Children', esp. 195-97, and Jones and Olsan, 'Performative Rituals for Conception and Childbirth'.

60 Finucane, *Rescue of the Innocents*, 11.

may illuminate his concern to provide these measurements to his readers (notably, he was not interested in the body of St. Henry at all). The vertical and horizontal lines on the last page of the printed legend, multiplied by a given number, result in the exact height and waist span of the saint: her waist would have been 48 centimetres and her height 140 centimetres – information essential for healing by 'measuring to a saint' (Figure 2.2). These sizes are quite unrealistic, as even Nonnosus remarks that she was apparently 'subtle and small'.[61] However, the given height of Cunigunde corresponds to the length of the healing belt still kept in Bamberg, which is 142 centimetres.[62] Although Nonnosus did not recount why these measurements would be useful to readers, I suggest that this detailed interest in the physical body of the healing saint was sparked by the 'measuring' practice.

The most popular girdle, belonging to the Virgin Mary and preserved in multiple examples across Europe, was believed to help with delivery pains in keeping with the notion of painless delivery by Mary herself.[63] In the same way, pregnant women sought the intercession of other holy mothers such as St. Anne, St. Elizabeth (the mother of John the Baptist), or St. Elizabeth of Hungary.[64] The identification of a 'medical specialization' of saints based on their legends was a recurring pattern, though not a rule. St. Margaret of Antioch, a widely venerated virgin, was also invoked during difficult childbirths; alternatively, her relics were used if accessible to a parturient woman. This association was presumably stimulated by a famous legend of St. Margaret coming out of a dragon's belly intact, which was perceived as analogous to a painless delivery.[65] Those saints who were not identified with motherhood, or with femininity at all, were also perceived as patrons

61 Nonnosus Stettfelder, *Dye Legend und Leben*, fol. 70r: 'Dy heilig junkfraw sant kungund ist gar subtils leibs gewesen und klein'.

62 Jung and Kempkens, *Gekrönt auf Erden und im Himmel*, 86 (cat. no. III-11).

63 Labour pain was 'normalized' and generally perceived as a consequence of original sin.

64 To my knowledge, there is no comprehensive study collecting and analysing these narratives of pregnant women seeking saints' help by invoking them or coming into contact with their relics (belts, girdles, tunics, or others) from the standpoint of the social history of religion and medicine. Exceptions are studies of medieval charms and prayers, including those used for childbirth. See Elsakkers, 'In Pain You Shall Bear Children'; Jones and Olsan, 'Performative Rituals for Conception and Childbirth'; Morse, 'Thys Moche More Ys Oure Lady Mary Longe'; and Skemer, 'Amulet Rolls' and *Binding Words*. This phenomenon is mentioned by Bartlett, *Why Can the Dead Do Such Great Things?*, and Harmening, 'Fränkische Mirakelbücher', while some isolated examples associated with St. Margaret of Antioch, St. Elizabeth of Hungary, St. Peter of Verona, and the cult of St. Thomas are analysed in the following publications: Krüger, 'Elisabeth von Thüringen und Maria Magdalena'; Larson, 'Who Is the Master of This Narrative?'; Powell, 'Miracle of Childbirth'; Prudlo, 'Mothers and the Martyr'.

65 Larson, 'Who Is the Master of This Narrative?'

Figure 2.2 Last page of the printed legend of Henry and Cunigunde with the measurements of Cunigunde's body

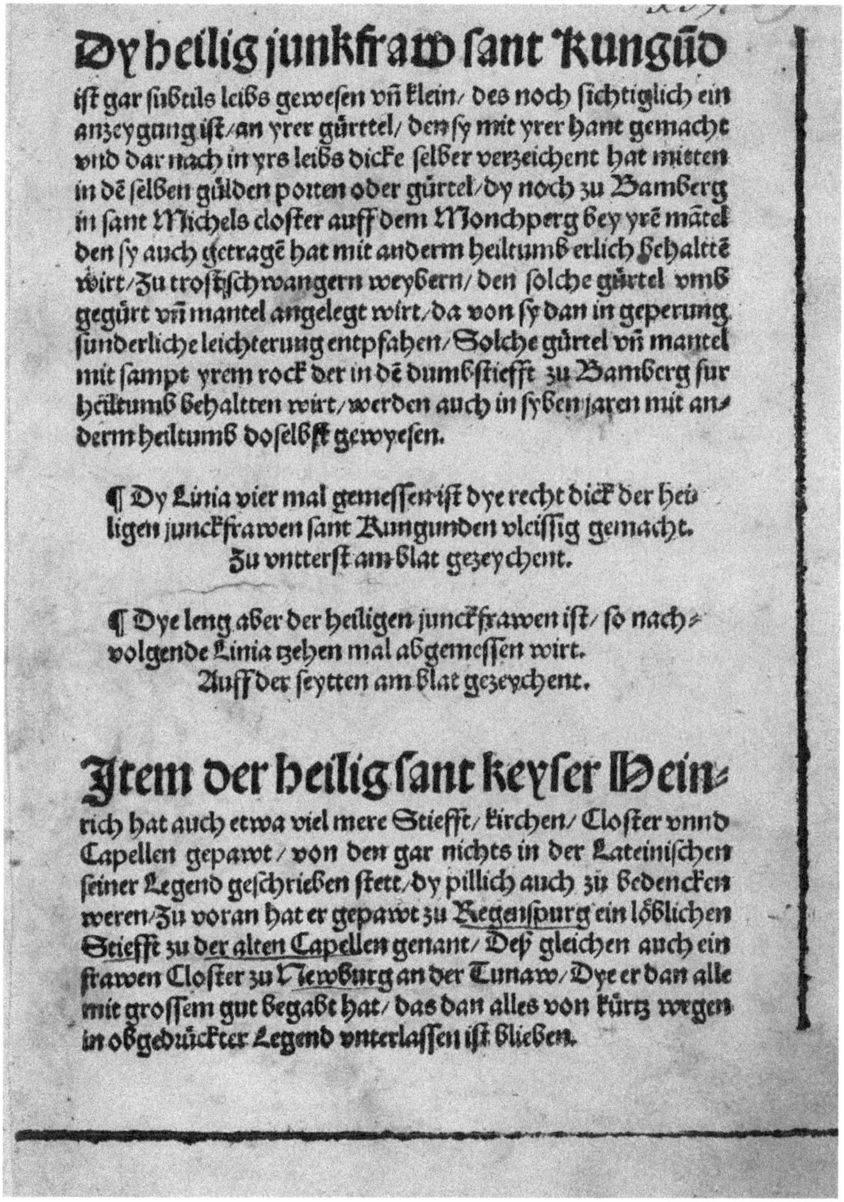

Dy heilig junkfraw sant Kungūd
ist gar subtils leibs gewesen vñ klein/ des noch sichtiglich ein
anzeygung ist/an yrer gürttel/ den sy mit yrer hant gemacht
vnd dar nach in yrs leibs dicke selber verzeichent hat mitten
in dē selben gülden porten oder gürtel/dy noch zu Bamberg
in sant Michels closter auff dem Monchperg bey yrē mātel
den sy auch getragē hat mit anderm heiltumb erlich behaltē
wirt/Zu trost schwangern weybern/ den solche gürtel vmb
gegürt vñ mantel angelegt wirt/da von sy dan in geperung
sunderliche leichterung entpfahen/Solche gürtel vñ mantel
mit sampt yrem rock der in dē dumbstiefft zu Bamberg fur
heiltumb behaltten wirt/werden auch in syben jaren mit an=
derm heiltumb doselbst gewyesen.

¶ Dy Linia vier mal gemessen ist dye recht dick der hei=
ligen junckfrawen sant Kungunden vleissig gemacht.
Zu vntterst am blat gezeychent.

¶ Dye leng aber der heiligen junckfrawen ist/ so nach=
volgende Linia zehen mal abgemessen wirt.
Auff der seytten am blat gezeychent.

Item der heilig sant keyser Hein=
rich hat auch etwa viel mere Stiefft/ kirchen/ Closter vnnd
Capellen gepawt/ von den gar nichts in der Lateinischen
seiner Legend geschrieben stett/dy pillich auch zu bedencken
weren/Zu voran hat er gepawt zu Regenspurg ein löblichen
Stiefft zu der alten Capellen genant/ Deß gleichen auch ein
frawen Closter zu Newburg an der Tunaw/Dye er dan alle
mit grossem gut begabt hat/ das dan alles von kürtz wegen
in obgedückter Legend vnterlassen ist blieben.

From Nonnosus Stettfelder, *Dye Legend und Leben des heyligen sandt Keyser Heinrich* (Bamberg: Pfeyll, 1511), fol. 70r. Bamberg, Staatsbibliothek, R.B. Inc. typ. E.1.

of female medicine. The belt of St. Gertrud of Nivelles, the belt of St. Foillan (kept in a monastery at Fosses-la-Ville), and the head of St. Sebaldus in Nuremberg were all brought to parturient women in order to ease their pains.[66] As Jane Tibbetts Schulenburg notes, giving birth was 'one of the major areas of medieval life in which saints were seen to be especially beneficial and assumed prominent, indispensable roles'.[67]

This evidence shows that the two spheres of 'professional' and 'religious' or 'folkloric' medicine intermingled and were often employed as complements to each other.[68] Miraculous healing deploying charms and relics was mentioned in late medieval medical treatises as a common medical practice. For example, Antonius Guainerius, a professor of medicine at the University of Pavia, recommended in his *Tractatus de matricibus* (1484) that parturient women appeal to St. Margaret of Antioch for help during childbirth: 'At the time of birth, it is good that the legend of the blessed Margaret be read, that she [the mother] has relics of the saints on her, and that you [apparently, the physician] carry out briefly some familiar ceremonies in order to please your patient and the old women'.[69] Lea Olsan also has shown that physicians acknowledged and rationalized the employment of charms in medieval therapy.[70] Hence one should reconsider the constructed division between 'holy medicine', deeply rooted in religious belief and local traditions, and professional medicine, whose practitioners grounded their knowledge in ancient and contemporary humoral theory.[71]

These multiple examples of saintly patronage over parturient women, evident especially in the late Middle Ages, correspond to practices formed around the cult of St. Cunigunde in Bamberg; they represent similar developments in the religious and medical practices surrounding childbirth. While the role of male physicians and midwives during childbirth remains a contested subject in the history of medieval medicine, it is clear that pregnant women regularly drew on different means of acquiring holy medicine.[72] It was not only an apparent lack of appropriate medical assistance that

66 Hillinus, 'Miracula sancti Foillani', 420 (2.12); the other examples mentioned in Harmening, 'Fränkische Mirakelbücher', 109-11.

67 Schulenburg, *Forgetful of their Sex*, 233.

68 McCleery, '"Christ More Powerful than Galen"?'

69 Cited in Lemay, 'Women and the Literature of Obstetrics and Gynecology', 197-98.

70 Olsan, 'Charms and Prayers in Medieval Medical Theory and Practice'.

71 Park, 'Medicine and Society', esp. 59-60, 82-83; McCleery, '"Christ More Powerful than Galen"?'

72 More on the involvement of physicians and midwives in women's healthcare can be found in the multiple publications of Green, including her 'Recent Work on Medieval Women's Medicine'.

created a demand for medicine of celestial origin, but also the belief in an intricate connection between bodily functions and religious practices. The Virgin Mary, St. Anne, or St. Margaret of Antioch acquired a wide-reaching reputation for their efficacy in the field of obstetrics, although most of the saints who acted as patrons to women were local figures. A similar demand might have triggered the rise of Cunigunde as a female healer, facilitated by the practical availability of her relics for devotees. Her overall popularity in Bamberg and over the territories of the bishopric made her an obvious choice when seeking divine intercession.

Another factor that may have prompted this shift in the focus of Cunigunde's cult from all-around healing to one that specialized in pregnancy could be her comparison to the Virgin Mary.[73] This development led to the rising popularity of Cunigunde as a local and regional saint, but also made her cult more attractive to a female following. However, this shift does not downplay the importance of Cunigunde and Henry for a more general clientele. At the same time that the obstetric specialization of Cunigunde intensified, pilgrims and local dwellers continued to use the couple's garments and other relics for various reasons. These objects continued to be exhibited regularly during the *Heiltumsweisung*. Under these circumstances, the practice of seeking the saintly assistance of Cunigunde when facing obstetric problems remained embedded within a broader healing purview in fourteenth- and fifteenth-century Bamberg.

Conclusion

Several historical and methodological conclusions can be drawn from this investigation of sanctity and the transformation of Cunigunde's cult. First, the specialization of a saint and her clientele should not be based solely on the content of miracle collections, which obviously reflect the agendas of their compilers. Such an approach neglects regional differences and temporal developments of the cult, as I have shown in the case of St. Cunigunde. The initial analysis presented here, following the footsteps of previous researchers, did not go beyond quantifying the data from the earliest miracle collections; that evidence revealed that Cunigunde's saintly capacities were presented as 'universal' or suitable for all kinds of clientele, from German queens to impaired beggars. This pattern stands in contrast to later developments of the cult, when Cunigunde appears to have become especially

73 Klauser, *Der Heinrichs- und Kunigundenkult*, 100-3, 138-40.

popular among female patrons, as documented by different sources. As a virgin saint, she became a promoter of miraculous healing among pregnant women and women with disorders of the reproductive system.

Second, the evidence suggests that the healing cult of Cunigunde became a renowned source of female healing in Bamberg and its environs by the fifteenth century. Specific healing practices were attributed to relics such as her belt and mantel, kept in the Benedictine monastery of Michelsberg, and the tunic housed in the Bamberg Cathedral. These two religious institutions controlled and regulated women's access to the healing objects and possibly benefitted from an intense flow of votive gifts. There is a clear resemblance between Cunigunde's healing objects and practices and those used in many other cults, such as those of St. Margaret of Antioch and St. Elizabeth of Hungary. These saints were well-known for their ability to ease childbirth pains and safeguard the devotee from disease. Yet it is important to recognize that, although the gender correlation between devotees and a saint may have been an important factor in generating obstetric specialization among saints, it was not a decisive one; belts, tunics, and other relics belonging to both male and female saints were credited with the same powers of easing childbirth and securing the health of an infant.

Finally, religious intervention, orchestrated by the cults of saints and the economy of relics, was an important source of healing and support for parturient women, especially considering that childbirth was not perceived as an event requiring medical assistance. The relief provided by the cult of saints worked as both miracle and medicine. The two categories of knowledge and experience were inseparable in matters of childbirth. I have argued that the pursuit of remedy from the cult of saints was not necessarily opposed to professionalized medicine as understood in the late medieval period. Continued investigation into patterns of interaction between miraculous and learned medicine, especially in the realm of medieval gynecology and obstetrics, may even dissolve the boundaries separating these categories.

Works Cited

Manuscripts

Bamberg, Staatsbibliothek, R.B. Msc. 120.
Brussels, Bibliothèque Royale de Belgique, MS 219-221.
Brussels, Bibliothèque Royale de Belgique, MS 3391-99.
Leipzig, Universitätsbibliothek, Rep. II 64.

Printed Works

Bartlett, Robert. *Why Can the Dead Do Such Great Things? Saints and Worshippers from the Martyrs to the Reformation* (Princeton, NJ: Princeton University Press, 2013).

Baumgärtel-Fleischmann, Renate. 'Die Kaisermäntel im Bamberger Domschatz', *Bericht des Historischen Vereins für die Pflege der Geschichte des ehemaligen Fürstbistums Bamberg*, 133 (1997), 93-126.

Cárdenas, Livia. *Die Textur des Bildes: das Heiltumsbuch im Kontext religiöser Medialität des Spätmittelalters* (Berlin: Akademie, 2013).

Corbet, Patrick. *Les saints ottoniens: sainteté dynastique, royale et féminine autour de l'an Mil* (Sigmaringen: Jan Thorbecke, 1986).

Cormack, Margaret Jean. 'Better Off Dead: Approaches to Medieval Miracles', in *Sanctity in the North: Saints, Lives, and Cults in Medieval Scandinavia*, ed. Thomas A. DuBois (Toronto: University of Toronto Press, 2008), 334-52.

'De S. Cunigunde Imperatrice', in *Acta sanctorum martii* 1, ed. Godfried Henschen and Daniel van Papenbroeck (Paris: Victor Palmé, 1865), 265-80.

Dick, Stefanie, Jörg Jarnut, and Matthias Wemhoff. *Kunigunde, consors regni: Vortragsreihe zum tausendjährigen Jubiläum der Krönung Kunigundes in Paderborn (1002-2002)* (Munich: Wilhelm Fink, 2004).

Duffin, Jacalyn. *Medical Miracles: Doctors, Saints, and Healing in the Modern World* (Oxford: Oxford University Press, 2009).

Elsakkers, Marianne. 'In Pain You Shall Bear Children (Gen 3:16): Medieval Prayers for a Safe Delivery', in *Women and Miracle Stories: A Multidisciplinary Exploration*, ed. Anne-Marie Korte (Leiden: Brill, 2001), 179-209.

Erasmus, Desiderius. *In Praise of Folly* (London: George Bickham, 1745).

Farrenkopf, Edmund Karl. *Breviarium Eberhardi cantoris: die mittelalterliche Gottesdienstordnung des Domes zu Bamberg, mit einer historischen Einleitung* (Münster: Aschendorff, 1969).

Finucane, Ronald C. *Miracles and Pilgrims: Popular Beliefs in Medieval England* (London: Rowman & Littlefield, 1977).

—. *The Rescue of the Innocents: Endangered Children in Medieval Miracles* (New York: St. Martin's Press, 1997).

Gilsdorf, Sean, ed. *Queenship and Sanctity: The Lives of Mathilda and the Epitaph of Adelheid.* (Washington, DC: Catholic University of America Press, 2004).

Goetz, Hans-Werner. 'Heiligenkult und Geschlecht: Geschlechtsspezifisches Wunderwirken in frühmittelalterlichen Mirakelberichten?', *Das Mittelalter*, 1 (1996), 89-111.

Goodich, Michael. *Miracles and Wonders: The Development of the Concept of Miracle, 1150-1350* (Aldershot: Ashgate, 2007).

—. 'Vision, Dream and Canonization Policy under Pope Innocent III', in *Pope Innocent III and his World*, ed. John Moore and Brenda Bolton (Brookfield: Ashgate, 1999), 151-63.

Green, Monica. 'Recent Work on Medieval Women's Medicine', in *Sexuality and Culture in Medieval and Renaissance Europe*, ed. Philip M. Soergel (New York: AMS Press, 2005), 1-46.

Guth, Klaus. 'Kaiserin Kunigunde: Kanonisation und hochmittelalterlicher Kult', *Würzburger Diözesangeschichtsblätter*, 62-63 (2001), 409-22.

Harmening, Dieter. 'Fränkische Mirakelbücher: Quellen und Untersuchungen zur historischen Volkskunde und Geschichte der Volksfrömmigkeit', *Würzburger Diözesangeschichtsblätter*, 28 (1966), 25-240.

Hillinus. 'Miracula sancti Foillani', in *Acta sanctorum octobris* 13, ed. Joseph van Hecke et al. (Paris: Victor Palmé, 1883), 417-26.

Jansen, Jürgen. *Medizinische Kasuistik in den 'Miracula sancte Elyzabet': Medizinhistorische Analyse und Übersetzung der Wunderprotokolle am Grab der Elisabeth von Thuringen (1207-1231)* (Frankfurt am Main: Lang, 1985).

Jones, Peter Murray and Lea T. Olsan. 'Performative Rituals for Conception and Childbirth in England, 900-1500', *Bulletin of the History of Medicine*, 89.3 (2015), 406-33.

Jung, Norbert and Holger Kempkens, eds. *Gekrönt auf Erden und im Himmel: Das heilige Kaiserpaar Heinrich II. und Kunigunde*, Veröffentlichungen des Diözesanmuseums Bamberg 26 (Bamberg: Vier-Türme-Verlag, 2014).

Justice, Steven. 'Did the Middle Ages Believe in their Miracles?', *Representations*, 103 (2008), 1-29.

Kee, Howard Clark. *Medicine, Miracle and Magic in New Testament Times* (Cambridge: Cambridge University Press, 1988).

Klauser, Renate. *Der Heinrichs- und Kunigundenkult im mittelalterlichen Bistum Bamberg* (Bamberg: Selbstverlag des historischen Vereins, 1957).

Korte, Anne-Marie. *Women and Miracle Stories: A Multidisciplinary Exploration* (Leiden: Brill, 2000).

Kræmer, Erik von. *Les maladies désignées par le nom d'un saint* (Helsingfors: Academic Bookstore, 1950).

Krüger, Klaus. 'Elisabeth von Thüringen und Maria Magdalena: Reliquien als Geburtshelfer im späten Mittelalter', *Zeitschrift des Vereins für Thüringische Geschichte*, 54 (2000), 75-108.

Kühne, Hartmut. *Ostensio reliquiarum: Untersuchungen über Entstehung, Ausbreitung, Gestalt und Funktion der Heiltumsweisungen im römisch-deutschen Regnum* (Berlin: De Gruyter, 2012).

Larson, Wendy R. 'Who Is the Master of This Narrative? Maternal Patronage and the Cult of St. Margaret', in *Gendering the Master Narrative: Woman and Power in the Middle Ages*, ed. Mary C. Erler and Maryanne Kowaleski (Ithaca, NY: Cornell University Press, 2003), 94-104.

Legendae sanctorum Henrici imperatoris et Kunigundis imperatricis (Brussels: Fratres vitae communis, 1484).

Lemay, Helen Rodnite. 'Women and the Literature of Obstetrics and Gynecology', in *Medieval Women and the Sources*, ed. Joel T. Rosenthal (Athens, GA: University of Georgia Press, 1990), 189-209.

Linke, Heinrich. *Beitrag zur Kulttopographie des Hl. Kaiserpaares Heinrich und Kunigunde: anlässlich des 1000-jährigen Bestehens für das Erzbistum Bamberg zusammengestellt* (Bamberg: n.p., 2007).

McCleery, Iona M. '"Christ More Powerful than Galen"? The Relationship Between Medicine and Miracles', in *Contextualizing Miracles in the Christian West, 1100-1500: New Historical Approaches*, ed. Matthew Mesley and Louise E. Wilson (Oxford: Oxford University Press, 2014), 127-54.

Metzler, Irina. *Disability in Medieval Europe: Thinking about Physical Impairment in the High Middle Ages, c.1100-1400* (London: Routledge, 2006).

Meyer, Carla. 'Die konstruierte Heilige: Kaiserin Kunigunde und ihre Darstellung in Quellen des 11. bis 16. Jahrhunderts', *Bericht des Historischen Vereins Bamberg*, 139 (2003), 39-101.

Morse, Mary. '"Thys Moche More Ys Oure Lady Mary Longe": Takamiya MS 56 and the English Birth Girdle Tradition', in *Middle English Texts in Transition: A Festschrift Dedicated to Toshiyuki Takamiya on his 70th Birthday*, ed. Simon Horobin and Linne R. Mooney (Woodbridge: York Medieval Press, 2014), 199-214.

Nonnosus Stettfelder. *Dye Legend und Leben des heyligen sandt Keyser Heinrich* (Bamberg: Pfeyll, 1511).

Olsan, Lea T. 'Charms and Prayers in Medieval Medical Theory and Practice', *Social History of Medicine*, 16.3 (2003), 343-66.

Park, Katharine. 'Medicine and Society in Medieval Europe, 500-1500', in *Medicine in Society: Historical Essays*, ed. Andrew Wear (Cambridge: Cambridge University Press, 1992), 59-90.

Petersohn, Jürgen. 'Die Litterae Papst Innozenz III. zur Heiligsprechung der Kaiserin Kunigunde (1200)', *Jahrbuch für fränkische Landesforschung*, 37 (1977), 1-25.

Powell, Hilary. 'The "Miracle of Childbirth": The Portrayal of Parturient Women in Medieval Miracle Narratives', *Social History of Medicine*, 25.4 (2012), 795-811.

Prudlo, Donald S. 'Mothers and the Martyr: The Unlikely Patronage of a Medieval Dominican Preacher', *Journal of the History of Sexuality*, 21.2 (2012), 313-24.

Ritchey, Sara. 'Caring by the Hours: The Psalter as a Gendered Healthcare Technology', in *Gender, Health, and Healing, 1250-1550*, ed. Sara Ritchey and Sharon Strocchia (Amsterdam: Amsterdam University Press, 2020), 41-66.

Schneidmüller, Bernd. 'Heinrich II. und Kunigunde: das heilige Kaiserpaar des Mittelalters', in *Kunigunde – consors regni: Vortragsreihe zum tausendjährigen Jubiläum der Krönung Kunigundes in Padeborn (1002-2002)*, ed. Stefanie Dick, Jörg Jarnut, and Matthias Wernhoff (Munich: Wilhelm Fink, 2004), 29-46.

Schulenburg, Jane Tibbetts. *Forgetful of their Sex: Female Sanctity and Society, ca. 500-1100* (Chicago: University of Chicago Press, 1995).

Sigal, Pierre-Andre. *L'Homme et le miracle dans la France medievale (XIe-XIIe siecle)* (Paris: Cerf, 1985).

Skemer, Don C. 'Amulet Rolls and Female Devotion in the Late Middle Ages', *Scriptorium*, 55 (2001), 197-227.

—. *Binding Words: Textual Amulets in the Middle Ages* (Philadelphia: Pennsylvania State University Press, 2006).

Vauchez, André. *Sainthood in the Later Middle Ages* (Cambridge: Cambridge University Press, 1997).

'Vita et miracula S. Cunegundis', in *Monumenta germaniae historica scriptores* 4, ed. Georg Pertz (Hanover: Hahn, 1841), 821-28.

Ward, Benedicta. *Miracles and the Medieval Mind: Theory, Record and Event, 1000-1215* (London: Scolar Press, 1982).

Wenz-Haubfleisch, Annegret. 'Der Kult der hl. Kunigunde an der Wende vom 12. zum 13. Jahrhundert im Spiegel ihrer Mirakelsammlung', in *Kunigunde: eine Kaiserin an der Jahrtausendwende*, ed. Ingrid Baumgärtner (Kassel: Furore, 1997), 157-86.

—. *Miracula post mortem: Studien zum Quellenwert hochmittelalter Mirakelsammlungen vornehmlich des ostfränkisch-deutschen Reiches* (Siegburg: Respublica, 1998).

Die weysung vnnd auszruffung des Hochwirdigen heylthumbs zu Bamberg (Bamberg: Johann Pfeil, 1509).

About the Author

Iliana Kandzha is a PhD candidate at Central European University. Her dissertation examines the medieval cults of the royal virgins St. Henry and St. Cunigunde, with an emphasis on their political and social dimensions. She received her BA in History from the Higher School of Economics in Moscow and an MA in Medieval Studies from Central European University.

Part 2

Producing and Transmitting Medical Knowledge

3 Blood, Milk, and Breastbleeding

The Humoral Economy of Women's Bodies in Medieval Medicine

*Montserrat Cabré and Fernando Salmón**

Abstract

In humoral physiology the pregnant body was considered capable of transforming menstrual blood into nourishment for the foetus. After childbirth, blood became breast milk. However, this harmonic continuum was threatened when the maternal body was unable to transform blood into milk: in the Hippocratic aphorism 5.40, when blood cannot be transformed in the breasts of women, it indicates madness. We analyse medieval interpretations of this condition through the commentaries of university masters who examined this textual and clinical reality. We discuss how humoral physiology – an extremely flexible system of thought – could only conceive of maternal bleeding breasts with recourse to madness. Disharmony in the maternal body not only disrupted the physiological routine but also the symbolic function of mothering.

Keywords: sex difference, humoral theory, medieval physiology, medieval medical commentaries, Hippocratic gynecological aphorisms, female madness

* It is our pleasure to acknowledge that during the research leading to this essay we have benefitted from the kind expertise of many colleagues. We would especially like to thank Marlen Bidwell-Steiner, Sandra Cavallo, Naama Cohen-Hanegbi, Giulia Ecca, Monica Green, Sergius Kodera, Oliver Overwien, Jutta Sperling, and Faith Wallis, as well as the participants in the 14 February 2018 Colloquium of Department II of the Max Planck Institute for the History of Science in Berlin. We are indebted to the editors of this volume, Sara Ritchey and Sharon Strocchia, for their unfaltering support and superb editorial skills that have eased the writing process while improving our work. Research funding has been provided by project HAR 2015-63995-P (MINECO/FEDER).

Ritchey, Sara & Sharon Strocchia (eds), *Gender, Health, and Healing, 1250-1550*. Amsterdam, Amsterdam University Press 2020
DOI: 10.5117/9789463724517_CH03

This essay aims to contribute to two rich and overlapping conversations in the history of medieval and early modern medicine in western Europe. First, it offers new perspectives on the ongoing discussion of the significance of physiology in premodern conceptions of the body, with a particular focus on sexual difference. Second, it enters into dialogue with a growing body of historiography concerned with the peculiarly flexible character of humoral epistemology: a highly successful theoretical framework for understanding the workings of human bodies that lasted for two millennia. These two conversations come together in our exploration of late medieval discussions of 'breastbleeding', or the phenomenon in which physicians understood menstrual blood as failing to properly transform into milk, therefore making the maternal body unable to lactate. The medical significance of this condition is presented in Hippocratic aphorism 5.40, one that has not garnered much scholarly attention. In this particular and theory-laden configuration, the breastbleeding of women is presented as a clinical sign of madness.

Transformation is key to humoral epistemology. The ability of bodies to transform substances explained how bodies worked, how they stayed healthy, and how the sexes expressed marked differences. In this essay, we explore humoral physicians' imaginings of the inability of women's bodies to successfully transform blood into milk or to purge it entirely, which inability, they asserted, could trigger toxic or other harmful consequences. We also show how the flexibility of the humoral epistemological frame allowed medieval physicians to reconcile the circumstances by which a toxic female body could coexist with a maternal one.

While recent historiographic developments are breathing new life into these issues, both lines of inquiry have long histories. Cultural approaches to the physiological aspects of humoral theory were pioneered in the 1980s, and it seems significant to acknowledge that historians interested in the history of women's bodies and of sexual difference played a leading role in developing this avenue of research.[1] The influential books by Joan Cadden and Barbara Duden are brilliant examples of this trend.[2] Classicists especially have contributed to the effort, and the historiography of emotions has provided fresh perspectives on the relationship between feelings and the comprehension of the inner workings of the body as perceived by patients and practitioners.[3] We still lack a full analysis tracing this historiographical

1 Pouchelle, *Corps et chirurgie*.

2 Duden, *Woman beneath the Skin*; Cadden, *Meanings of Sex Difference*.

3 Nutton, 'Humoralism'; King, *Hippocrates' Woman*. On emotions, see Rublack, 'Fluxes'.

engagement, as Harold Cook has noted in a recent review, but it seems undeniable that interest in the history of physiology has grown markedly in the past few years.[4] Two important collective works, *Blood, Sweat and Tears: The Changing Concepts of Physiology from Antiquity into Early Modern Europe* and *The Body in Balance: Humoral Medicines in Practice*, are testimony to a renewed impetus that draws on earlier work but involves new conceptualizations.[5]

Many of these fresh perspectives on the value of studying past modes of physiological thinking have been fuelled by a lively debate around the 'one-sex' model. The 'one-sex' model was proposed by Thomas Laqueur in 1990 and was met with an immediate and persistent success that continues to the present day.[6] Laqueur's thesis promoted the idea that, until the eighteenth century, there was a unitary view of sex difference based on a set of homologies between the male and female bodies and that, therefore, the 'two-sex model' should be considered an invention of modern medicine. Laqueur's theory was based on his understanding that Galen had proposed female genitalia as simply an interior inversion of male genitalia, which failed to descend due to women's lack of heat. This proposition was based on morphological similarities, with the ovaries, for example, appearing to look much like the testes.

Despite its enormous popularity, Laqueur's thesis was questioned by premodernists from the very beginning. In a lucid review published soon after the publication of *Making Sex*, Katharine Park and Robert Nye pointed out that one of the main pitfalls of Laqueur's thesis was its basic interpretative dependence on anatomy, which Laqueur understood as a fundamentally materially embodied enterprise.[7] Park and Nye called attention to the extent to which Laqueur overlooked the metaphysical basis of the premodern understanding of the sexes and the fact that the medical and natural philosophical ground of this understanding was humoral physiology, rather than anatomy or bodily form.[8] Almost twenty years later, Park took issue again with Laqueur's thesis. This time, Park demonstrated the explanatory weakness of a *longue durée* model that failed to engage with the Middle Ages. Her critique reinforced Cadden's earlier insight regarding the limited understanding of how Galenic anatomical

4 Cook, review of *Blood, Sweat and Tears*.

5 Hortsmanshoff et al., eds., *Blood, Sweat and Tears*; Horden and Hsu, eds., *Body in Balance*.

6 Laqueur, *Making Sex*.

7 The textual rather than material technologies behind medieval learned anatomical knowledge have been explored by Salmón, 'Body Inferred'.

8 Park and Nye, 'Destiny is Anatomy'.

knowledge, on which the 'one-sex' model was based, was transmitted in the medieval period.[9]

Park and Nye's review essay has been the most comprehensive and widely cited critique of Laqueur's model for three decades. Later critics of Laqueur's thesis have furthered their arguments regarding the epistemological importance of humoral knowledge in premodern conceptions of the body generally, and of sex difference in particular. For example, Michael Stolberg has questioned Laqueur's model based on the early modern physiology of menstruation.[10] Most recently, Helen King has used humoral theory as the axis along which to reconstruct diverse modes of explanation of sex difference during antiquity and the Renaissance.[11] It should come as no surprise, then, that these studies come from historians who recognize the broad analytical significance of the study of humoral physiology.[12] However, many critiques of Laqueur's use of source material and his oversimplified interpretations have failed to engage with the Middle Ages. Consequently, they are not only inadequate when it comes to fully exploring the weaknesses of his two-millennia model, they also fail to acknowledge and therefore to investigate the flexible nature of humoral physiology itself and the dynamic, adaptable character that accounts for its success.

Within this wide historical and historiographical framework, the aim of this essay is modest. Taking one central purpose of the female body as an example, it seeks to show how function, rather than form, was crucial to the medieval medical understanding of human bodies and sex difference. At the same time, it demonstrates the way in which the notion of transformation was key to the humoral epistemology that prevailed in explaining the workings of human bodies and sex difference in learned medical circles.

Blood and Milk: A Healthy Harmony

Medieval authors of medical and natural philosophical treatises expressed an abiding interest in sex difference, which they often situated in the function of

9 Park, 'Cadden, Laqueur, and the "One-Sex" Body'; Park, 'Medicine and Natural Philosophy', 96-98.

10 Stolberg's criticism of Laqueur nevertheless recognized the need to examine historical anatomy. See his contribution to the 'Critiques and Contentions' section of the 2003 *Isis* issue dedicated to the 'one-sex body' controversy in Stolberg, 'Woman Down to her Bones'; Stolberg, 'Menstruation and Sexual Difference'.

11 King, *One-Sex Body on Trial*.

12 King, 'Introduction'.

the uterus. One particular focus of concern was manifested in discussions of the physiology of blood. Menstrual blood was considered to be the purgation that all women, cold in nature, required. Menstruation was understood as providing the function of cleansing or purging women's bodies of the residual superfluities that their overall lack of heat prevented them from consuming or refining into semen.[13] In the Galenic and Salernitan traditions, menstruation was seen in a positive light, since its regular occurrence ensured women's health and fertility. Indeed, therapeutic handbooks, treatises on women's health, and all types of domestic books are full of recipes to avoid retention of the menses and to provoke 'the flowers', as menstruation was often called. When conception occurred, it was understood that the superfluous blood was retained so that it could be processed as nutrition, first for the fetus, and then after birth for the newborn baby.[14] Belle Tuten, for example, has pointed to the endurance of this view from the Hippocratic texts to the early Middle Ages, even when there was no agreement on how the connection worked anatomically; furthermore, her essay in this volume demonstrates that, at least by the later Middle Ages, domestic and vernacular practitioners shared with academic physicians an understanding of the critical relationship between blood and milk in the fluid humoral economy.[15] Following in the footsteps of their ancient predecessors, medieval physicians believed that there was a passage for the blood to flow from the womb to the breasts, where it would be transformed into milk. While addressing Galen's commentary on the Hippocratic aphorism 5.39, the Florentine physician Taddeo Alderotti (1206/1215-1295) offers the standard medieval view of the physiology of blood and milk.[16] He divides his own commentary into five parts, tackling the issue in the last two:

> On the fourth part he [Galen] says almost as a conclusion that since the flesh of the breasts is not bloody but white, the wetness of the blood arriving at the breasts necessarily turns into a white substance, that is milk. And the bigger the amount of the bloody wetness that runs to the

13 For an overview of medical and natural-philosophical approaches to sexual difference, see Cadden, *Meanings of Sex Difference*.

14 Green, 'Flowers, Poisons and Men'.

15 Tuten, 'Lactation and Breast Diseases in Antiquity', and Tuten, 'Care of the Breast', this volume.

16 Medieval textual traditions normally do not number the aphorisms and Renaissance and modern editions differ slightly in their numbering. For the sake of clarity, we follow the convention commonly used by both ancient and medieval scholars, including Hanson, 'Aphorismi 5.28-63', and Vázquez Buján, 'La transmisión latina'.

> breast, the higher the production of milk, as we see it happens in the eighth and ninth month after conception. And this is about the fourth part. In the fifth and last part he says that the generation of milk from the blood arriving at the breasts may occur without conception, namely when retained menstrual blood is transformed, for some part of the blood that must be evicted through menstruation reaches the breasts and is converted into milk. Therefore take the truth of this aphorism in this way: because the cause of the generation of milk is due to a past or a present conception, to a present or a recent childbirth or due to the retention of menstruation, if a woman is not pregnant at present nor has been pregnant in the recent past and there is milk in her breasts, it follows necessarily that this is a sign of menstrual retention.[17]

To further theorize this transformation, medieval physicians conceived of a passage between the uterus and the breasts, which can be seen in a variety of medical and natural philosophical sources. For example, in a section on the process of feeding the fetus in the womb, the *Secreta mulierum*, or 'Secrets of Women', a popular treatise on generation and 'women's nature', postulates the existence of a direct, physical channel connecting the fluids of the breast to those of the uterus:

> The child is enclosed in the womb by a natural power which is hidden in the complexion of the fetus. The first thing that develops is a certain vein or nerve which perforates the womb and proceeds from the womb up to the breasts. When the fetus is in the uterus of the mother her breasts are hardened, because the womb closes and the menstrual substance flows to the breast. Then this substance is cooked to a white heat, and it is called the flower of woman; because it is white like milk it is also called the milk

17 Thaddaeus Florentinus, *Expositiones*, fol. 140vb: 'De quarta dicit quasi concludendo quod cum caro mamillarum not sit sanguinolentam sed alba, necesario convertit humiditatem sanguineam venientem ad eam in substantiam albam que est lac et quanto in maiori abundantia currit talis humiditas sanguinea ad mamillas, tanto magis multiplicatur lac, sicut videmus fieri in 8º et nono mense conceptionis. Et hoc de quarta. De quinta el ultima dicit quod talis generatio lactis ex sanguine veniente ad mamillas potest fieri sine conceptione, scilicet quando menstrua retinentur transmutatur, enim aliqua pars sanguinis quod debebat expelli per menstrua ad mamillas et convertitur in lac. Collige igitur causam veritatis aphorismi hoc modo: cum generatio lactis non possit fieri nisi aut propter conceptionem preteritam aut presentem vel preteritum partum vel propter retentionem menstruorum, si aliqua mulier non est pregnans in presenti neque peperit in preterito proximo, sequitur necesario quod habitus lactis significet retentionem menstruorum'. The English translation of the Greek lemma in Hippocrates, *Aphorisms*, 169: 'If a woman has milk when she neither is with child nor has had a child, her menstruation is suppressed'.

> of a woman. After being cooked in this way, it is sent through the vein to the womb, and there the fetus is nourished with its proper natural food. This vein is the umbilical cord which is cut off by the midwives at birth, and thus we see newborn babies with their cord tied with a piece of iron.[18]

This passage demonstrates the importance in medieval physiology of the ability of a woman to seamlessly transform blood to milk, a process that was vital to the health of the baby. Women's bodies were thus imagined as nutritive and life-giving, qualities that, as Eva-Maria Cersovsky shows in her contribution to this volume, played a key role in naturalizing feminine compassion and caregiving.[19]

And yet, this way of thinking about women as a source of nutriment and care existed side by side with a trend that sustained opposing beliefs. In the second half of the thirteenth century, the influence of Aristotelianism as well as a revival of the Plinian tradition in learned circles helped to develop and spread a physiological view of female bodies that linked the centrality of menstrual blood to women's potential for venom.[20] This conception of the female body as noxious was alive in diverse social and cultural contexts, both in popular and elite circles, and it was not infrequent that both notions coalesced in the very same intellectual and textual traditions, as Monica Green has shown.[21] These contradictory perceptions of the female body as both dangerous and generative were current in certain university settings well into the sixteenth century.[22]

Among the most learned and philosophically sophisticated efforts aligned with the noxious view were those put forward by university physicians who struggled to explain a disease in which venomous menstrual blood played a key role. This endeavour was fully developed by two Spanish physicians who devoted monographs to the topic, both written in Latin. Diego Álvarez

18 Lemay, ed., *Women's Secrets*, 109. The Latin critical edition of this paragraph differs slightly from Lemay's translation, which was made from the Lyon 1580 edition; see Barragán, *El 'De secretis mulierum'*, 384-88, lines 125-44. Thirteenth-century readers' engagement with this particular section of the text is attested in Green, *Making Women's Medicine Masculine*, 246, n. 47.

19 Cersovsky, '*Ubi non est mulier*'.

20 The *Secreta mulierum* tradition is full of warnings against women on the grounds of their venom; see Lemay, ed., '*Women's Secrets*'. To mention one medical practitioner's contention, the fourteenth-century English surgeon John Ardene thought that if a practitioner had sexual intercourse with a menstruating woman just before treating his patients, it could interfere with the healing of their wounds, as could the breath of menstruating women. See Green, 'Flowers, Poisons and Men', 57.

21 Green, *Making Women's Medicine Masculine*, 204-45.

22 Park, *Secrets of Women.*

Chanca, a learned physician and a committed explorer who accompanied Columbus on his second trip to the Indies, published the *Tractatus de fascinatione* in 1499. A second treatise was published in 1530 by Antonio de Cartagena, a professor of medicine at the University of Alcalá de Henares. They defined a new disease called *fascinatio*, which was considered to afflict people of weak complexions, typically children, who became seriously ill and could even die as a result.[23]

The most significant feature of this illness was its production by a human agent, whose poisonous complexion precipitated the expulsion of venomous vapours through the eyes, thus contaminating the air. A weak body then absorbed the corrupted air through the pores of the skin or directly through the eyes, making the person sick. According to this explanation, if sick bodies were necessarily weak, inflicting bodies had the ability to produce dangerous venom that did not harm themselves. Women's bodies were accorded that very capacity: menstrual blood, which had long constituted the physiological axis defining the female body, came to be seen as a poisonous substance. According to these physicians, effluent menstrual blood made women potentially dangerous. Nevertheless, the cessation of menses – what we now call menopause – did not improve this condition because old female bodies lost their previous capacity to expel the poison externally; therefore, venomous blood remained inside elderly women's bodies all the time, not only during their periods. In keeping with this explanation, Chanca and Cartagena offered treatments for the *fascinated* sick. Their remedies involved control of the six non-naturals and they offered advice for preventing the illness as well. They did not, however, make any attempt to treat the agents of the illness, that is, the *fascinating* women themselves.

The interest of these Spanish physicians in fully explaining and constructing this illness was a theoretical novelty. Nevertheless, the cultural certitude that a human agent, specifically a woman, could inflict harm on another body without apparent direct physical intervention was not new. The pre-existing social phenomenon upon which their medical explanation was constructed was known in the Middle Ages as the 'evil eye'. Sudden illnesses and deaths of children and other people with weakened bodily constitutions were explained as a result of the evil sight of women, particularly old women. While popular traditions blamed women without theorizing the causes of the evil eye, academic physicians built a whole new rational explanation for the causes of the disease. In so doing, physicians relied on ancient medical

23 Salmón and Cabré, 'Fascinating Women'. A modern edition of the treatises is published in Sanz Hermida, *Cuatro tratados médicos*.

theories, as they often did. Both learned and vernacular audiences thus shared a generalized contempt for women, a misogyny that is increasingly reflected in the domain of natural philosophy. It was in these circles that it became possible to develop a physiological view of women's bodies as venomous on account of their menstrual blood.

Despite the attention and detail given to physiological theories explaining the causes of *fascinatio*, a paradox became apparent. This negative, poisonous view of menstruation necessitated harmonization with the maternal body, the *only* body capable of generating and welcoming human life. Indeed, there were successful efforts to provide a coherent theory that could integrate both generative and toxic views of the female body. For example, Gregor Reisch's *Margarita philosophica* (*The Philosophical Pearl*) provides a significant attempt to elaborate and reconcile these issues. Written by a Carthusian monk between 1489 and 1496 and published in 1503, the *Margarita philosophica* contained an abbreviated abstract representing an 'epitome of the whole philosophy'. While not intended as a course book for university students, it was in fact used at certain institutions, although it never became part of a formal curriculum. Written in a straightforward educational tone and cast as a dialogue between a master and pupil, the *Margarita* was wildly popular. Following its initial publication in 1503, the book saw at least twelve more editions during the sixteenth century.

The *Margarita* was the first printed handbook among university disciplines to endorse the integrated theory of female bodies and to achieve widespread popularity. Chapter 39 of Book 9 of the *Margarita* is devoted to reconciling the apparently contradictory capacities of the female body to generate and to harm.[24] Aptly titled 'On the nourishment of the foetus in the mother's womb: on the afterbirth, and on the noxiousness of the woman's menstrual blood', the chapter explained each of these issues in turn:

> Master: In the woman pregnant with a conception, the usual menses cease to flow and are divided into three parts, of which the first moves to the breasts in which it is cooked into a milky substance; the second is fully digested in the liver of the mother; and the third, which is a superfluity, stays until the time comes for it to be expelled. From the first, the child is nourished when it is born, from the second the foetus in the womb begins to be fed and enlarged from the day of motion; but it takes it not through the mouth but through the veins which are in the umbilicus (by

24 For an Arabic commentary on the possibility of reconciling these two views, see Selove and Batten, 'Making Men and Women', 257.

> which veins it is also joined to the mother). But since this menstrual blood is very well digested, it leaves no superfluities in nourishing the foetus except a little urine, which is received among the membranes around the afterbirth and is expelled together at the birth.[25]

Here, we see the master focusing on female bodily difference through an explanation of function. The menstrual blood appears in three different forms and serves different functions. As the instructional dialogue continues, the master reconciles the nurturing maternal body with the noxious one:

> Pupil: What do you call the afterbirth?
> Master: A little bag in which the foetus is contained, and it is born with the bag following [*sequendo*] it, whence also it receives the name [*secundina*]; this is attached to the womb through the cotyledons. There is another small skin [*panniculus*] whose name is biles, which, enveloping the middle part of the foetus, receives the urinal water from the umbilical vein. There is also a third skin which they call abgas, which surrounds the whole foetus. This little bag is more necessary than all the others, in that it protects the foetus from noxious things, especially from undigested menstrual blood, which if it touches the unprotected foetus, would destroy it instantly, since menstruating women by sight alone both draw red spots on a new mirror, and could stain a delicate infant. Whence also sometimes some drops from the blood, touching the infant cause red spots on the infant, which is not to be erased even by flaying the skin. This blood does not exist in men because of their stronger heat which digests superfluous things, and if anything is left over it passes into the hairs.[26]

The idea of the conversion or transformation of the menstrual blood into milk enabled the generative faculty and the noxious capacity of the female body to be integrated into a single physiological explanation in which its positive and negative abilities could co-exist within a *healthy* female body. As Gianna Pomata has observed, early modern medicine developed a positive imaginary for the maternal body that focused on a harmonious *continuum* between different reproductive organs, the uterus and the breasts, and their different physiological functions, such as generation and breastfeeding.[27] This harmonious continuum rested upon the transformation of blood

25 Quoted in Cunningham and Kusukawa, eds. and trans., *Natural Philosophy Epitomised*, 152.
26 Ibid., 153.
27 Pomata, 'La meravigliosa armonia'.

into milk, a connection that prevailed in humoral theory until the rise of experimental physiology.[28] But what happened if conversion did not occur? Medieval physicians were concerned about the failure of the maternal body to conform to this harmonious view.

Breastbleeding: Disruption and Illness

The Hippocratic *Aphorisms*, a most revered text attributed to the 'father of medicine', explicitly addressed this disorder. In one of the terse statements belonging to the gynecological group of aphorisms, the disruption of the regular transformation of the blood that fulfilled the function of nursing is understood as a sign of illness: 'When blood collects at the breasts of a woman, it indicates madness'.[29] The sentence therefore established a direct relationship between insanity and the lack of harmony in a woman's lactating body.[30]

Galen, the most influential commentator on the work, approached the aphorism in his usual systematic way. First, he summarized his own opinions on the gynecological aphorism, explaining that blood arrived at the breasts and is transformed there into nourishing milk. Second, Galen expressed his amazement at Hippocrates' assertion that when this does *not* happen, the physician must be aware that he is facing a case of *mania*, that is, a type of madness involving a state of crazed fury and agitation. Galen's perplexity is based on his long clinical experience, since he writes that he has never seen a case like this. However, he respects Hippocrates' authority and concludes that if this condition is addressed in the text, it is because it is a real clinical entity that Hippocrates had witnessed; therefore, there had to be an explanation for this phenomenon. And in fact, he offers a physio-pathological rationale to explain this possibility. In normal conditions, the relative coldness of the breasts facilitates the conversion of the blood into milk. However, in the case of excess heat in the blood, this process cannot

28 Orland, 'White Blood and Red Milk', and Orland, 'Why Could Early Modern Men Lactate?'

29 Aphorism 5.40, Hippocrates, *Aphorisms*, 169.

30 The condition finds a certain ungendered analogy in *Epidemiae* 2.6.32, where it is stated that blood gathering at the breasts foretells madness; see Hanson, 'Aphorismi 5.28-63', 286. However, this book of *Epidemics* was unknown in Latin translation until the late fifteenth or early sixteenth century; Kibre, ed., *Hippocrates Latinus*, 138. In addition, all the interpreters of aphorism 5.40 that we discuss, from Galen to Amatus Lusitanus, consistently understand the meaning of Hippocrates' sentence as the failure of a woman's body to convert blood into milk, attested by breastbleeding.

take place and the vapours produced by the overheated blood rise to the head, producing *mania*.[31]

Medieval physicians learned about this condition in their regular engagement with the *Aphorisms*, one of the most widely read and commented upon works in the history of medical learning. The textual nature of the aphoristic genre made it particularly suitable for teaching as well as for exegesis and offered ample room for interpretation. Indeed, many extant copies of the Latin versions of the *Aphorisms*, both with and without Galen's exposition of the text, contain readers' annotations that vary from little notes to significant commentaries. Commenting upon texts was a highly valued epistemological and teaching tool in medical scholasticism. Medical masters made their mark in discussions of this condition by offering their sound logical reasoning on the Hippocratic statement and on Galen's thinking about it, as he was the most influential of its commentators.

The transmission of the Hippocratic *Aphorisms* in the medieval Latin West is well attested, since the work figured among the core collection of five texts known as the 'Articella', which shaped, with later additions, Western medical education from the twelfth century onwards.[32] Many details of the *Aphorisms*' textual history remain murky, however. Throughout the early Middle Ages, the text circulated both independently and accompanied by a commentary of dubious authorship, in versions based on the so-called 'old ravenata', a Latin translation made from the Greek in Ravenna probably in the mid-sixth century.[33] In the late eleventh century, it was newly retranslated from the Greek within the Salernitan circle of Alfanus (d. 1085) with the aim of Hellenizing the text.[34] The Greco-Latin tradition was enriched in the twelfth century with versions often accompanied by commentaries, including Burgundio of Pisa's (d. 1198) partial translation that, by 1314, was completed by Niccolò da Reggio (*fl.* 1308-45).[35] Moreover, as part of his major project to establish a Galenic perspective on medicine, Constantine the African (d. 1098/99) translated Galen's commentary on the *Aphorisms* from the Arabic, seemingly using an existing translation of the lemmata (the headings or titles of the aphorisms; singular: 'lemma') from

31 Hippocrates [cum commentum Galieni], *Liber aphorismorum*, fol. 33vb.

32 Green, 'Gloriosissimus Galienus', 326-27.

33 For recent work on the history of this tradition, see Haverling, 'On Textual Criticism', and Vázquez Buján, 'La transmisión latina'.

34 Wallis, 'Why Was the "Aphorisms" of Hippocrates Retranslated'.

35 Burgundio translated Books 1-4, thus leaving aside the gynecological section. Kibre, *Hippocrates Latinus*, 32; see also 'In Hippocratis Aphorismos tradotto da Burgundio da Pisa', in *Galeno*.

the Greek.[36] As Monica Green has recently suggested, this translation was apparently the first of Constantine's Galenic translations from the Arabic and the second in popularity after the *Tegni*.[37] Although this translation of Galen's commentary on the *Aphorisms* seems to have enjoyed limited circulation during the long twelfth century, it became very influential afterwards, since in the second quarter of the thirteenth century, it appeared in the expanded version of the 'Articella' known as the 'ars commentata', which was the core text of the medical curriculum.[38] From this point on, generations of university medical students learned and discussed the Hippocratic *Aphorisms* through the prism of Galen.[39]

Aphorism 5.40 proved to be an enigmatic statement. Learned medicine took issue with the description of the very condition, endorsing various interpretations that did not emphasize the idea of 'accumulation' or 'collection' of blood in the breasts as the original Greek stated, but rather its lack of conversion, its bleeding or exit from the nipple. This is the reading given by some of the twelfth-century Salernitan masters in the common gloss preserved in the so-called Digby commentary. While wondering about the phenomenon, the anonymous commentator describes the effluence of blood: when blood comes out from a woman's breast, why does it happen? ('quando de mamillas mulieris sanguis exit, unde hoc fit?').[40] The question points the aphorism in a certain direction, and the following exegesis clarifies this point. The commentary that follows explains that, in normal conditions, the blood that arrives at the breast turns into milk; if it is excessively hot, however, it cannot be converted into milk. The vapour that is generated by this blood then ascends to the brain producing *mania*, a certain type of madness. Here, insanity is the result of the incapacity of a maternal body to transform blood into milk for the purpose of lactation, and the mechanism is similar to the interpretation given by Galen. An analogous explanation

36 'In Hippocratis Aphorismos tradotto da Burgundio da Pisa', in *Galeno*.

37 Galen's *Tegni* or *Microtegni* or *Ars medica* (*Technē iatrikē*) was a summary of the main principles of Galen's system of medicine. Various versions of the text were in circulation in the Latin Middles Ages but the most commonly read were two twelfth-century translations, the so called *translatio antiqua* done from the Greek and a *translatio arabica* that contained the commentary of Ali ibn Ridwan; O'Boyle, *Art of Medicine*, 92-95.

38 Green, 'Gloriosissimus Galienus'. We are indebted to Monica Green for her expert advice on this question.

39 On the medical university curriculum from 1250 on, see O'Boyle, *Art of Medicine*.

40 Oxford, Bodleian Library, Digby 108, fol. 62v: 'Sanguis si habilis fuerit in lac convertitur sed si ad eo fervidus est ut mutari in lac non possit cum mamille sint nervose per mediocritatem nervorum, fumus acutus ascendens inde et cerebrum inficiens facit maniam subtrahatam ergo sanguis'.

is provided by Archimatheus Salernitanus (*fl.* second half of the twelfth century), who fears the same illness if the ordinary process of conversion occurring in women's breasts does not take place; in addition, he identifies the nerves and arteries that channel the blood into the brain.[41] Here it becomes evident how attention to function problematizes any suggestion that medieval constructions of gender were dominated by a monolithic one-sex model. The functions of menstruation and lactation were critical to medieval explanations of sex difference and the kinds of diseases to which women were uniquely susceptible.

Medieval Latin renderings of this aphorism consistently transmit in the lemma the notion of blood conversion, not the idea of blood collection: that is, they appeal to the harmonic flow of blood that must be transformed in the maternal body. In many of the extant commentaries, the full renderings of the lemmata of the aphorisms are not presented; in such cases the idea of transformation is provided in the explanation itself.[42] Indeed, the lemmata of the different medieval versions explicitly included the verb *convertitur*. In medieval Latin, the aphorism was transmitted as 'Mulieribus quibus ad mamillas sanguis convertitur maniam significat' ('When blood is converted in the breasts of women, it means madness'). In other words, the original Greek word συστρέφεται, which conveyed the idea of collection or accumulation, was transliterated in medieval Latin as *συσ-con/τρέφεται-vertitur*: *convertitur*.[43] This meaning seems to be peculiar to the medieval Latin versions, as the Syriac and Arabic traditions of the *Aphorisms* retain the sense of 'collection'.[44] The presence of transliterations from the Greek is not rare in medieval Latin translations of the text.[45] However, this example involves an obvious error in the meaning of the sentence. Its persistence throughout the centuries shows that the epistemological framework through which the female body was understood prevailed over the literal interpretation of the

41 Archimatheus Salernitanus, *Erklärungen*, 107.

42 Cambridge, Gonville & Caius College, 111 (180), fol. 109ra: 'Mulieribus quibus etc. Quomodo sanguis fluit ad mamillas docuit in precedenti afforismorum et quomodo mutetur in lac in hoc autem docet et si tamen veniat non mutetur in lac maniam significat'. ('In women who etc. The way in which the blood arrives at the breasts and how it is converted into milk is taught in the previous aphorism. This one teaches that if it arrives there but it cannot be converted into milk, this is a sign of madness.')

43 We are indebted to Giulia Ecca for her expert help on this matter and for her generosity in sharing her work-in-progress Italian translation of the original Greek aphorism and of Galen's commentary.

44 Oliver Overwien has kindly provided us this information.

45 For other instances, see Wallis, 'Why Was the "Aphorisms" of Hippocrates Retranslated', 183-86; and Vázquez Buján, 'La transmisión latina', 215.

words.[46] The correct meaning of the statement (that blood is *not* converted) was clear to anyone who had already read the previous aphorism as well as Galen's commentary on it, which deals with a pathological aspect of the ordinary transformation of blood into milk.[47] Indeed, it would be clear to anyone familiar with the physiology of the production of breast milk, and it is in this context that it was understood. The continuing presence of this philological slip in the Latin medical tradition therefore highlights the misogynistic drive of a medical system that tends to pathologize the precarity of the maternal body, always subject to potential toxicity and mania.

Since the text was a basic tool for learning medicine, medieval copies of the *Aphorisms* not infrequently bear readers' annotations, including those of university students who wrote marginal or interlinear notes that show a significant engagement with the text. These anonymous annotations correct the odd literal meaning of the lemma by adding a '*non*' to the '*convertitur*' or by providing further clarification that 'it is not converted into milk'.[48] Several instances testify to the exposition of 'Mulieribus quibus ad mamillas' in the context of university medical education. Teaching in Montpellier, Bernard de Angarra (*fl.* 1290-1320) included its discussion in the list of questions on the *Aphorisms* that he elaborated for use in his classroom. Aligning himself with Galen in regard to the rarity of the phenomenon, his concern was to explain how the blood would ascend from the breasts to the brain.[49] Writing some years earlier in the 1280s, Taddeo Alderotti, a committed teacher at the studium of Bologna, penned a thorough exposition

46 Examples of copies from different traditions: 'Mulier cui in mammis sanguis conuertitur, mannia, hoc est insania, significa[n]t' (eighth-ninth century), Vázquez Buján, 'La transmisión latina', 220; 'Mulieribus quipus [*sic*] ad ma[millas] san[guis] conver[titur, maniam significat]', Archimatheus Salernitanus, *Erklärungen*, 107 (twelfth century); 'Mulieribus quibus ad mamillas sanguis convertitur, maniam significat', Cambridge, Peterhouse, 247, fols. 2r, 105v (thirteenth century); 'Mulieribus quibus ad mamillas sanguis convertitur, maniam significat', Vienna, Österreischische Nationalbibliothek, 2328, fol. 23va-b (1321); 'Mulieribus quibus ad mamillas sanguis convertitur, maniam significat', Erfurt, Biblioteca Amploniana, F 278, fol. 201va (fourteenth century); 'Mulieribus quibus convertitur sanguis ad mamillam maniam significat' (1428/29), Paschold, *Die Frau und ihr Körper*, 194; 'Mulieribus quibus ad mamillas sanguis convertitur maniam significat', Hippocrates [cum commentum Galieni], *Liber aphorismorum*, fol. 33vb (1483).

47 5.39. 'If a woman have [*sic*] milk when she neither is with child nor has had a child, her menstruation is suppressed'; in Hippocrates, *Aphorisms*, 169.

48 Two thirteenth-century examples: 'cum non convertit in lac', Cambridge, Peterhouse, 247, fol. 2r; and 'et non convertitur in lac', Cambridge, St. John's College, D 24, fol. 51va.

49 Erfurt, Biblioteca Amploniana, F 290, fol. 99vb. On Bernard de Angarra's teaching at Montpellier, see McVaugh, 'In a Montpellier Classroom'.

of the *Aphorisms* with Galen's commentary using Constantine's translation. He complained about its quality but insisted that this was the most commonly used translation, although he acknowledged that there were other, better ones available.[50] When addressing the Latin aphorism he drew particular attention to its odd rendering, probably considering that in a teaching context it was important to note the erroneous formulation of the authoritative text. After acknowledging the inconsistency of the aphorism as it stood, he suggested two philological reflections. First, that a 'not' is missing in the formulation, so that adding a '*non*' would show the real meaning of Hippocrates's sentence, clarifying that it is when the blood is 'not' transformed into milk that we can speak of madness. He also presented another option that respected the text as it was. Taddeo contended that '*con-vertitur*' might mean to turn itself into something contrary to its own nature. Since blood arriving in the breasts had to turn into milk naturally, which did not happen in this case, *convertitur* would be the right wording since it means that the blood that reaches the breast remained there as blood. This is a typical piece of scholastic rhetoric that seems not to have been taken very seriously by Taddeo himself, who instead favoured the simplicity of introducing the missing 'not'.

In addition to his philological concern, Taddeo tackled the question of the veracity of the aphorism, something that Galen addressed directly. He concludes that the aphorism is true because its consequence is true – unconverted blood in the breast produces *mania* – even if the antecedent (in scholastic jargon) is very rare: that is, it is only infrequently the case that blood is excessively hot, thus making its transformation into milk impossible. In fact, although Taddeo takes different possibilities into consideration, the physiological explanation he offers of the transformation of the blood is much the same as Galen's, with one exception. He notes that the vapours of menstrual blood are more prone to producing *mania*, a process that parallels the explanation given to fascination, where the corrupted vapours of menstrual blood rise to the head and are expelled through the eyes. In both conditions (mania and fascination), it is the failure of menstrual blood to comply with its functions that causes pathology.

Taddeo's positive assessment of the aphorism's validity is further reinforced by his amendment of Constantine's translation that points its reading in a certain direction. Taddeo says that the failure to transform blood into milk may be a sign of 'future madness' ('maniam futuram'); that is, interpreting the possibility of madness as a future prognosis rather

50 Kibre, *Hippocrates Latinus*, 32.

than as a present diagnosis. By introducing this change, he developed a more substantial rationale for the veracity of the Hippocratic statement, thereby alleviating the doubt that earlier commentators, including Galen, had expressed.[51] This interpretation was shared by other thirteenth-century readers who added the word 'future' above the word 'mania' ('maniam scilicet futuram') in copies of the text they were reading.[52]

The explanation of deferred mania proved to be convincing to later commentators as well. Writing in Ferrara in 1403, Jacopo da Forlì (*c.*1360-1414) commented upon 'Mulieribus quibus ad mamillas' without questioning its veracity, although adding some precision to it. He based his judgments upon what 'many authors say' without acknowledging their identity, with the exception of Ibn Sīnā (Avicenna), whose medical encyclopedia, the *Canon of Medicine*, shaped medieval medical theory and practice on both sides of the Mediterranean basin.[53] Avicenna systematized Galenic physiopathology, devoting one section to the anatomy of the breasts and the generation of milk from blood. He detailed different pathologies involving the excessive or scarce production of breast milk and explained its different qualities in direct relation to the diverse qualities of blood.[54] So closely was Avicenna associated with mammary pathologies that he is depicted offering instruction on a disembodied breast in a fourteenth-century miniature illuminating those chapters of his work (Figure 3.1). Jacopo followed these basic lines of argumentation but also engaged with an earlier chapter of the *Canon* devoted to mental alterations, in which the accumulation of blood in women's breasts is explicitly noted as a sign of *mania*.[55] Avicenna does not mention the Hippocratic aphorism but simply lists the sign and explains that the pathological condition is produced when the blood is corrupted by excessive heat. However, the most influential commentator of the *Canon*, Gentile da Foligno (d. 1348), did connect this passage directly with aphorism 5.40. Rendering its lemma in full, Gentile explained that since the breasts are a cold organ, they fail to transform excessively hot blood into milk, instead producing vapours that rise to the brain.[56]

Jacopo da Forlì provided the common physiological explanation of the mechanism underpinning mania, in which hot fumes rose from the breasts

51 Thaddaeus Florentinus, *Expositiones*, fol. 141vb.

52 Cambridge, St. John's College, D 24, fol. 51va.

53 Siraisi, *Avicenna in Renaissance Italy*.

54 Avicenna, *Liber canonis*, bk. 3, fen 12, fol. 209vb-210va: 'De mammilla et dispositionibus eius, et est tractatus unus'.

55 Ibid., bk. 3, fen 1, tract. 4, ch. 16, fol. 149va: 'De signis manie universalibus et specierum eius'.

56 Gentile da Foligno, *Tertius canonis Avicennae*, fol. 83va-b.

Figure 3.1 Avicenna as an Eastern master demonstrating the breast to a male student

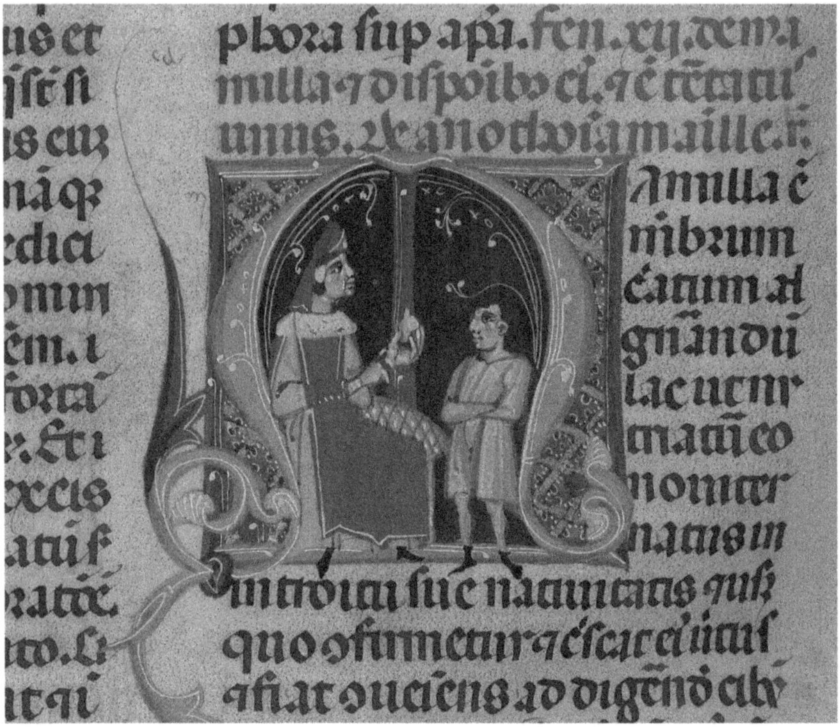

Illuminated initial of a fourteenth-century copy of the Latin translation by Gerard of Cremona of Avicenna's *Canon*, bk. 3, fen 12, 'De mamilla', probably from a Swabian workshop. Vatican City, Biblioteca Apostolica Vaticana, Urb. Lat. 241, fol.166vb, detail. © 2019 Biblioteca Apostolica Vaticana. Reproduced by permission. All rights reserved.

to the brain as a result of unconverted blood. In addition, he postulated that this process could happen with any accumulation of blood in the superior part of the body. In his view, however, it remained a gendered phenomenon because it occurred more frequently in women, due to the presence of veins that provided passageways to the breasts from the womb. He qualified the veracity of the aphorism ('ad veritatem aphorismo') on various conditions: the amount of blood that reaches the breast; the quality of the blood; and the relative strength of the brain to repel the ascending fumes. By taking into account the characteristics of the blood, whether it was pure hot blood or mixed, he opened up the mental consequences of the ailment so that they were no longer restricted to mania but expanded to include any state of mental alteration.[57]

57 Jacopo da Forlì, *Expositio super libro aphorismorum*, fol. 73va-b.

Jacopo's works were highly esteemed by contemporaries and his commentary on the Hippocratic *Aphorisms* was printed as early as 1473, followed by several reprints. Ugo Benzi (1376-1439), the philosopher and physician with whom he was in personal contact, explicitly quoted Jacopo's commentary when writing his own.[58] We know that Jacopo used Constantine's version of the *Aphorisms*, but it is likely that Ugo was familiar with both the Greek and the Latin versions.[59] As Tiziana Pesenti has shown, Benzi's mentor Santasofia used a collated version of both, and the Greek-Latin version enjoyed considerable fortune in certain Italian schools in the later fourteenth century.[60] For Ugo, the correct interpretation of the Hippocratic aphorism needed to be grounded in evidence of the emission of blood through the breast in sufficient quantity and in a continuous manner ('ab ipsis mamillis sanguis exprimatur in notabili quantitate et perseveranter'). He contended that lack of transformation or collection of blood in the breast was a sign of madness only in these circumstances, as inferred from the aphorism's phrasing. Ugo devoted ample discussion to the question of whether it was appropriate to use the category of *mania* in this case, concluding that it should be used in a wide sense.[61]

Hence medieval Latin readers of the 'Mulieribus quibus ad mamillas' confronted the puzzling aphorism in different ways. First, they interpreted its meaning, in particular the word *conversio*, within the theoretical frame of humoral physiology that understood women's blood as a transformative nourishing substance. Second, they imagined plausible theoretical explanations for the sentence. Third, they adapted their understanding of the statement by transposing the prognostic sign of breastbleeding from the present to the future. Finally, some authors expanded the condition itself by widening the concept of *mania* to encompass any mental disease, as the illness caused by the inability of the blood to become nourishing milk. Importantly, none of the late medieval interpreters of the text questioned its veracity on observational grounds, as Galen had done; nor did they discuss any specific case involving the condition. Those reading Galen's commentary reported on his perplexity; like him, they gave the statement credence because they fundamentally trusted Hippocrates' statement.

However, there are reasons to think that the connection between failure to transform blood into milk, on the one hand, and women's madness, on the other, may have been perceived as a real clinical threat in the Middle Ages.

58 Benzi, *Expositio super Aphorismos*, fol. 128r-va.

59 Touwaide, 'Jacopo da Forlì', 281a.

60 Pesenti, *Marsilio Santasofia*, 448-49.

61 Benzi, *Expositio super Aphorismos*, fol. 128rb-va.

Indeed, the learned surgeon Lanfranc of Milan (d. before 1306) reported such a case in his surgical manual when expounding on diseases of the breasts. Commenting on the Hippocratic aphorism that apostemes may occur as a result of blood that cannot be converted into milk ('sanguinem attractum qui non potest in lac converti'), he explicitly mentioned mania as a possible result of the condition. Lanfranc offered different treatments that he had used to good effect, including topical remedies applied to the breast, cupping glasses, phlebotomy in the basilic or saphena vein, and a dietary regimen. He also recounted an eyewitness case of a noblewoman suffering from a breast aposteme, who ignored his treatment and favoured one suggested by a lay surgeon. Withdrawing his services, Lanfranc predicted that the woman would become manic and after three days, she did indeed die of frenzy.[62] A thorough study of medieval surgical handbooks may unearth similar cases now buried in sections on apostemes.

For now, we can say that physicians' centuries-long engagement with this Hippocratic aphorism continued into the early modern world. Indeed, the Portuguese Jewish physician Amatus Lusitanus (1511-1568), professor at the University of Ferrara, appealed explicitly to the aphorism when reporting his own clinical experience. In his case histories that inaugurated a new genre of medical writing, Amatus recounts several instances of lactating women whose breasts bled abundantly ('sanguis illi effluere coepit copiosissime'). A dedicated Galenist, Amatus was very aware of Galen's lack of clinical familiarity with this condition, but on this issue he aligned himself with Hippocrates. In addition, he described an effective treatment that could prevent lactating women who failed to convert their blood into milk from falling into insanity: the extraction of blood from the saphena vein in the foot.[63]

Exploring how medieval physicians engaged with works that communicated the foundations of humoral epistemology over many centuries highlights the dynamism of medieval medical thought. At the same time, studying physicians' exegeses on issues peculiar to the female body reveals the complex, creative ways in which they imagined and created the reality of gendered pathologies. The medieval economy of women's bodies was flexible in its ability to harmonize noxious, killing capacities with a maternal, healthy normality. However, disharmony within the physiology of maternity could

62 Lanfranc of Milan, *Cyrurgia*, fol. 194va. The case is cited in Green, *Making Women's Medicine Masculine*, 93.

63 Amatus Lusitanus, *Curationum medicinalium*, centuria 2, curatio 21, fols. 41v-42r. On this work in the context of the development of early modern medical observation and empiricism, see Pomata, 'Sharing Cases'.

find no place except in pathology. If a venomous female body was culturally plausible within the framework of women's sanity, bleeding breasts could not be conceived without recourse to the disorder of madness. They not only disrupted female physiological normativity but also, perhaps more importantly, the symbolic function of mothering.

Works Cited

Manuscripts

Cambridge, Gonville & Caius College, 111 (180).
Cambridge, Peterhouse, 247.
Cambridge, St. John's College, D 24.
Erfurt, Biblioteca Amploniana, F 278.
Erfurt, Biblioteca Amploniana, F 290.
Oxford, Bodleian Library, Digby 108.
Vienna, Österreischische Nationalbibliothek, 2328.

Printed Works

Amatus Lusitanus. *Curationum medicinalium centuriae duae, prima et secunda* (Paris: Sebastianum Nivellium, 1554).

Archimatheus Salernitanus. *Erklärungen zu den hippokratischen Aphorismen*, ed. with introd. by Hermann Grensemann (Hamburg, 2005), https://web.archive.org/web/20150205033503/http://www.uke.de/institute/geschichte-medizin/downloads/institut-geschichte-ethik-medizin/ArchimAphEdition.pdf (accessed 15 July 2019).

Avicenna. *Liber canonis tocius medicinae* (Venice, 1527). Repr. in Brussels: Collectaneis Medicinae Historia, 1971.

Barragán Nieto, José Pablo. *El 'De secretis mulierum' atribuido a Alberto Magno: estudio, edición crítica y traducción* (Porto: Féderation Internationale des Instituts d'Études Médiévales, 2012).

Benzi, Ugo. *Expositio super Aphorismos Hippocratis et Galieni* (Venice: Bonetus Locatellus, 1498).

Cadden, Joan. *Meanings of Sex Difference in the Middle Ages: Medicine, Science, and Culture* (Cambridge: Cambridge University Press, 1993).

Cersovsky, Eva-Maria. '*Ubi non est mulier, ingemiscit egens*? Gendered Perceptions of Care from the Thirteenth to Sixteenth Centuries', in *Gender, Health, and Healing, 1250-1550*, ed. Sara Ritchey and Sharon Strocchia (Amsterdam: Amsterdam University Press, 2020), 191-214.

Cook, Harold. Review of *Blood, Sweat and Tears: The Changing Concepts of Physiology from Antiquity into Early Modern Europe*, ed. Manfred Hortsmanshoff, Helen King, and Claus Zittel, *Renaissance Quarterly*, 67.3 (2014), 980-82.

Cunningham, Andrew and Sachiko Kusukawa, eds. and trans. *Natural Philosophy Epitomised: A Translation of Books 8-11 of Gregor Reisch's Philosophical Pearl (1503)* (Farnham: Ashgate, 2010).

Duden, Barbara. *The Woman beneath the Skin: A Doctor's Patients in Eighteenth-Century Germany* (Cambridge: Harvard University Press, 1991).

Galeno: catalogo delle traduzioni latine, ed. Stefania Fortuna, www.galenolatino.com/ (accessed 11 July 2019).

Gentile da Foligno. *Tertius canonis Avicennae cum amplissima Gentilis Fulginis expositione* (Venice: H. Octavianus Scotus, 1522).

Green, Monica. 'Flowers, Poisons and Men: Menstruation in Medieval Western Europe', in *Menstruation: A Cultural History*, ed. Andrew Shail and Gilliam Howie (Basingstoke: Palgrave MacMillan, 2005), 51-64.

—. 'Gloriosissimus Galienus: Galen and Galenic Writings in the Eleventh- and Twelfth-Century Latin West', in *Brill's Companion to the Reception of Galen*, ed. Petros Bouras-Vallianatos and Barbara Zipser (Leiden: Brill, 2019), 319-42.

—. *Making Women's Medicine Masculine: The Rise of Male Authority in Pre-modern Gynaecology* (Oxford: Oxford University Press, 2008).

Hanson, Ann E. 'Aphorismi 5.28-63 and the Gynaecological Texts of the *Corpus Hippocraticum*', in *Magic and Rationality in Ancient Near Eastern and Graeco-Roman Medicine*, ed. H.F. Hortsmanshoff and M. Stol in collaboration with C.R. van Tilburg (Leiden: Brill, 2004), 277-304.

Haverling, Gerd V.M. 'On Textual Criticism and Linguistic Development in the Late Latin Translation of the Hippocratic Aphorisms', in *Body, Disease and Treatment in a Changing World: Latin Texts and Contexts in Ancient and Medieval Medicine*, ed. David Langslow and Brigitte Maire (Lausanne: Éditions Bibliothèque d'Histoire de la Médecine et de la Santé, 2010), 105-18.

Hippocrates. *Aphorisms*, in *Hippocrates*, ed. G.P. Gold, trans. W.H.S. Jones, vol. 4 (Cambridge: Harvard University Press, 1992).

— [cum commentum Galieni]. *Liber aphorismorum*, in *Articella* (Venice: Hermann Liechtenstein, 1483), fols. 9ra-45vb.

Horden, Peregrine and Elisabeth Hsu, eds. *The Body in Balance: Humoral Medicines in Practice* (New York: Bergham, 2013).

Hortsmanshoff, Manfred, Helen King, and Claus Zittel, eds. *Blood, Sweat and Tears: The Changing Concepts of Physiology from Antiquity into Early Modern Europe* (Leiden: Brill, 2012).

Jacopo da Forlì. *Expositio super libro aphorismorum Hyppocratis* [lib. I-VI], in *Commentum Galienus super libro aphorismorum Hypocratis: expositio Jacobo*

Forlivianensis et Marsilius de Sancta Sophia super libro aphorismorum Hypocratis (Pavia: Michaelem et Bernardinum de Garaldis, 1501), fols. 2ra-85rb.

Kibre, Pearl, ed. *Hippocrates Latinus: Repertorium of Hippocratic Writings in the Latin Middle Ages*, rev. ed. (New York: Fordham University Press, 1985).

King, Helen. *Hippocrates' Woman: Reading the Female Body in Ancient Medicine* (London: Routledge, 1998).

—. 'Introduction', in *Blood, Sweat and Tears: The Changing Concepts of Physiology from Antiquity into Early Modern Europe*, ed. Manfred Hortsmanshoff, Helen King, and Claus Zittel (Leiden: Brill, 2012), 1-25.

—. *The One-Sex Body on Trial: The Classical and Early Modern Evidence* (Farnham: Ashgate, 2013).

Lanfranc of Milan. *Cyrurgia*, in *Cyrurgia Guidonis de Cauliaco et Cyrurgia Bruni, Teodorici, Rolandi, Lanfranci, Rogerii, Bertapalie* (Venice: Bernardinum Venetum de Vitalibus, 1519), fols. 166va-210vb.

Laqueur, Thomas. *Making Sex: Body and Gender from the Greeks to Freud* (Cambridge, MA: Harvard University Press, 1990).

Lemay, Helen Rodnite, ed. *Women's Secrets: A Translation of Pseudo-Albertus Magnus' De Secretis Mulierum with Commentaries* (Albany, NY: State University of New York Press, 1992).

McVaugh, Michael. 'In a Montpellier Classroom', in *Professors, Physicians and Practices in the History of Medicine: Essays in Honor of Nancy Siraisi*, ed. Gideon Manning and Cynthia Klestinec (Cham, Switzerland: Springer, 2017), 29-48.

Nutton, Vivian. 'Humoralism', in *Companion Encyclopedia of the History of Medicine*, ed. William Bynum and Roy Porter, vol. 1 (London: Routledge, 1993), 281-91.

O'Boyle, Cornelius. *The Art of Medicine: Medical Teaching at the University of Paris, 1250-1400* (Leiden: Brill, 1998).

Orland, Barbara. 'White Blood and Red Milk. Analogical Reasoning in Medical Practice and Experimental Physiology (1560-1730)', in *Blood, Sweat and Tears: The Changing Concepts of Physiology from Antiquity into Early Modern Europe*, ed. Manfred Hortsmanshoff, Helen King, and Claus Zittel (Leiden: Brill, 2012), 443-78.

—. 'Why Could Early Modern Men Lactate? Gender Identity and Metabolic Narrations in Humoral Medicine', in *Medieval and Renaissance Lactations: Images, Rhetorics, Practices*, ed. Jutta Sperling (Farnham: Ashgate, 2013), 37-54.

Park, Katharine. 'Cadden, Laqueur, and the "One-Sex" Body', *Medieval Feminist Forum*, 46 (2010), 96-100.

—. 'Medicine and Natural Philosophy: Naturalistic Traditions', in *The Oxford Handbook of Women and Gender in Medieval Europe*, ed. Judith M. Bennett and Ruth M. Karras (Oxford: Oxford University Press, 2013), 84-100.

—. *Secrets of Women: Gender, Generation, and the Origins of Human Dissection* (New York: Zone Books, 2006).
Park, Katharine and Robert Nye. '"Destiny is Anatomy": Essay Review of Thomas Laqueur's *Making Sex*', *New Republic* (18 February 1991), 53-57.
Paschold, Chris E. *Die Frau und ihr Körper im medizinischen und didaktischen Schrifttum des französischen Mittelalters* (Pattensen: Horst Wellm, 1989).
Pesenti, Tiziana. *Marsilio Santasofia tra corti e università* (Treviso: Antilla, 2003).
Pomata, Gianna. 'La meravigliosa armonia: il rapporto fra seni ed utero dall'anatomia vascolare all'endocrinologia', in *Madri: storia di un ruolo sociale*, ed. Giovanna Fiume (Venice: Marsilio, 1995), 45-81.
—. 'Sharing Cases: The *Observationes* in Early Modern Medicine', *Early Science and Medicine*, 15 (2010), 193-236.
Pouchelle, Marie-Christine. *Corps et chirurgie à l'apogée du Moyen Âge* (Paris: Flammarion, 1983).
Rublack, Ulinka. 'Fluxes: The Early Modern Body and the Emotions', *History Workshop Journal*, 53.1 (2002), 1-16.
Salmón, Fernando. 'The Body Inferred: Knowing the Body through the Dissection of Texts', in *A Cultural History of the Human Body in the Medieval Age*, ed. Linda Kalof (Oxford: Berg, 2010), 77-97.
Salmón, Fernando and Montserrat Cabré. 'Fascinating Women: The Evil Eye in Medical Scholasticism', in *Medicine from the Black Death to the French Disease*, ed. Roger French, Jon Arrizabalaga, Andrew Cunningham, and Luis García-Ballester (Aldershot: Ashgate, 1998), 53-84.
Sanz Hermida, Jacobo. *Cuatro tratados médicos renacentistas sobre el mal de ojo* (Valladolid: Junta de Castilla y León, Consejería de Educación y Cultura, 2001).
Selove, Emily and Rosalind Batten. 'Making Men and Women: Arabic Commentaries on the Gynaecological Hippocratic Aphorisms in Context', *Annales Islamologiques* 48.1 (2014), 239-62.
Siraisi, Nancy G. *Avicenna in Renaissance Italy: The Canon and Medical Teaching in Italian Universities after 1500* (Princeton, NJ: Princeton University Press, 1987).
Stolberg, Michael. 'Menstruation and Sexual Difference in Early Modern Medicine', in *Menstruation: A Cultural History*, ed. Andrew Shail and Gilliam Howie (Basingstoke: Palgrave Macmillan, 2005), 90-101.
—. 'A Woman Down to her Bones: The Anatomy of Sexual Difference in the Sixteenth and Early Seventeenth Centuries', *Isis*, 94 (2003), 274-99.
Thaddaeus Florentinus. *Expositiones in arduum aphorismorum Ipocratis* (Venice: Lucantonio Giunta, 1527).

Touwaide, Alan. 'Jacopo da Forlì', in *Medieval Science, Technology and Medicine: An Encyclopedia*, ed. Thomas Glick, Steven J. Livesey, and Faith Wallis (New York/London: Routledge, 2005), 281.

Tuten, Belle S. 'Care of the Breast in the Late Middle Ages: The *Tractatus de passionibus mamillarum*', in *Gender, Health, and Healing, 1250-1550*, ed. Sara Ritchey and Sharon Strocchia (Amsterdam: Amsterdam University Press, 2020), 119-37.

—. 'Lactation and Breast Diseases in Antiquity: Medical Authorities on Breast and Health Treatment', *Quaestiones Medii Aevi Novae*, 19 (2014), 159-86.

Vázquez Buján, Manuel Enrique. 'La transmisión latina de los *Aforismos* hipocráticos en el códice *Paris, BNF, Latin* 11218', *Revue d'Histoire des Textes*, n.s., 13 (2018), 195-243.

Wallis, Faith. 'Why Was the "Aphorisms" of Hippocrates Retranslated in the Eleventh Century?', in *Vehicles of Transmission, Translation, and Transformation in Medieval Textual Culture*, ed. Robert Wisnovsky, Faith Wallis, Jamie C. Fumo, and Carlos Fraenkel (Turnhout: Brepols, 2011), 173-93.

About the Authors

Montserrat Cabré is Professor of the History of Science at the University of Cantabria, Santander (Spain), and director of the Office for Gender Equality and Social Responsibility. Her research focuses on medicine and sexual difference as well as on women's health practices in the Middle Ages.

Fernando Salmón is Professor of the History of Science in the medical school at the University of Cantabria, Santander (Spain). His research focuses on medieval medical scholasticism and he is currently general editor of the *Arnaldi de Villanova Opera medica omnia* (AVOMO).

4 Care of the Breast in the Late Middle Ages

The *Tractatus de passionibus mamillarum*

*Belle S. Tuten**

Abstract

The *Tractatus de passionibus mamillarum*, a short treatise written in fifteenth-century Italy, details treatments for women who experienced painful breast engorgement while lactating. It is primarily a translation of a chapter concerning the breast taken from the *Lilium medicine* of the Montpellier physician, Bernard de Gordon. The author of the *Tractatus*, however, eliminates most of Bernard's commentary. The treatments are simple combinations of herbs, minerals, and liquids meant to be applied to the skin as plasters or poultices. This essay contextualizes the *Tractatus* within the historiography and literature of breastfeeding and provides a brief transcription and translation of its original recipe. It argues that the *Tractatus* represents a 'hybrid' form of healthcare and body knowledge that bridged household and academy.

Keywords: breastfeeding, recipe books, breast disease, household medicine, Bernard de Gordon

* This project was generously supported by a Boston Medical Library fellowship in the History of Medicine at the Countway Library of Medicine, Harvard University. Thanks especially to Jack Eckert for his assistance. I owe great thanks to Rossella Bonfatti, who provided the first draft of the transcription of the Boston text and a translation into modern Italian and English. I also thank Luke Demaitre for providing generous information on Bernard de Gordon, as well as the editors of this volume.

Ritchey, Sara & Sharon Strocchia (eds), *Gender, Health, and Healing, 1250-1550*. Amsterdam, Amsterdam University Press 2020
DOI: 10.5117/9789463724517_CH04

> First of all, note that there are many and different problems of women's breasts, which mostly cause a decrease in milk, whether by excess, or by too much milk, or by coagulation, that is curdled milk, which cause the breast swelling and pain. In addition, hot apostemes and cold apostemes and nodes and glands and hardness and ulcers and corrosion and fistulae and excessive growth are formed in the breasts.
>
> – *Tractatus de passionibus mamillarum*, Venice, Biblioteca Nazionale Marciana, Latin VII 40, fol. 19r[1]

The *Tractatus de passionibus mamillarum* appears in two fifteenth-century manuscripts and addresses an unusual topic: care of the breast, especially the nursing breast.[2] It is largely extracted from the *Lilium medicine* of Bernard de Gordon (*c*.1270-1330), a practising physician who taught at the University of Montpellier. The *Tractatus* is an Italian adaptation of his work, interspersing some original material and the work of other writers.[3] In choosing particular paragraphs from Bernard's work, the anonymous translator avoided technical information related to the humors and medical philosophy. He also added brief, practical information from the work of other writers, such as Ibn Sīnā and Ibn Rushd.[4] The treatise, comprising four folios in total, contains twenty-seven recipes designed to be applied topically to the skin, but presents no remedies to be taken internally. As a result, the *Tractatus* appears to have been written for everyday practical use by readers who possessed little or no formal medical learning. The *Tractatus* does not fit neatly into the category of learned medicine, but neither is it a work of empirical or experiential writing. Rather, it is a hybrid: based on a

1 'Nota prima che molto sono li passione de li mamille e diversi li quali maxima mente sono diminutione de late. E tropo exuberantia overo tropo quantitate de late. e coagulatione i chagiamente de late. Dala quale coagulatione nase ala mamilla inflatione e dolore. Anchora naseno in ella mamilla apostema calda e apostema freda. E nodi e glandoli e dureza e ulceri e corossioni E fistula E tropo acresimento de le mamille'.

2 Venice, Biblioteca Nazionale Marciana, Latin VII 40 (BNM VII 40), is described in Valentinelli, *Bibliotheca manuscripta ad S. Marci Venetiarum*, 5: 92-94. The second manuscript of the *Tractatus* is Boston, Harvard University, Francis A. Countway Library of Medicine, Boston Medical Library MS 38 (BML 38).

3 Demaitre, *Doctor Bernard de Gordon*, 52-53. The *Lilium medicine* was translated into multiple languages, but there is no known Italian version, despite printed Latin versions disseminated from Venice in the late fifteenth century. This small section adapted from the *Lilium* is, as far as I am aware, the only Italian version that is extant; Demaitre, 'Bernard de Gordon', 106; pers. commun., Luke Demaitre, 2 December 2017.

4 For reasons addressed below, the author was likely male and will be referred to in this essay by the pronouns 'he/him/his'.

Latin medieval text, it contains interpolations and original material that make it an empirical work as well.

The *Tractatus* is significant not only because of its subject but also because of its late fifteenth-century date. Renaissance readers, increasingly literate in the vernacular, created a demand for literature about health and wellness. As Julia Gruman Martins' essay in this volume shows, vernacular translations responded to local circumstances and the needs of specific markets, thus altering medical knowledge in the process of disseminating it.[5] At the same time, the fifteenth century was a turning point when male university-trained physicians absorbed women's health within their purview. Many authors turned their attention to women's bodies out of concern for fertility and dynastic purity, taking as their sources traditional learned Greek and Arab authors of previous generations. After the publication in 1513 of Eucharius Rösselin the Elder's *Rosengarten*, 'the first Early Modern midwifery manual', male-authored handbooks on women's health and fertility as well as works about health and diet regimens began to proliferate in the ensuing centuries.[6] These works claimed authority over knowledge about women's health. Writers such as Michele Savonarola (d. 1469) cautioned their female readers to rely on male physicians rather than ignorant midwives.[7] Male writers also addressed household affairs and family concerns in great detail and in increasing numbers.[8]

The *Tractatus* is thus representative of an escalating male medical interest in domestic affairs that would affect progeny, such as the wellbeing and supply of wet nurses. It was written at the inception of these major changes to vernacular discourses surrounding the family, marriage, and women's healthcare. More specifically, it reflects the increasing medicalization of the breast as a site of care for ensuring maternal and infant health and the delicate balance of the fluid humoral economy, a matter taken up elsewhere in this volume by Montserrat Cabré and Fernando Salmón.[9] To draw out the significance and context of the *Tractatus*, it is necessary to discuss the history of the care of the breast in medical literature, then the content of the treatise itself as an artefact of both learned and empirical medical writing.

5 Martins, 'Understanding/Controlling the Female Body'.

6 Whaley, *Women and the Practice of Medical Care*, 93-97, quote at 95; Cavallo and Storey, *Healthy Living*, 13-24.

7 Green, *Making Women's Medicine Masculine*, 25-26, 246-47. See also the materials cited in Sheridan, 'Whither Childbearing', 239-42.

8 See, for example, Barbaro, *Wealth of Wives*; Cavallo and Storey, *Healthy Living*, 13-15.

9 Cabré and Salmón, 'Blood, Milk, and Breastbleeding'.

The Breast in Earlier Medical Literature

The early writers of the Hippocratic corpus and the Greco-Roman period sometimes addressed the care of nursing women and provided remedies for breast diseases. The Hippocratic treatise, *On the Nature of the Child*, explained that when a woman became pregnant, the weight of the growing uterus pressed liquid out of the food in her stomach, which made its way through the flesh to her breasts to be concocted into breast milk.[10] Later, Galen argued in *On the Usefulness of the Parts of the Body* that the breasts and uterus were connected by vessels that carried menstrual blood from the uterus to the breasts.[11] The late first- or early second-century CE Greek writer Soranus of Ephesus went further than previous authors by writing a treatise on gynecology that addressed the choice and care of a wet nurse and the care of the nursing woman.[12] This text made its way into Latin via the work of Caelius Aurelianus in the fifth century CE and the work of Muscio in the sixth, and both authors included midwives among their intended audiences. Encyclopedists of late antiquity writing in Greek, such as Paul of Aegina and Oribasius, also borrowed material from Soranus, Hippocrates, Galen, and Dioscorides and included their remedies for breast complaints. These remedies made their way into Arabic treatises such as Ibn al-Jazzār's (895-979) *Zād al-musāfir wa-qūt al-hādir* (Provisions for the traveller and nourishment for the settled), which influenced many of the Salernitan writers on women's health. Treatment of breast complaints also made up the twelfth fen of the third book of Avicenna's *Canon of Medicine*, which exerted considerable influence over European writers of the high Middle Ages.[13] Among the Salernitans, however, only John of St. Paul included information on breast care or breast diseases.[14]

The emergence of the medical community at Montpellier in the thirteenth and fourteenth centuries provided more opportunities for medical writers to address the care of the breast, but in general, these writers concentrated more on interventions for serious problems than on remedies for nursing mothers. Montpellier writers on surgery such as Henri de Mondeville (1260-1316) and Guy de Chauliac (1300-1368) included various therapies for breast diseases such as apostemes and very brief mentions of other breast problems.[15] Similarly,

10 Lonie, *Hippocratic Treatises*, 13.

11 On this topic see Tuten, 'Lactation and Breast Diseases in Antiquity', 165-66.

12 Soranus of Ephesus, *Maladies des femmes*.

13 Siraisi, *Avicenna in Renaissance Italy*, 19-40.

14 Green, *Making Women's Medicine Masculine*, 40-41.

15 Henri de Mondeville, *La chirurgie*, ed. Pagel, tract. 3, doct. 2, cap. 18, 496-97; Guy de Chauliac, *Inventarium sive Chirurgia magna*, tract. II, doct. 2, cap. 5, 121-22.

writers on anatomy described the breast as part of their sections on the chest, but these descriptions were often very brief, and writers of medical compendia such as Gilbertus Anglicus (1180-1250) concentrated primarily on cancer when they discussed the breasts.[16] In illustrated texts, diagrams of the female anatomy focused on the uterus and its fetal contents, depicting women's breasts without commentary or concern.[17] Bernard de Gordon's section on the breast was the most complete discussion of breastfeeding from this period.

The low priority given to nursing breasts in texts by a majority of learned authors could suggest a number of different possibilities. Perhaps the breasts, located on the body's surface, and generally subject to few pathological conditions of interest to learned physicians, were simply not a priority for writers who were increasingly curious about the 'secret parts' of women, the vagina and uterus. As Katharine Park notes, 'The precarious nature of fatherhood, and thus of the family itself, centred on the uterus, the dark, inaccessible place where the child's tie with its father was created, its sex determined, and its body shaped'.[18] Fertility was a highly charged social issue, affecting family lines, inheritance, familial identity, and sexual mores. By contrast, nursing was so naturalized as a female activity and so closely associated with infant care that most learned writers left the care of the breast to women, rather than diverting their attention away from the all-important concern of fertility. Most likely, breastfeeding knowledge passed from woman to woman and is mostly lost to us. It is possible that Bernard de Gordon, in compiling remedies for the *Lilium medicine*, picked up some of the empirical knowledge and practical remedies that were shared in personal exchanges. Since both Bernard de Gordon and the writer of the *Tractatus* found such remedies sufficiently important to transmit, they present a rare opportunity to examine remedies that were likely to have been used by nursing mothers.

Manuscripts

Two manuscripts contain the only surviving exemplars of the *Tractatus de passionibus mamillarum*: one is conserved in Venice, the other in Boston.

16 Gilbertus [Anglicus], *Compendium medicinae*, fols. cciii, cccxxxi. On cancer in the medieval context see Demaitre, 'Medieval Notions of Cancer'.

17 Green, 'Bodily Essences', 159.

18 Park, *Secrets of Women*, 25. See also Pouchelle, *Body and Surgery in the Middle Ages*, 133-39; Green, 'From "Diseases of Women" to "Secrets of Women"'.

Manuscript Latin VII 40 of the Biblioteca Nazionale Marciana, in Venice, is a medical miscellany of 116 folios bearing the owner's name, Ianellus of Martinengo, suggesting that it originates at least in part in Lombardy. This manuscript also bears the date 1466.[19] The manuscript is a true miscellany in that it contains both complete copied works and variable content that must have been added over time.[20] Following eighteen folios of assorted recipes in Latin, the *Tractatus* is the first complete work in the codex (fols. 19r-21r), and it is trailed by five more folios of recipes. A variety of texts follow the recipes, including a verse titled 'Signs of death', along with selections from the work of Arnau of Villanova (*c.*1240-1311) assembled under the title, 'Liber brevis tractatus'.[21] This patchwork of excerpts is followed by a series of passages from other writers, including brief references to Galen and Hippocrates. Seventeen more folios of recipes ensue, capped by a boldly handwritten index. The last work in the miscellany, placed after the index, is the *De quinta essentia* of John of Rupescissa (*c.*1310-1370), an alchemist and eschatological prophet who believed that the human body could be cured of diseases through the use of alchemy.[22] This work is carefully inscribed and is separated from the rest of the miscellany by a series of blank folios.

In contrast, Boston Medical Library 38 is a miscellany consisting of 106 folios. A remedy for 'la lepra novella' (possibly syphilis) on one folio probably dates it after 1495.[23] It is written on carefully ruled pages, with rubricated initials and headings, in a uniform hand, and appears to have been copied all at one time. The work begins with John of Rupescissa's *De quinta essentia*, an inclusion that attests to the growing popularity of alchemical practices across Europe *c.*1500.[24] It is followed by a short treatise on surgery in Latin, the bulk of which derives from Constantine the African's version of Alī ibn al-'Abbās al-Majusi's (Haly Abbas's) *Pantegni*.[25] The *Tractatus*, here titled the *Tractatus pulcherrimus de passionibus mamillarum*, begins on folio 76r with an incipit, and continues in Italian until it switches into a series of recipes, first in Italian, then in Latin, on folio 79v. The part of the manuscript that follows the *Tractatus* has some missing leaves, as the Latin and Italian recipe section breaks off unexpectedly. It continues with a work called

19 BNM VII 40, fol. 100r.

20 See Eckhardt and Starza Smith, 'Emergence of the English Miscellany', 1-3.

21 The 'Signs of death' text bears a close resemblance to the one printed in De Renzi, ed., *Collectio salernitana*, 5: 62.

22 DeVun, *Prophecy, Alchemy, and the End of Time*, 60-62.

23 BML 38, fol. 103v. On syphilis see Quétal, *History of Syphilis*, 11-12.

24 Principe, *Secrets of Alchemy*, 69-72.

25 Pagel, 'Eine bisher Unveröffentlichte Lateinische Version der Chirurgie der Pantegni'.

the *Virtutes septem herbarum*, attributed here to Alexander the Great.[26] An edition of Michael Scot's *Astrologia* follows, rendered loosely into Italian, and the manuscript ends with a set of instructions for administering phlebotomy.[27] The manuscript is very clean of marks, stains, and deletions, with the exception of a large stain on one of the folios.[28]

Although the two manuscripts are significantly different from one another, they are closely related in that both contain the *Tractatus de passionibus mamillarum* and Rupescissa's *De quinta essentia*. In both manuscripts, *De quinta essentia* is attributed not to John of Rupescissa but to the Catalan philosopher Raymond Llull (*c.*1232-1315).[29] The language of the *Tractatus* in the two manuscripts is significantly different, but the structure and contents are identical. However, the differences are significant enough to argue that they are both copies of another lost exemplar, one that most likely contained both *De quinta essentia* and the *Tractatus*.

Content of the *Tractatus*

The *Tractatus* inherited much of its content and structure from Bernard de Gordon's *Lilium medicine*. Bernard's chapters described body parts and their diseases by following a pattern: a definition of the part in question, and the names and types of the diseases of that part, followed by a description of the anatomy of the affected organ.[30] His chapter on the breast begins by describing problems arising from either too little or too much milk. He then goes on to explain that the conditions of the breast were dependent on the amount of blood in the body, which could be affected by diet, exercise, and phlebotomy when necessary.[31] The author of the *Tractatus*, however, adapted only part of this section: he translated only the opening list of conditions more or less verbatim from Bernard, and echoed his promise to treat the subject briefly.[32] Bernard's lengthy definitions of good and bad

26 On the *Virtutes septem herbarum secundum Alexandrum Imperatorem*, see Thorndike, 'Latin Pseudo-Aristotle', 241-42.

27 Wilson, 'Catalogue', 150-57.

28 BML 38, fols. 63v-64r.

29 BNM VII 40, fol. 100r; BML 38, fol. 1r. Many works of alchemy were attributed to Llull in the fifteenth century, including a version of *De quinta essentia*; Principe, *Secrets of Alchemy*, 71-72.

30 Demaitre, *Doctor Bernard de Gordon*, 55-56.

31 Bernard de Gordon, *Lilium medicine*, in Munich, Bayerische StaatsBibliothek, MS Clm 13019, fol. 67v.

32 BNM VII 40, fol. 19r; BML 38, fol. 76r.

blood and their effect on milk were left out. So were all his references to phlebotomy, which was never recommended in the *Tractatus*.

In the *Lilium medicine*, Bernard explained that both hot and cold causes could lead to an over-abundance of milk, which caused both swelling and curdling in the breasts. He advised his reader to remember that, 'Everything which reduces seed reduces milk.'[33] The author of the *Tractatus* chose to omit Bernard's philosophical statements in favour of a very straightforward list of problems, with these headings: 'Against the clotting of milk from a hot cause' and 'from a cold cause'.[34] Similarly, Bernard's next section, which covered medications to suppress milk altogether, was largely omitted, which suggests that suppressing milk was not a topic of interest for the author of the *Tractatus*.[35] It is likely that the author of the *Tractatus* was part of an upper-class household that employed wet nurses for the children of the house, so he may not have thought that suppressing milk was worth discussing. Instead, the author concentrated on the problems of the breast that resulted from nursing. For example, he opted to copy a brief set of instructions on how to distinguish distension in the breast from an aposteme or abscess: 'in this case, the coagulation of milk can be discerned from an aposteme, because the swelling [of a coagulation] covers the whole breast, and causes it to be glossy [from distension], while an aposteme is primarily in one part'.[36] Medical writers in the Middle Ages attributed breast engorgement to milk 'curdling' or 'becoming cheese', which was likely a reflection of their experience observing animal milk in their everyday lives.[37]

The remedies that the author of the *Tractatus* adapted from Bernard were all external applications such as plasters and unguents placed on the breasts. For example, in the section on remedies for milk curdling in the breast from a hot cause, the *Tractatus* prescribed the following recipe translated from Bernard: 'Take equal parts cabbage juice, blackberry juice, purslane

33 *Lilium medicine*, fol. 67v: 'Omnia igitur que parvificant semen et parvificant lac'.

34 BNM VII 40, fol. 19r-v; BML 38 fol. 76r-v: 'Contra caseatione lactis a causa calida'; 'Contra caseatione lactis a causa frigida'.

35 Fildes, *Breasts, Bottles and Babies*, 47. Bernard himself had argued that women should breastfeed their own children, which was not the practice among upper-class Italian urban households.

36 BNM VII 40, fol. 19r: 'Anchora sapia che la caseatione delo late in dele mamille e molto differente dala apostema dele mamille. e se cognosce in questo modo zoe che lo tumore o vero inflatione fato per late caseato sie equal mente per tuta la mamilla, cum alchuna luciditate. E la apostema e sola mente in alchuna parte dela mamilla e non in tuta la mamilla'.

37 Tuten, 'Lactation and Breast Diseases in Antiquity', 170. The idea originally comes from Soranus.

juice, rose oil, and white vinegar, and mix them with enough barley flour to make a plaster. And the plaster will be more effective if you add a little bit of ground myrrh and saffron, because these are warm substances and they will better penetrate the cold ones. And this plaster should be placed on the breast when warm.'[38] In the next section, on cold causes for milk curdling, the author included 'the following liniment that can resolve the curdling of milk from either cause, hot or cold, supposing a good health regimen. Take vinegar, white wine and cool water, and boil them together for a little while.' The resulting mixture could be dropped on the breasts when still warm. 'This recipe you have from master Bernard de Gordon in his chapter "On the abundance of milk".'[39] These recipes, which used common household ingredients, followed the normal humoral practice of warming 'cold' conditions and cooling 'hot' conditions, although the plasters recommended in the *Tractatus* were always applied warm.

In general, the author of the *Tractatus* translated the recipes taken from Bernard simply and literally. The author of the Boston manuscript, however, sometimes added experiential information to Bernard's recipes. For example, in a recipe in which Bernard called for 'a small quantity of sandalwood', the author added the recommendation to use 3 drams.[40] He also elaborated on a recipe for a plaster by including the practical advice that 'this kind of poultice needs to be placed directly on the breasts and bound [with a bandage] as best you can, but not too tightly'.[41] In a recipe for the healing of fistulas, the author of the Boston manuscript added the comment, 'This is a remedy made for the fistulas of the breasts that often happen to women, especially when they give birth the first time, and it's

38 BNM VII 40, fol. 19r-v, 'Adoncha sela caseatione delo late fera per tropo caliditade poede cum questi remedii. zoe prima fa questo emplastro. Tole suce de verze. Suco de morela, Suco de porcelaga, olio rosato, Aceto biancho, e de tuti igual mente e meseda cum quelli tanta farina dorzo quanta basta afare lo emplastro. Et piu vertuoso sera lo dito emplastro se secho in corpararay alchuna pocheta quantitade de mirra pesta e de sofrano pesto. per che questi cosi caldi farano lialti cosi fredi melio penetrare. Et questo tale emplastro se de metere caldo actual mente in sula mamilla'.

39 Ibid., fol. 19v, 'Preterea sapia che questa embrocatione vale a resolvere la caseatione delo late in dele mamille fata da qualunque casone o vero calda o vera freda che la sia e mitigal lo dolore elo tumore, supposito che sia lo bono rezimento dela vita. zoe. Tole aceto, vino biancho, e aqua frescha, e fali bolire in pocho in sema e possa li dite cose temperata mente caldi fali cazere in sula mamilla in pocho da alto. Et questo remedio tu lay da m bernardo de gordonio in delo capitolo delatropo habundantia delo late'.

40 BML 38, fol. 78r.

41 Ibid., fol. 76v: 'E questo tal impiastro se die metere caldo actualmente sopra la mamilla e ligare a melio che poy che non sia tropo streta la ligatam'.

a very beautiful secret.[42] These adjustments made the recipes clearer and easier to administer, suggesting that the author had used or seen these recipes or perhaps even experimented with them. It is curious that these interpolations occur in the manuscript that bears the least physical evidence of having been used; it provides evidence that the Boston manuscript was a copy of a different version than the Venice manuscript. The suggestions also make clear that the *Tractatus* was practical and intended to make the work of Bernard accessible to a wider audience.

After the section on clotting milk, the contents of the *Tractatus* mirrored Bernard's chapter, with more sections translated verbatim. After clotting were remedies for apostemes, and then what he describes as 'nodes and glands and hard places', and then corrosion, ulcers, and fistulas – a broad listing of all the problems that could arise in a woman's breast.[43] Excerpting directly from the *Lilium medicine* then ended, but the treatise's list of recipes did not.[44] The *Tractatus* had no clear terminus in either manuscript; it was followed in both by a remedy for an ulcerated wound and one against worms in children. Each manuscript then devolved into a different series of recipes for a wide array of complaints, including postpartum bleeding, intestinal worms, and insomnia. The scribe of BML 38 liked to end his completed texts with the pious remark, 'Laus Deo', but in the *Tractatus*, this expression is absent. The treatise merely trailed off.[45]

Although the *Tractatus* was based principally on the work of Bernard de Gordon, he was not the only author cited. Dispersed among the adaptions from the *Lilium medicine*, the author included one brief section conveying bits of advice and recipes from other canonical authors:

> Serapion says that the juice of the dwarf elder does not allow the milk to clot in the breast. Almansor says that the best remedy for the pain of the breast with swelling is a fresh egg yolk applied to the breast with greasy wool. Avicenna says that earthworms ground up with myrrh and a decoction of calamint and raw anise act against the obstruction of milk in the breasts, making it flow easily and not letting it curdle.[46]

42 Ibid., fol. 79v: 'E questo he remedio fato contra le fistole de le mamille che spesso acade a le done maxime quando perturisseno la prima fiata, et he secreto bellissimo'.

43 *Lilium medicine*, fols. 67v-68v: 'et nodi et glandule et duricies et ulcera, et corrosio et fistula et nimia mamillarum augmenacio [...]'.

44 BNM VII 40, fol. 22r; BML 38, fol. 79v.

45 For example, BML 38, fols. 44v, 101v.

46 BNM VII 40, fols. 19v-20r: 'Serapione dise che lo suco deli ebuli non lasa acagiare lo late in deli mamille: E Almansore dise che alo dolore deli mamille cum inflatione lo rosolo delo ouo

Here, the author of the *Tractatus* refers to three works widely known in fifteenth-century Latin translations: *On simples* by Serapion the Younger (*fl.* thirteenth century), a medicinal botany book written in the twelfth or thirteenth century; the *Book for Almansor* by Muhammad ibn Zakariyah al-Razi (854-925), known as Rhazes in Latin; and the *Canon of Medicine* of Ibn Sīnā (980-1037), known as Avicenna. Latin versions of all three works by these medical authorities were printed in Italy in the fifteenth and early sixteenth centuries.[47] The attributions, however, are questionable.[48] I have been unable to find any references to the use of an egg yolk on wool in the *Book for Almansor*; nor does Ibn Sīnā's *Canon* mention the use of earthworms for breast problems, although they are prescribed for other conditions.[49] There is a brief recipe credited to the breast-aposteme section of Guglielmo da Saliceto's *Practica*, but the *Practica* contains a similar recipe only in the section devoted to the armpits.[50] These discrepancies raise the question of where the author of the *Tractatus* obtained his information. It is likely that these attributions resulted from uncritical copying from another source that was at least one level removed from the original works. The inclusion of these names, however, indicates the importance that the author attributed to earlier Arabic authorities and his attempt to integrate his own translation into the discourse of learned medicine fashionable in the fifteenth century. The inclusion of these authors probably indicates a desire to cite their writings, even incorrectly, as a way of increasing the authority of the *Tractatus*.[51]

In addition to the recipes borrowed from the *Lilium medicine*, the *Tractatus* also contains one original recipe (Figure 4.1 and Table 4.1). This recipe differs from the material adapted from Bernard de Gordon in several

frescho meso sula mamilla cum lana susia e ultimo remedio. Et Avicena dise che li lumbrici terestri cum mirra e decoctione de calamento ede anesi crudi vale ala opilatione delo late in dela mamilla e falo molto ben covere e non lo lassa acogiare'.

47 See Siraisi, *Avicenna in Renaissance Italy*, 64, 178, n. 8.

48 Serapion's work, for example, did advise that dwarf elder was good for correcting milk coagulation, but in the stomach rather than in the breast; when he discussed treating the coagulation of milk in the nursing breast, he recommended that human sweat be mixed with rosemary oil and used as an ointment; Serapion the Younger, *De simplicibus medicinis opus*, ch. 274, 'De ebulo et sambuco', 183; ch. 456, 'De sudore', 107 (see Averroes, *In hoc volumine*).

49 Avicenna, *Canon of Medicine* (*Al-Qanun fi'l-Tibb*), vol. 2, bk. 3, fen 12, 1166-68. Sigerist, 'Mediaeval Medical Texts', 106, cites an example of earthworms used in breast remedies; the recipe is found in Vendôme, Bibliothèque municipale 175, fol. 101r.

50 BNM VII 40, fol. 21r: 'Et questo emplastro scive M. Guelmo placentino in dela sua praticha in delo capitulo deli apostemi deli mamille'. See Guglielmo da Saliceto, *Chirurgie de Guillaume de Salicet*, 86.

51 Green, *Making Women's Medicine Masculine*, 246-47.

Figure 4.1 An original recipe from the *Tractatus de passionibus mamillarum*

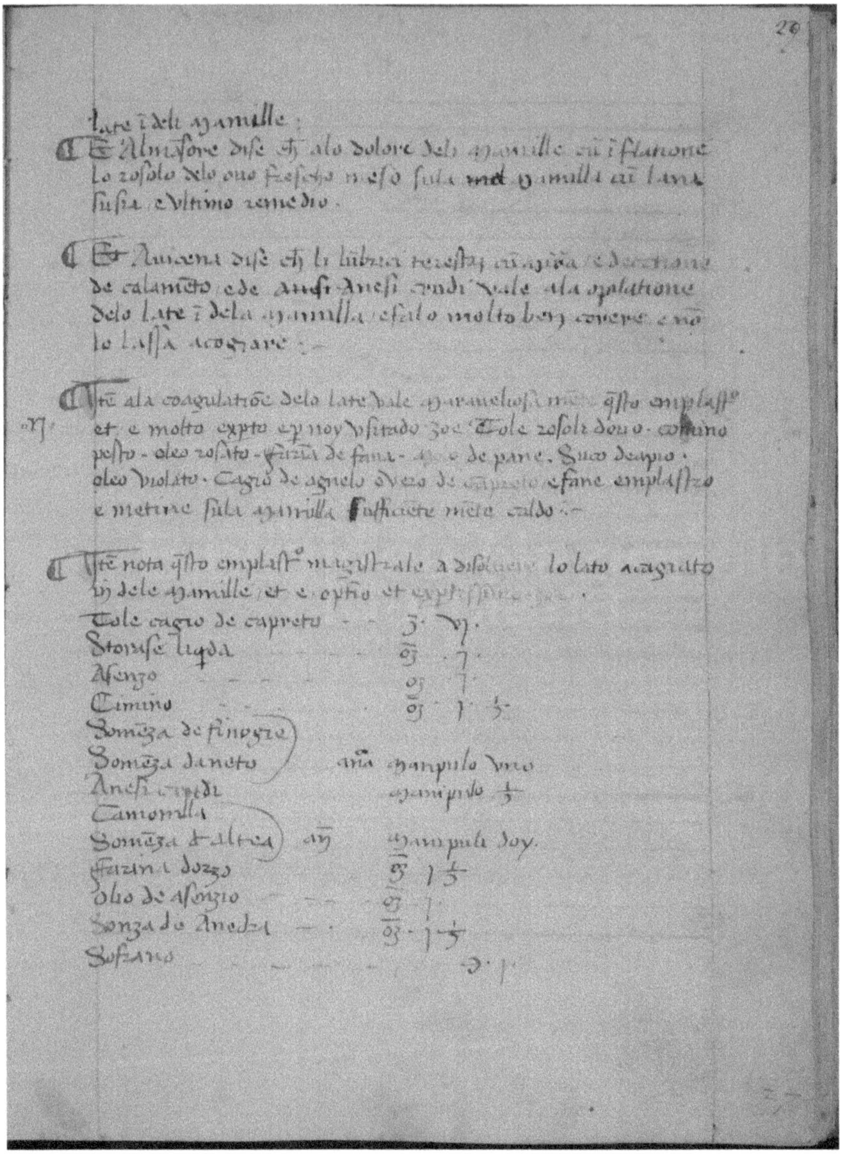

Venice, Biblioteca Nationale Marciana, MS Latin VII 40, fol. 20r. Used by permission.

Table 4.1 Transcription of an original recipe from the *Tractatus de passionibus mamillarum*

Item nota questo emplastro magist[er]iale a disolvere lo lato acagiato in dele mamille et e optimo et expertissimo. zoe	
Tole cagio de capreto - - -	ʒ vi
Storase liquida- - - -	oz̄1
Asenzo - - - -	oz 1
Cimino - - - -	oz̄1 1/ↄ
Somenza de finogre	an̄a manipulo uno
Somenza daneto	
Anesi crudi	manipulo 1/ↄ
Camomilla	
Somenza d altea	oz̄ manipuli doy
Farina dorzo - - -	oz̄ 1 1/ↄ
Olio de asenzio - - -	oz̄1
Sonza de anedra - - -	oz̄1 1/ↄ
Sofrano	э 1.
Vino biancho quanto basta e fane emplastro e azonze in pocholin di aceto e possa metere suli mamille tempera mente caldo.	
Item, note this masterful plaster that dissolves curdled milk in the breast and it is the best and the most proven, this way:	
Take kid rennet - - -	6 drams
Liquid storax resin- - - -	1 ounce
Wormwood - - - -	1 ounce
Cumin - - - -	1.5 ounce
Fenugreek seed	one handful each
Dill seed	
Raw anise	½ handful
Chamomile	
Marshmallow seed	two handfuls each
Rice flour - - -	1.5 ounce
Oil of wormwood - - -	1 ounce
Duck fat - - -	1.5 ounce
Saffron	1 scruple
White wine, as much as you like, and make a plaster and add a small amount of vinegar and you can place it on the breast at a warm temperature.	

Following Venice, Biblioteca Nazionale Marciana, MS Latin VII 40, fol. 20r-v.

ways. The formatting, for example, is different for this recipe in the Venice manuscript (though not in the Boston manuscript). In general, in both manuscripts Bernard's recipes were copied in paragraph format, just as they appeared in Bernard's work. The original recipe in the Venice manuscript, however, was written out in columns with the amount of each ingredient clearly labelled. This choice may suggest that the recipe was copied from a source that used the different format, and possibly even that it was put into practice.[52] This recipe also included comments that argued for its superiority based on empirical testing: 'In addition, note this masterful plaster for dissolving curdled milk in the breast; it is the best and most proven'.[53] The recipe calls for storax resin, kid rennet, and duck fat, in addition to a large selection of herbs, seeds, and flours. Although these ingredients were commonplace, the use of animal sources distinguished this recipe from those prescribed by Bernard, who utilized only plant oils (usually violet, sesame, or rose) or wine as the liquid binder for his plasters, rather than animal fats.

Although the ingredients listed in the original recipe were slightly different from those found in Bernard's recipes, they still bore a strong connection to learned humoral theory. All of the ingredients listed in the original recipe were discussed in Avicenna's *Canon*, where he identified them according to hot and dry qualities (with the exception of barley flour, which was used as a base and binder for the plaster). These ingredients included wormwood, cumin, fenugreek, dill, anise and saffron, among others.[54] Plasters made with bean or barley flour date back to the Hippocratic authors and to Dioscorides.[55] Particularly representative of such recipes is fenugreek, which still enjoys a reputation as a galactagogue among some nursing mothers today.[56] These commonalities suggest that, although the author was possibly transmitting an original recipe, the recipe still adhered to basic humoral theory.

Although it is not possible to know for certain, the author of the treatise probably was male. Scholars have established that, although female literacy was rising in the fifteenth century, women were less likely to command the facility in Latin required to translate Bernard de Gordon, since they could

52 The two recipes that end the *Tractatus* in the Venice manuscript also use this format.

53 BNM VII 40, fol. 20r: 'Item note questo emplastro magistrale a disolvere lo lato acagiato in dele mamille et e optimo e expertissimo'.

54 Avicenna, *Canon of Medicine* (*Al-Qanun Fi'l-Tibb*), vol. 2, *passim*.

55 Dioscorides, *De materia medica*, 130, 136.

56 Sim et al., 'Use, Perceived Effectiveness and Safety of Herbal Galactagogues'; Dioscorides, *De materia medica*, 134.

not access the kinds of institutions where Latin was taught.[57] Searching for learned medical advice for use by an upper-class household, the writer may have been prompted to select Bernard de Gordon's instructions from the *Lilium medicine* because the section on the breast had the advantage of both brevity and practicality. Although affluent fifteenth-century Italian households showed great familiarity with vernacular medical texts, as Sheila Barker and Sharon Strocchia observe elsewhere in this volume, few works concentrated on the care of the breast; hence there was not a wide selection from which to choose.[58]

The audience for the *Tractatus* is likely to have been composed of women living in well-off urban or courtly households, possibly in extended households where more than one woman was lactating or nursing children at the same time. Certainly by the seventeenth century, noble Roman households maintained a staff of wet nurses when several children needed suckling.[59] If the target audience for this manuscript consisted primarily of female caregivers, it is worth considering how the *Tractatus* might have bridged the perceived divide between learned and experiential medicine. Mary Fissell has argued that studying the history of women in healthcare problematizes, and sometimes even eradicates, this difference: if our questions start 'at the bedside of the sufferer, attending to the physical labour entailed in the care of the sick', it is easy to imagine the recipes in the *Tractatus* being tested and prepared by women and then that knowledge subsequently circulated within familiar circles.[60] Both their ease of preparation and the ready availability of everyday ingredients argue that the recipes in the *Tractatus* belonged to the world of household medicine, which provided the first resort for many conditions in the late medieval and Renaissance period.[61] Premodern households often developed their own internal regimens and narratives of health, which contributed to unique family and local histories. Montserrat Cabré has shown that, given the nature and *longue durée* of women's domestic work, the oral and written transmission of recipes resulted in long periods of relevance and use.[62] The hybrid nature of the *Tractatus*, which contains both empirical investigation and learned tradition, suggests a

57 Green, 'Gendering the History of Women's Healthcare', 495.

58 Barker and Strocchia, 'Household Medicine for a Renaissance Court'.

59 Castiglione, 'Peasants at the Palace'.

60 Fissell, 'Introduction', 10-11.

61 Strocchia, 'Introduction', 498-500.

62 Cabré, 'Women or Healers?', 23-24, argues that 'women's health actions form a continuum that runs from the ordinary to the occupational, from gratuitous therapeutic attention to paid acts of health care'.

particular relevance in this kind of familial environment, where women's caregiving, cooking, and learning converged.

Understood in this way, the *Tractatus de passionibus mamillarum* provides a window into the healthcare of nursing women associated with upper-class fifteenth-century Italian households. It is of interest both for its subject matter – the female breast, an under-represented topic in the medical writing of the period – and for its practical, straightforward approach to breast problems. Both as a written work and as a physical artefact, it is a hybrid of learned Latin medicine and empirical testing; its multiple copies suggest a passing of knowledge from one household to another. As such, it blurs the lines dividing learned and experiential medicine.

Works Cited

Manuscripts

Boston, Francis A. Countway Medical Library of Harvard Medical School, Boston Medical Library MS 38.

Munich, Bayerische StaatsBibliothek, MS Clm 13019.

Venice, Biblioteca Nazionale Marciana, MS Latin VII 40.

Printed Works

Averroes [Ibn Rushd] et al. *In hoc volumine continentur insignium medicorum Ioan. Serapionis Arabis De simplicibus medicinis opus praeclarum & ingens, Averrois Arabis, De eisdem liber eximius, Rasis filii Zachariae, de eisdem opusculum perutile, incerti item autoris de centaureo libellus hactenus Galeno inscriptus, dictionum arabicarvm iuxta atq[ue] latinarum index valde necessarius, in quorum emendata excusione, ne quid omnino disyderaretur Othonis Brunfelsii singulari fide & diligentia cautum est* (Argentorati [Strasbourg]: Georgius Ulricher, 1531).

Avicenna [Ibn Sīnā]. *The Canon of Medicine (Al-Qanun Fi'l-Tibb)*, ed. Laleh Shah Bakhtiar and Jay R. Crook, trans. O.C. Gruner and Mazhar H. Shah, vol. 2: *Natural Pharmaceuticals* (Chicago: Great Books of the Islamic World/ KAZI Publications, 2012).

Barbaro, Francesco. *The Wealth of Wives: A Fifteenth-Century Marriage Manual*, ed. and trans. Margaret L. King (Tempe, AZ: Arizona Center for Medieval and Renaissance Studies, 2015).

Barker, Sheila and Sharon Strocchia. 'Household Medicine for a Renaissance Court: Caterina Sforza's *Ricettario* Reconsidered', in *Gender, Health, and Healing,*

1250-1550, ed. Sara Ritchey and Sharon Strocchia (Amsterdam: Amsterdam University Press, 2020), 139-65.

Cabré, Montserrat. 'Women or Healers? Household Practices and the Categories of Health Care in Late Medieval Iberia', *Bulletin of the History of Medicine*, 82 (2008), 18-51.

Cabré, Montserrat and Fernando Salmón. 'Blood, Milk, and Breastbleeding: The Humoral Economy of Women's Bodies in Late Medieval Medicine', in *Gender, Health, and Healing, 1250-1550*, ed. Sara Ritchey and Sharon Strocchia (Amsterdam: Amsterdam University Press, 2020), 93-117.

Castiglione, Caroline. 'Peasants at the Palace: Wet Nurses and Aristocratic Mothers in Early Modern Rome', in *Medieval and Renaissance Lactations*, ed. Jutta Gisela Sperling (Aldershot: Ashgate, 2013), 79-99.

Cavallo, Sandra and Tessa Storey. *Healthy Living in Late Renaissance Italy* (Oxford: Oxford University Press, 2013).

Demaitre, Luke E. 'Bernard de Gordon et son influence sur la pensée médicale aux XIVe et XVe siècles', in *L'Université de médicine de Montpellier et son rayonnement (XIIIe-XVe siècles)*, ed. Daniel Le Blévec (Turnhout: Brepols, 2004), 103-31.

—. *Doctor Bernard de Gordon, Professor and Practitioner* (Toronto: Pontifical Institute of Mediaeval Studies, 1980).

—. 'Medieval Notions of Cancer: Malignancy and Metaphor', *Bulletin of the History of Medicine*, 72 (1998), 609-37.

De Renzi, Salvatore, ed. *Collectio Salernitana: ossia documenti inediti, e trattati di medicina appartenenti alla scuola medica*, 5 vols. (Naples: Dalla tipografia del Filiatre-Sebezio, 1852).

DeVun, Leah. *Prophecy, Alchemy, and the End of Time: John of Rupescissa in the Late Middle Ages* (New York: Columbia University Press, 2009).

Dioscorides. *De materia medica*, trans. Lily Y. Beck (Hildesheim: Olms/Weidmann, 2005).

Eckhardt, Joshua and Daniel Starza Smith. 'Introduction: The Emergence of the English Miscellany', in *Manuscript Miscellanies in Early Modern England*, ed. Joshua Eckhardt and Daniel Starza Smith (Aldershot: Ashgate, 2014), 1-16.

Fildes, Valerie A. *Breasts, Bottles and Babies: A History of Infant Feeding* (Edinburgh: Edinburgh University Press, 1986).

Fissell, Mary E. 'Introduction: Women, Health, and Healing in Early Modern Europe', *Bulletin of the History of Medicine*, 82.1 (2008), 1-17.

Gilbertus [Anglicus]. *Compendium medicinae* (Lyon: n.p., 1510).

Green, Monica. 'Bodily Essences: Bodies as Categories of Difference', in *A Cultural History of the Human Body in the Middle Ages*, ed. Linda Kalof (Oxford: Berg, 2010), 149-72.

—. '"Cliff Notes" on the Circulation of the Gynecological Texts of Soranus and Muscio in the Middle Ages (2017)', www.academia.edu/7858536/Monica_H._Green_Cliff_Notes_on_the_Circulation_of_the

—. 'From "Diseases of Women" to "Secrets of Women": The Transformation of Gynecological Literature in the Later Middle Ages', *Journal of Medieval and Early Modern Studies*, 30.1 (2000), 5-40.

—. 'Gendering the History of Women's Healthcare', *Gender & History*, 20.3 (2008), 487-518.

—. *Making Women's Medicine Masculine: The Rise of Male Authority in Pre-modern Gynaecology* (Oxford: Oxford University Press, 2008).

Guglielmo da Saliceto. *Chirurgie de Guillaume de Salicet, achevée en 1275*, ed. Paul Pifteau (Toulouse: Saint-Cyprien, 1898).

Guy de Chauliac. *Inventarium sive Chirurgia magna*, ed. Michael R. McVaugh (Leiden: Brill, 1997).

Henri de Mondeville. *Die Chirurgie des Heinrich von Mondeville (Hermondaville) nach Berliner, Erfurter und Pariser Codices zum ersten Male*, ed. Julius Pagel (Berlin: Hirschwald, 1892).

Lonie, Iain M., ed. *The Hippocratic Treatises, "On Generation," "On the Nature of the Child," "Diseases IV": A Commentary*, Ars Medica 2 (Berlin: De Gruyter, 1981).

Martins, Julia Gruman. 'Understanding/Controlling the Female Body in Ten Recipes: Print and the Dissemination of Medical Knowledge about Women in the Early Sixteenth Century', in *Gender, Health, and Healing, 1250-1550*, ed. Sara Ritchey and Sharon Strocchia (Amsterdam: Amsterdam University Press, 2020), 167-88.

Pagel, Julius. 'Eine bisher unveröffentlichte lateinische Version der Chirurgie der Pantegni nach einer Handschrift der Königl. Bibliothek zu Berlin', *Archiv für klinische Chirurgie*, 81 (1906), 735-86.

Park, Katharine. *Secrets of Women: Gender, Generation, and the Origins of Human Dissection* (New York: Zone Books, 2006).

Pouchelle, Marie-Christine. *The Body and Surgery in the Middle Ages*, trans. Rosemary Morris (New Brunswick, NJ: Rutgers University Press, 1990).

Principe, Lawrence M. *The Secrets of Alchemy* (Chicago: University of Chicago Press, 2013).

Quétel, Claude. *History of Syphilis*, trans. Judith Braddock and Brian Pike (Baltimore: Johns Hopkins University Press, 1990).

Serapion the Younger. *De simplicibus medicinis opus*. See under Averroes [Ibn Rushd] et al.

Sheridan, Bridget. 'Whither Childbearing: Gender, Status, and the Professionalization of Medicine in Early Modern France', in *Gender and Scientific Discourse in Early Modern Culture*, ed. Kathleen P. Long (Aldershot: Ashgate, 2010), 239-58.

Sigerist, Henry E. 'Mediaeval Medical Texts in Manuscripts of Vendôme', *Bulletin of the History of Medicine*, 14 (1943), 68-113.

Sim, Tin Fei, H. Laetitia Hattingh, Jillian Sherriff, and Lisa B.G. Tee. 'The Use, Perceived Effectiveness and Safety of Herbal Galactagogues during Breastfeeding: A Qualitative Study', *International Journal of Environmental Research and Public Health*, 12.9 (September 2015), 11050-71.

Siraisi, Nancy G. *Avicenna in Renaissance Italy: The Canon and Medical Teaching in Italian Universities after 1500* (Princeton, NJ: Princeton University Press, 1987).

Soranus of Ephesus. *Maladies des femmes*, ed. Paul Burguière, Danielle Gourevitch, and Yves Malinas, 4 vols. (Paris: Les Belles Lettres, 1988).

Strocchia, Sharon T. 'Introduction: Women and Healthcare in Early Modern Europe', *Renaissance Studies*, 28.4 (2014), 496-514.

Thorndike, Lynn. 'The Latin Pseudo-Aristotle and Medieval Occult Science', *Journal of English and Germanic Philology*, 21 (1922), 229-58.

Tuten, Belle Stoddard. 'Lactation and Breast Diseases in Antiquity: Medical Authorities on Breast Health and Treatment', *Quaestiones Medii Aevi Novae*, 19 (2014), 159-86.

Valentinelli, Joseph, ed. *Bibliotheca manuscripta ad S. Marci Venetiarum*, 6 vols. (Venice: Ex Typographia Commercii, 1868-73).

Whaley, Leigh Ann. *Women and the Practice of Medical Care in Early Modern Europe, 1400-1800* (New York: Palgrave Macmillan, 2011).

Wilson, William Jerome. 'Catalogue of Latin and Vernacular Alchemical Manuscripts in the United States and Canada', *Osiris*, 6 (1939), 1-836.

About the Author

Belle S. Tuten is Charles A. Dana Professor of History at Juniata College in Huntingdon, Pennsylvania. Her work concentrates on views of the female breast in medieval medicine and culture.

5 Household Medicine for a Renaissance Court

Caterina Sforza's *Ricettario* Reconsidered

Sheila Barker and Sharon Strocchia

Abstract

Household recipe books were the most prevalent form of women's authoritative medical writing in Renaissance Europe. Among the most significant female-authored collections from fifteenth-century Italy was that of Caterina Sforza (1463-1509), Countess of Imola and Forlì. Two recently discovered manuscripts shed new light on her creative praxis and the practical knowledge she collected, developed, and tested. We argue that Caterina's vast miscellany of 'secrets' must be read intentionally within the context of a household economy writ large, simultaneously serving the health needs and political objectives of a Renaissance court. These discoveries highlight the authority of experiential knowledge within the domestic realm and beyond. Since the manuscripts were subjected to censorship, we interrogate the later reclassification of some of Caterina's authoritative knowledge as heterodox.

Keywords: recipe books, pharmacy, cosmetics, experimentation, magic, censorship

The study of household recipe books in late medieval and early modern Europe has sparked enormous interest in recent years. These troves of practical knowledge were the most common form of women's medical writing in Renaissance Europe, often providing the textual basis for female medical authority.[1] Recent studies have shown that recipe books played a

1 The literature on late medieval and early modern recipe books is extensive. Works pertinent to this discussion include Cabré, 'Women or Healers?'; Leong, 'Making Medicines'; Leong and Pennell, 'Recipe Collections'; Laroche, *Medical Authority*.

Ritchey, Sara & Sharon Strocchia (eds), *Gender, Health, and Healing, 1250-1550*. Amsterdam, Amsterdam University Press 2020
DOI: 10.5117/9789463724517_CH05

key role in the practice of household medicine, which remained the primary mode of caring for the sick until the nineteenth century.[2] Often organized in eclectic ways, recipe books offered valuable guides to healing as well as good household management. Bundled together in these compendia were a wide variety of recipes ranging from medicaments, cosmetics, and culinary secrets to instructions for making ordinary household products such as ink, soap, and stain remover.[3] The impressive range of activities encompassed by recipe collections testifies to the complex skills needed to govern an early modern household. In the sometimes idiosyncratic ways they curated their collections, female householders found opportunities to display both their prudence and intellectual interests.

As indicators of their authors' active pursuits, the recipe books compiled by women also testify to female engagement with early modern cultures of experimentation. It was not uncommon for affluent women to try out medical recipes in order to improve their smell, texture, taste, and shelf life, or to adapt them in line with available ingredients. Nor was it unusual for makers to test homemade remedies on themselves and family members to determine their efficacy, using informal procedures of their own making.[4] Recipe books thus provided a vital medium for recording, tracking, and annotating experiments in 'kitchen physic'. These texts register patterns of careful observation within a cognitive framework that, by the late fifteenth century, was increasingly oriented toward the empirical.[5] As Belle Tuten shows elsewhere in this volume, vernacular recipe collections also document how the intersection of learned and experiential medicine created hybridized forms of knowledge and care practices.[6] At the same time, recipes enjoyed a rich social life. The treasured recipes of expert practitioners circulated among far-flung correspondents as well as local communities of practice. In both cases the recipes functioned as a currency of exchange that could be put to use in making valued products such as ointments, electuaries, distillates, and perfumes, which in turn could be gifted as a mark of favour.[7]

2 Pelling, 'Thoroughly Resented?', argues for the fundamental importance of household healing in the early modern period. For recent bibliography, see Blumenthal, 'Domestic Medicine', and LeJacq, 'Bounds of Domestic Healing'.

3 The term 'secret' was used in several senses in early modern recipe books. Eamon provides a synthetic explanation in 'Appearance, Artifice, and Reality', 132-34, and a more expansive discussion in 'How to Read a Book of Secrets'.

4 Leong and Rankin, 'Testing Drugs and Trying Cures'.

5 Long, *Artisan/Practitioners*; Smith, *Body of the Artisan*.

6 Tuten, 'Care of the Breast'.

7 Rankin, *Panaceia's Daughters*; Leong and Pennell, 'Recipe Collections', 133-34.

Given that early modern recipe books encompassed such a broad swath of practical knowledge, it is not surprising that they were handed down from generation to generation as family heirlooms.[8] Recipe books could be included in the dowries of Italian artisans' daughters, for instance, since they frequently contained valuable trade secrets.[9] Similarly, noble brides who entered into dynastic marriages transported familial recipe collections in their trousseaux; in so doing, they facilitated the circulation of medical knowledge and practices across political and linguistic boundaries.[10] The recipe archives of English gentlewomen – perhaps the most avid of all early modern collectors – track their complex involvement in Atlantic knowledge exchange as well as the importation of new drugs from the Americas.[11] As these texts moved between generations and across cultural spaces, they acquired new layers in the form of additional recipes and practical tips inserted by current users. Some early modern recipe books were customized by the addition of paratextual aids like indices and marginal notations. Still others bridged the gap between manuscript and print by incorporating handwritten extracts copied from published works.[12]

One of the best-known and most significant female-authored recipe books produced in Renaissance Italy was compiled by Caterina Sforza (1463-1509), the Countess of Imola and Forlì in Italy's strategic Romagna region. The natural daughter of the Milanese duke Galeazzo Maria Sforza and his mistress Lucrezia Landriani, Caterina was groomed for court life despite her illegitimacy. Her marriage at age 14 to Girolamo Riario, the nephew of Pope Sixtus IV, reflected a common strategy for affiliating fifteenth-century Italian courts through webs of marital alliances. As she matured, Sforza became an avid prince-practitioner who sustained keen interests in medicine, alchemy, and botany while shuttling between residences in Milan, Rome, Florence, and her own dominion. Like other early modern noblewomen, she used recipes and remedies as a form of currency within a broad epistolary network. Her medical correspondents encompassed noble relations, local apothecaries, political agents, and irregular practitioners, including a Roman Jewish empiric named Anna. Sforza's massive compendium of 454 recipes, the so-called *Experiments*, integrated the fruits of hands-on experimentation

8 Rankin, 'Exotic Materials'.

9 Trivellato, 'Guilds, Technology and Economic Change'.

10 Barker, 'Contributions of Medici Women'.

11 Snook, 'English Women's Writing'.

12 Leong, 'Herbals she peruseth'.

with secrets procured from extensive court contacts across Europe.[13] The vast majority of recipes in her collection were medicinal in nature. They included pills and powders to cure fevers; unguents to treat gout, tumours, sciatica, and wounds; distillates to relieve infections; poison antidotes and elixirs to strengthen the body; and techniques to resolve stubborn reproductive problems. Like other vernacular recipe books discussed by Julia Gruman Martins in this volume, Sforza's *ricettario* evokes a compendial imagination in which beauty secrets, veterinary medicine, and the transmutation of metals all coexist in the same practical arena.[14] Several recipes were rendered either in cipher or in Latin to better preserve their secrecy.

Throughout the collection, Sforza attested to the efficacy of various remedies by noting that they had been tried and tested by her own hand, using such phrases as 'proven remedy', 'truly tested and proven', and 'proven and certain'. Only after repeating a procedure multiple times and trying it out could she and other household practitioners be assured of the desired result. Although we still know little about these testing methods, they undoubtedly engaged the senses to a significant degree. In the course of producing and evaluating remedies, expert practitioners not only relied on written instructions but also gauged changes in colour, texture, and smell as indicators of how materials reacted to heat and manipulation. This type of experimentalism was one of the most significant ways by which the body and the natural world could be known in the early modern period. By foregrounding the value of first-hand knowledge, experimentation opened up robust channels of knowledge production for Renaissance women with inquiring minds who otherwise were barred from participation in professional and intellectual guilds. Recipe books thus served as a mode of intellectual inquiry and investigative practice for both genders, and their collective wisdom could be shared within family groups and other trusted circles. It was partly due to their experimental nature that these treasuries of knowledge became such a powerful way for women to establish their healing authority and enable their participation in discourses of natural philosophy.

The history of this remarkable recipe collection, which has been called 'a foundational text in the history of pharmacology', nevertheless remains shrouded in mystery.[15] The original codex, written in Sforza's own hand,

13 *Experimenti de la Ex.ma S.r Caterina da Furlj*. This volume has been studied in the context of Sforza's scientific activities by Ray, *Daughters of Alchemy*, 14-45; Fiumi and Tempesta, 'Gli "experimenti" di Caterina Sforza'; Viroli, *Caterina Sforza*, 207-11; Graziani and Venturelli, *Caterina Sforza*, 150-59.

14 Martins, 'Understanding/Controlling the Female Body'.

15 Ray, *Daughters of Alchemy*, 14.

has been lost. It has long been thought that her *ricettario* survived only in a unique copy, currently housed in a private archive in Ravenna, where it is inaccessible to the public. This copy was transcribed from the original, perhaps around 1525, by Lucantonio Cuppano (1507-1557), a trusted lieutenant serving in the army of Sforza's only son, Giovanni de' Medici (1498-1526). This Medici commander, often known by the nickname 'delle Bande Nere', had inherited the manuscript collection from his mother.[16] A devoted Medici steward, Cuppano reportedly began making a copy of these 'most treasured things' as a useful pastime while stationed in garrison. The temporary misplacement of the original codex in 1525 while Giovanni's military company resided in Rome may have given its owner added impetus to make a duplicate.[17] Marked with the initial 'C' on its cover, Cuppano's transcription forms the basis of the published edition of Sforza's *ricettario*. That edition, issued in 1893, serves as the platform for all scholarly studies of her experimental activities to date.

Recently, however, a previously unstudied manuscript copied from other segments of Sforza's production has been unearthed in the Florentine National Library, along with a separate partial index referencing yet another set of her recipes.[18] These two manuscripts, also produced by Cuppano, add significantly to what the published edition reveals of Sforza's interest in medicine and science. The principal manuscript, designated by the initial 'B' on its cover, adds over 400 recipes to her known corpus; throughout the essay, we refer to this codex as the B volume. The second text, called here the Palatino index, provides a partial index to what may be yet another transcribed volume of Sforza's vast repository of recipes, one that to this day remains unidentified.[19] This new evidence suggests that Caterina devised

16 For Cuppano's biography, see Coppi da Gorzano, 'Il conte Lucantonio Coppi detto Cuppano'.

17 'Lettere di Giovanni de' Medici', at 127, dated 29 December 1525: 'Ci trovamo manco nelli forzieri a Roma uno libro scritto a mano di ricette di più et varie cose operate: che sensa falla nisuno lo ritroviamo, chè in ogni modo lo volemo'. ('We find missing from the strongboxes in Rome a handwritten book of recipes for many and various working things; we must find it because, one way or another, we want it.')

18 Florence, Biblioteca Nazionale Centrale di Firenze (BNCF), Magliabechiana (Magl.) XV 14; and BNCF, Palatino 1021, fols. 51r-55v. This discovery was first published by Barker, 'Contributions of Medici Women'.

19 The Palatino index might bear some relation to BNCF, Magl. XV 58, whose title page reads: 'In questo libro si notaronno per [loss] Lucantonio di Ysodoro Cuppano da Montefalcho servitor dello Illustrissimo Signor Giovanni de' Medici mio singularissimo patrone alcune memorie, de' libri della Eccellentissima Madama Caterina da Forli, matre di ditto mio signore, quale memorie la maggior parte erano di mano di ditta Madama et ditti libri erano a presso del Signor mio Illustrissimo e per passar tempo io ne trascrisse bona parte di essi, maxime per esser estimate cose rarissime'. ('In this book are noted by [*loss*] Lucantonio di Ysodoro Cuppano da Montefalcho,

and recorded well over a thousand recipes, more than double the previously known number. The new Florentine manuscripts not only confirm the fact that the duchess was among the most sophisticated knowledge-makers of her day, they also highlight the growing authority wielded by experiential knowledge both within and outside the domestic realm.

Besides expanding the scope of Sforza's empirical interests, this new information foregrounds the domestic nature of her recipe collection. Caterina has been seen as a forerunner of the 'new science' that transformed early modern Europe.[20] While her experimental bent is not at issue, we argue that this kind of praxis was central to Renaissance household medicine itself, although it was conducted with far greater resources and dedication in her case. Caterina's vast miscellany of recipes must be read more intentionally within the context of a household economy writ large – one that simultaneously served both the immediate health needs and the political objectives of a Renaissance court. Of particular interest are the ways in which Sforza's encyclopedic compendium reflected the practical demands of managing a great household. Renaissance courts employed a wide variety of personnel, ranging from courtiers, ladies-in-waiting, and secretaries to servants, stable hands, and jesters; this was true even of Forlì, a relatively small court. Despite the availability of university-trained physicians at Renaissance courts, consorts like Caterina assumed responsibility for the well-being of their intimates, staff, and guests as part of their domestic duties.[21] Building on the observation made by Cordula Nolte elsewhere in this volume that mothers and daughters in affluent German families typically played key roles in domestic care, it would seem that these activities reinforced the superior status of well-born women with respect to the other members of their households.[22] It appears that Caterina's many overlapping roles – including wife, mother, duchess, and regent from 1484 to 1499 – tilted her collection toward the broad gamut of practical matters encountered in everyday court life.

servant of the Most Illustrious Lord Giovanni de' Medici, my most singular patron, several memoranda from the books of the Most Illustrious Lady Caterina da Forlì, mother of my said master; the majority of these memoranda were from the hand of the said lady, and these books were kept by my Most Illustrious Lord. And to pass the time, I have transcribed a large part of them, especially since they are esteemed as the rarest things.') Like the C volume, this codex bears on its cover page the key to Caterina's substitution cipher.

20 Ray, *Daughters of Alchemy*.

21 While court medicine has attracted considerable attention in recent years, we still know little about how Italian noblewomen engaged in medical decision-making, interacted with court physicians, or facilitated the circulation of medical knowledge within court settings. For now, see Barker, 'Christine of Lorraine', and Strocchia, *Forgotten Healers*, 14-49.

22 Nolte, 'Domestic Care in the Sixteenth Century'.

Because Sforza's responsibilities encompassed both the political and the managerial, her recipe collection was similarly complex and wide-ranging. Recorded immediately next to each other are simple tips for conserving household resources, such as making vinegar from wine, alongside such bellicose features of Renaissance statecraft as defending against artillery, defeating one's enemies, and avoiding capture.[23] The inclusion of multiple recipes to treat various gynecological and obstetrical problems must be linked to the responsibilities she and other consorts exercised toward their close female attendants and other women at court. Similarly, Caterina's interest in equine medicine and the farrier's art also should be situated within the ambit of a princely consort's domestic duties. Even her alchemical recipes for metal working focus on such practical matters as making steel weapons, creating caustic compounds to dissolve metals, and adding weight to coinage in order to enhance the value of currency. Far from being haphazard or scattershot, her compendium of recipes speaks directly to the demands of Renaissance court life in all of its diversity. Lifting up the practical household nature of Sforza's collection does nothing to diminish its experimental qualities; instead, it highlights how early modern noblewomen seized the opportunities created by the empirical turn.

Like the recipes in the published volume, the recipes recorded in the B volume utilize multiple explanatory frameworks – humoral, alchemical, divine, and occult – in an eclectic combination that was consonant with contemporary healing practices across Renaissance Europe. However, the discovery of the B volume is a boon to the study of Caterina's recipes not only because it gives a more accurate understanding of the astonishing quantity she collected, but also because this text exhibits the clear traces of deliberate and methodical censorship.[24] The text was considerably pared down, mostly through a process of mechanical excision, after Cuppano completed his faithful and uncritical transmission of Caterina's secrets. As will be explained below, there is no doubt that this partial destruction of the text was carried out explicitly for the purpose of removing the recipes involving magic.

After briefly exploring the history of the B volume recipe collection, we analyse its content by focusing on a few of the hundreds of medical recipes that form its bulk. We shed further light on the nature and scope of this

23 BNCF, Magl. XV 14, fol. 21r. The recipes numbered 90, 132, and 303 dealing with these matters have been excised, so their folio numbers are unknown.

24 Published by Pasolini, Cuppano's manuscript C volume is not available for public consultation. Centuries before Pasolini made his transcription, this volume seems to have been purged by censors of its magic recipes.

collection by placing Caterina's recipes in the context of fifteenth-century household medicine as it was practised both at Italian courts and in the homes of the merchant classes – a subject that remains surprisingly understudied. The essay argues that Caterina's secrets, despite being exceptionally encyclopedic in their range, were united by their utility and pragmatic nature, an observation that applies just as well to the magic recipes that were expunged from her codices. The partial censorship of her intellectual legacy signalled momentous changes in the parameters used to define not only religious orthodoxy but also medicine and science. Belonging to the earliest strands of the long Medici genealogy of experimentation, Sforza's recipe book continued to be consulted over many decades and, when necessary, reshaped in conformity with changing epistemological boundaries.

The Manuscripts

A brief physical description of these newly identified materials is in order, especially since the manuscript on which the published version is based remains unavailable. The B volume consists of 151 numbered folios, including the index. The first 88 folios were numbered sequentially in the upper right corner in the original brown ink; a modern archivist renumbered all pages in pencil in 1917.[25] The spine bears the title 'Secrets of medicine and alchemy', while the unnumbered front flyleaf declares Cuppano to be the manuscript's owner.[26] As mentioned earlier, the manuscript bears a large initial B on the front cover (Figure 5.1). It was standard Tuscan accounting practice to identify codices that formed part of a longer series by assigning each volume a sequential capital letter. As major-domo of Giovanni de' Medici's extensive military household, Cuppano would have been responsible for record-keeping, and thus undoubtedly was familiar with this practice.[27] Hence the Florentine B codex almost certainly shares the same origins as the published C volume, and precedes it in the sequence of production.[28]

25 BNCF, Magl. XV 14, unnumbered backboard. We utilize the modern folio numbers throughout this essay.

26 Ibid. The title given on the spine reads: 'Segreti di medicina e d'alchimia' ('Secrets of medicine and alchemy'), while the unnumbered front flyleaf announces: 'Hic liber est Domini Lucantonio de Cuppanis' ('This book belongs to Messer Lucantonio de Cuppano').

27 On the standardization of accounting practices, see Goldthwaite, 'Practice and Culture of Accounting'.

28 Further evidence that both the B and C volumes were produced under almost identical circumstances comes from the similar notations on their parchment covers. On the first it is

Figure 5.1 Front cover of Sforza's recipe book marked with initial 'B'

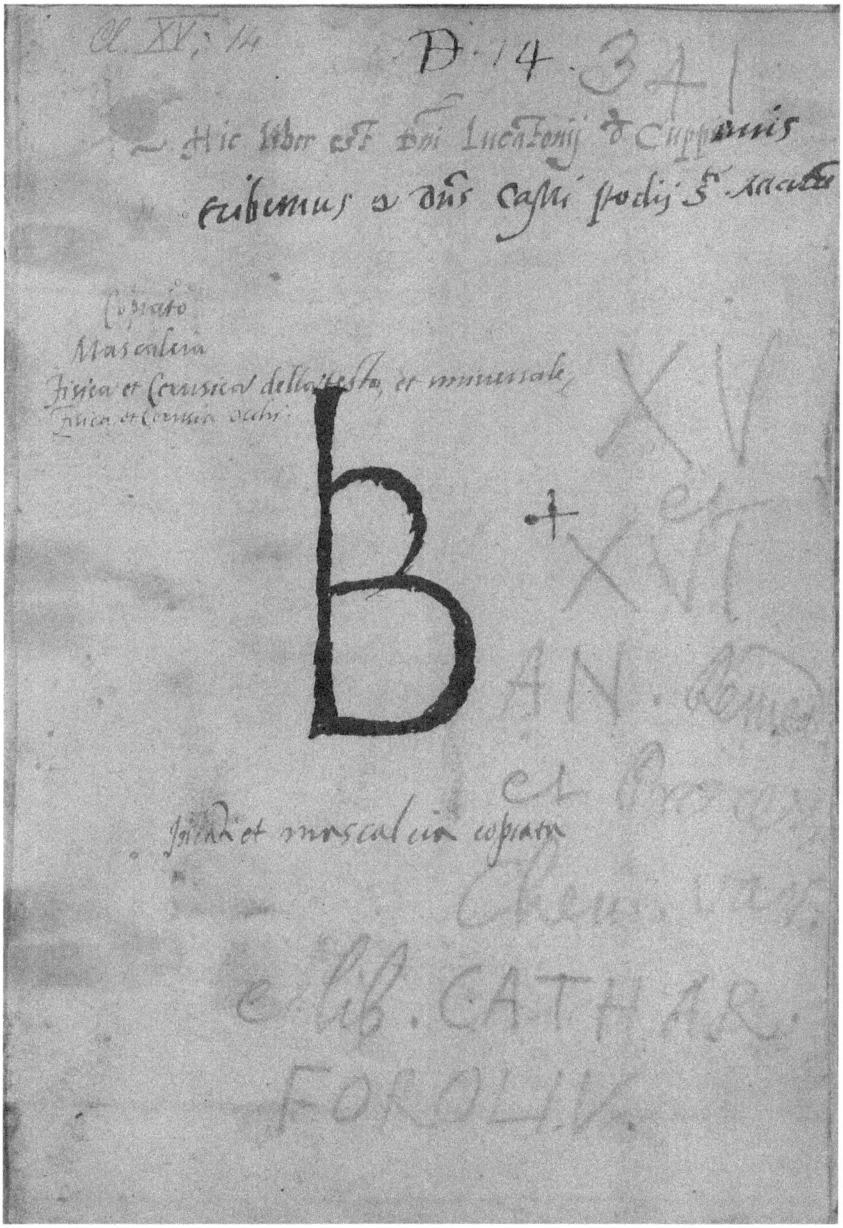

Florence, Biblioteca Nazionale Centrale di Firenze, Magl. XV 14, unfoliated. By permission of Ministero per i beni e le attività culturali/ Biblioteca Nazionale Centrale di Firenze.

In fact, Cuppano offers testimony to a multivolume project in his preface to the B volume. Written in the shape of an inverted triangle that evokes a printed frontispiece is the following declaration: 'Here begins the copy of the second book extracted from the original books of the Illustrious Lady Caterina of Forlì. The first book is designated by the letter A and this second book by the letter B, just as is the aforesaid original, of which this is a copy'.[29] In light of this reference, it is possible that the Palatino index refers to part of the now-lost A volume of Sforza's *ricettario*, the first in the sequence of his transcription project.

At first glance, the ordering of recipes collected in the B volume seems devoid of any discernible pattern. This random method of compilation was common in Renaissance recipe books and may have reflected Sforza's actual practice to some extent. Throughout her adult life, Caterina reportedly kept a blank journal with her at all times, in which she could make notes and record recipes on a running basis.[30] Each recipe bore a short title indicating its function; on occasion, Sforza included the recipe's provenance, especially when the original maker enjoyed a prominent reputation.[31] This random arrangement meant that some type of paratextual aid was useful for pinpointing a specific recipe quickly. Indeed, the adoption of paratextual aids – indices, marginal notes, extracts – became increasingly commonplace in vernacular manuscripts throughout Europe after 1500.[32]

Whether Caterina's original recipe collection included numeration, indices, or some other apparatus is unknown, but it seems likely that Cuppano reproduced the recipes in the same random order in which he found them. The reasoning is simple: if Caterina had organized her recipes with a clear logic, Cuppano would not have ignored that logic in favour of chaos. In any case, when Cuppano produced the transcriptions for the B volume, he numbered each of the 423 recipes sequentially, and he used these numbers to cross-reference the recipes in his index. By comparison, the published

written, 'incanti et mascalcia copiata' ('spells and the farrier's art [have been] copied'), while on the second, written by the same hand, it says, 'copiati l'incanti' ('the spells [have been] copied').

29 BNCF, Magl. XV 14, unnumbered front flyleaf: 'Incomenza la copia del secondo libro cavati dalli originali delli libri della Ill.ma S.ra Madama Caterina de Furli, il quale primo libro è segnato a Lettera A et questo libro secondo è segnato a lettera B si come se il predetto originale del quali questo è la copia'.

30 Fiumi and Tempesta, 'Gli "experimenti" di Caterina Sforza', 139.

31 For instance, BNCF, Magl. XV 14, recipe no. 233, fols. 51v-53r: 'Questa è la recetta che adoperava Papa Bonifatio innanzi che egli fusse papa e guadagnò molto con essa'. ('This is the recipe that Pope Bonifatio used before he became pope, and he profited much from it.') The recipe enabled the practitioner to transform four small pearls into a single large one of greater value.

32 Leong, '"Herbals she peruseth".'

C codex contains 454 recipes, which are mostly medicinal in nature. The Palatino index augments the scope of her collection still further. Although this index only covers recipes beginning with the letters M to T – less than half the alphabet – it carries numbers up to 931, suggesting it once organized that number of additional recipes. If our hypothesis is correct that the Palatino index represents just a fragment of the missing A volume, then the A volume alone might have spanned as many as 2,000 recipes.

The idiosyncratic organization of the index contained in the B volume and the Palatino index is identical, as is the scribal hand, strongly suggesting that both indices were created by Cuppano. The indices are organized according to two criteria. First, they are arranged alphabetically according to their names (which usually describe either the formula type or the complaint they address). Thus, under the letter A we find 'acque' (distilled waters) and under V 'veleno' (poison) and 'vermi' (worms). Then, the recipes gathered under each letter are subdivided into five epistemic categories: medicines ('medicine'), hygiene and beauty products ('lisci'), incantations ('incanti'), equine remedies ('mascalcia'), and alchemy ('alchimia') (Figure 5.2). Of the 423 recipes, 207 recipes (49 per cent of total) were classified as medicines; 110 (26 per cent) were considered to be alchemical; 48 (11 per cent) regarded hygiene and beauty; 39 (9 per cent) concerned charms and spells; and 19 (4 per cent) targeted equine ailments. With this categorical breakdown in mind, we turn now to the contents of the collection itself.

Household Medicines for a Renaissance Court

To understand the household nature of Sforza's *ricettario*, the multilayered character of Renaissance courts must be taken into account. While courts have been studied most frequently as complex political entities, they were also great households whose members were bound by ties of kinship and dependence. The vast range of personnel employed at fifteenth-century Italian courts suggests that these were communities for sharing knowledge about an equally vast range of concerns. The 195 staff members on the Milanese court payroll in 1463 ran the gamut from secretaries, cooks, and musicians to stewards and comptrollers who handled provisioning and expenditures. They also ranged from persons of rank to young serving boys who slept on the floor.[33] Given this extensive scope of court personnel, it is not surprising that the household recipe book of a female ruler like Sforza had an equally capacious reach.

33 Lubkin, *Renaissance Court*, 29-30.

Figure 5.2 Index page in B volume showing taxonomy of recipes

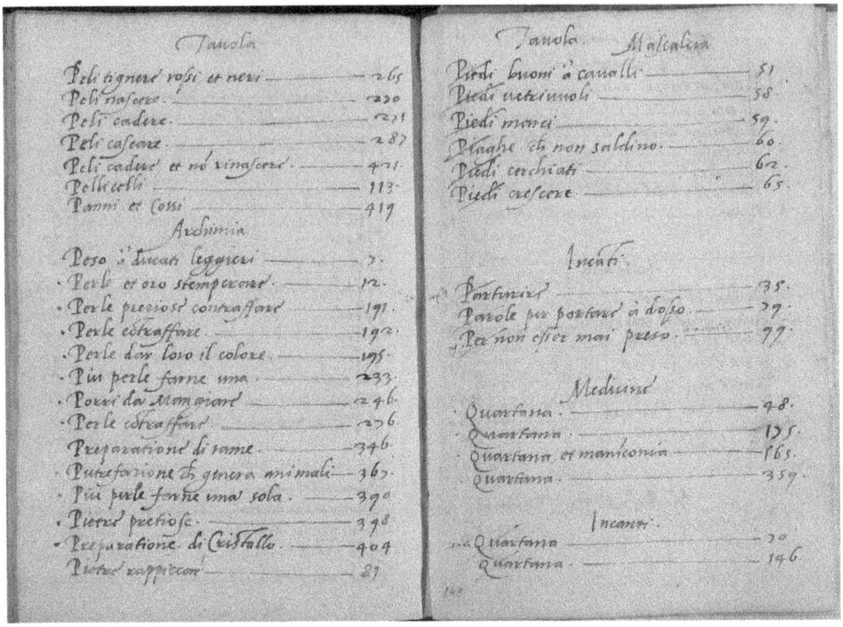

Florence, Biblioteca Nazionale Centrale di Firenze, Magl. XV 14, fols. 147v-148r. By permission of Ministero per i beni e le attività culturali/Biblioteca Nazionale Centrale di Firenze.

At the heart of the court was the princely household, staffed by intimates and attendants who performed vital functions of everyday life. Members of this *domus* provided care, companionship, and the benefit of experience; they had access to intimate court spaces as well as to the body of the prince, his consort, and children. Although fifteenth-century Italian courts varied considerably in size, the number of personnel comprising the inner household could be substantial. In 1463, before Galeazzo Maria Sforza became duke of Milan, his personal household consisted of forty staff members, including five gentlemen, twelve chamberlains, a chaplain, a barber, and various footmen. After he assumed the ducal throne in 1466, his private household swelled to several hundred persons who enjoyed varying degrees of access to his person.[34]

Renaissance consorts generally maintained their own households that were distinct from the princely retinue. These households were modelled along customary domestic lines in that they incorporated the care of young children. Attending the needs of Italian consorts, dowager duchesses, and

34 Ibid.

their children was a large cadre of women, ranging from well-born court ladies and personal attendants to matrons, wet nurses, and other caregivers. Members of this inner circle frequented the intimate chambers of the court, making them privy to certain confidences, both personal and political. Appointments to these positions customarily belonged to consorts themselves, as did authority over other private household matters. Scholars have shown that these domestic arrangements provided an important source of power and patronage for noblewomen. Consorts like Bianca Maria Visconti, wife of the Milanese duke Francesco Sforza, satisfied some of the many demands incurred through kinship and friendship by dispensing these offices as political favours.[35] These private households were smaller in size than those of their husbands or sons, but could still be significant. Bianca Maria counted some ten to twenty female attendants in the latter years of her husband's reign; another two dozen women cared for the nine princely offspring. Similarly, nineteen or twenty women, including Turkish and Albanian slaves, attended Barbara of Brandenburg, Duchess of Mantua (d. 1481).[36]

The importance of this female entourage helps to explain Sforza's inclusion of numerous remedies devoted to issues of reproduction and female sexuality. These recipes addressed relatively commonplace conditions, such as ways to induce menstrual flow or relieve labour pains, as well as more urgent situations such as expelling a stillborn fetus from the womb.[37] This kind of practical knowledge would have enabled Sforza to circulate informal medical advice within her entourage while giving her a platform for informed decision-making when interacting with court physicians. Recipes for understanding the full range of reproductive matters extended to betting on the sex of an unborn child, which became a popular pastime at the Medici court in the mid-sixteenth century.[38] Being adept at court management also meant being skilled in the arts of deception, since much of Renaissance court life pivoted on social perception and appearances. It may not be surprising that Sforza included several useful recipes for making a woman who was not a virgin appear to be virginal.[39]

As consort and regent, Caterina also exercised duty of care with respect to other staff members who served the court in more quotidian roles, while

35 Covini, 'Tra patronage e ruolo politico', 260-61.

36 Welch, 'Women as Patrons and Clients'.

37 BNCF, Magl. XV 14, nos. 104 and 105 (fol. 21v), nos. 109 and 110 (fol. 22r), no. 157 (fol. 28v), no. 161 (fol. 29v), no. 188 (fol. 36v), and no. 312 (excised).

38 BNCF, Palatino 1021, nos. 116 and 118. On gambling habits, see Baker, '*Dux ludens*'.

39 BNCF, Magl. XV 14, nos. 22-23 (fol. 7v).

contemporary notions of hospitality gave her responsibility for the well-being of guests and diplomatic visitors during her fifteen-year regency. Renaissance courts differed considerably in the degree to which they subsidized medical care for staff and visitors, but there is no doubt that this type of assistance could be put to political uses both inside and outside the court.[40] While we know relatively little about Sforza's actual practice in this regard, including her interactions with court physicians, it is clear that her encyclopedic collection of recipes prepared her for every eventuality. Recipes included in the B volume ran the gamut from poison antidotes and plague remedies to febrifuges and analgesics for sciatica and gout. Caterina recorded secrets for treating all manner of wounds, various respiratory and digestive ailments, and 'cures' for cancer and melancholy. The sheer range of health needs registered in her collection speaks volumes about her perceived managerial role in running a great household – one in which healthcare might take on decidedly political overtones.

Beauty Secrets

Although beauty products were the targets of frequent moralizing attacks throughout the Renaissance, they played a significant role in maintaining health and hygiene.[41] Italian court women were renowned for making cosmetics, perfumes, and grooming products. Sforza's adoptive mother, Bona of Savoy, who married Galeazzo Maria the same year Caterina was born, manufactured a wide array of items for personal use and to give as gifts. Similarly, Caterina's contemporary Isabella d'Este proclaimed herself to be 'unsurpassed by any perfumer in the world'.[42] The proliferation of recipes for cosmetics and scented waters in vernacular recipe books of the fifteenth century signals the rising status of these gifts circulating between and among European courts.

The predilection of court ladies for grooming and cleansing products was diffused more widely thanks to the well-heeled merchant wives who imitated their tastes. By participating in the same culture of cosmetics and hygiene as their aristocratic superiors, these city women gained access to a basis for the exchange of gifts and knowledge with court society, which in turn allowed them to distinguish themselves among their peers and

40 Dean, 'Court and Household'; Strocchia, *Forgotten Healers*, 45-49.

41 Cabré, 'Beautiful Bodies'.

42 Quoted in Ray, *Daughters of Alchemy*, 36.

enhance their own social standing. In 1447, for instance, the Florentine widow Alessandra Strozzi capitalized on the connections her banker-son Filippo had established with the Neapolitan court when she asked him to obtain a favourite soap and face water on behalf of her daughter Caterina.[43] Because they were usually composed of readily available and affordable ingredients, and because they were well adapted to the patterns of exchange in female sociability, products aimed at hygiene and beautification quickly attained a prominent place in the surviving correspondence and recipe collections of early modern Italy. By tracking written references to the circulation of these products as well as the sharing of their formulas, we can map the flow of medical knowledge and practices between Italian courts and urban populations, especially from a gendered perspective.

At the same time, the exchange of beauty secrets initiated by court women marked the structural vulnerability of Renaissance consorts, most of whom operated with scant financial resources in an era of growing magnificence.[44] Renaissance noblewomen not only purveyed these secrets and their recipes as a form of self-fashioning, but they also used them as a way to significantly expand their gift-giving potential. Bona of Savoy – an important trendsetter in this area – frequently had little cash on hand to reward attendants for services well-rendered or to consolidate networks of favour within and beyond the Milanese court. Her cosmetic items were graciously received in lieu of money because they functioned as symbolic tokens of the recipient's social capital and access to a seat of power. Moreover, owing to their material qualities, these gifts could visibly ennoble the recipient's body, whether through the transformative effect of suddenly lightened hair, a delicate and unblemished complexion, a waft of heavenly fragrance, or a flash of a white smile.[45] Health-giving items such as perfumes, cosmetics, and grooming products also could be regifted to extend secondary tiers of rewards and preference. Nor were these products just for women. Sforza's *ricettario* included grooming products for men too, such as tinctures for darkening the hair and beard that enhanced the illusion of perpetual, youthful virility.

Given this context, it is not surprising that the first six recipes recorded in the B volume concerned beauty products, mainly face creams to remove freckles, spots, and wrinkles. The inclusion of these recipes in particular points to the emergence of the skin as an increasingly important social and aesthetic marker in fifteenth-century courts. The next three recipes

43 Strozzi, *Letters*, 33.
44 Covini, 'Tra patronage e ruolo politico', 274-77.
45 Welch, 'Women as Patrons and Clients', 26.

delineate alchemical processes for changing the colour or weight of ordinary metals, which appear to address completely different concerns. Despite their seemingly odd juxtaposition, all ten recipes are closely linked by both the nature of their ingredients and their ultimate objectives. All ten rely on the use of cleansing and purifying agents – some more caustic than others – to alter surface appearances through chemical interactions.[46] These common intentions and desired outcomes point to hidden threads of connectivity underlying the organization of Caterina's recipes that transcend a simple taxonomy.

Veterinary Medicine

The inclusion of recipes concerned with veterinary medicine clearly distinguishes Sforza's collection from recipe books kept by Italian merchant families like the Bardi and Rosselli, which made no mention of animal treatments of any kind. In recording these secrets, Caterina took a pragmatic approach to animal husbandry. Of particular interest was the health of her stables. For centuries horses had been essential to daily transport and the conduct of warfare, but by the mid-fifteenth century these beautiful but costly animals had become increasingly important to the ceremonial splendour that defined Renaissance court culture. Over the course of the sixteenth century, the art of horsemanship developed into a significant court spectacle, culminating in the grand equestrian ballets of the baroque period.[47] In Caterina's day, the size of Italian princely stables indexed the splendour of the court. In 1475 the Milanese court, which exercised such a formative influence on Caterina's thinking, maintained at least ninety horses in its stables. Suitable steeds were so expensive – some costing as much as 40 ducats – that many Milanese courtiers borrowed mounts from the ducal stables for ceremonial occasions. Caring for these valuable animals demanded numerous personnel: twenty-nine men served the ducal stables alone, ranging from the stable master to farriers and stable hands.[48]

Hence it is not surprising that Sforza sought to protect these important court assets by including equine remedies in her therapeutic arsenal. Still, she showed a decidedly practical bent in selecting from the vast repertoire of remedies devoted to equine medicine. Caterina dedicated nineteen recipes

46 BNCF, Magl. XV 14, fols. 1r-3v.

47 Goethals, 'Patronage Politics of Equestrian Ballet'.

48 Lubkin, *Renaissance Court*, 130; Covini, 'Tra patronage e ruolo politico', 257-58.

(4 per cent of the total) in the B codex solely to the farrier's art of shoeing horses ('mascalcia'). This was a recognized subfield of expertise, one that merited separate classification by Cuppano. The proper care of horses' hooves enjoyed a long history dating back to Hippocrates, who reportedly wrote a treatise on this subject. Medieval Arabic and Latin authors augmented this field by incorporating materials on surgical interventions, wound care, and remedies for parasites. One of the most influential works on *mascalcia* circulating in Caterina's day was the Latin treatise written *c.*1340 by the Roman veterinarian Lorenzo Rusio, farrier to Cardinal Napoleone Orsini. This treatise circulated broadly in both manuscript and print form. An illuminated copy of Rusio was made for the court of Ferrara in 1425; a printed vernacular version appeared as early as 1486, followed by numerous editions in Italian and other languages issued throughout the sixteenth century.[49]

In selecting equine remedies, Sforza addressed common problems that would help keep her stables in top form. In so doing, she melded the arts of court management with experimental praxis. Among the recipes she registered were those intended 'to make a horse's hooves perfect' and to harden the hooves of a horse displaying 'bad, glass-like hooves'. She also gathered remedies to treat diverse equine ailments such as intestinal worms as well as those aimed at fattening up sick animals. Her remedy to staunch the bleeding in a ruptured vein crossed the boundaries between animal and human health since, according to Caterina, it worked equally well in both people and horses.[50] Importantly, all but one of these equine remedies bore the title 'esperimento', underlining the empirical orientation of Sforza's creative praxis. It is doubtful that she tested each of these recipes herself, yet their inclusion helped the duchess validate practical knowledge claims and build social capital as a careful steward of household resources.

Household Alchemy: Distillation as Technology and Practice

Lawrence Principe has observed that alchemy had two main purposes in Renaissance Europe: transmuting metals and making medicines.[51] Yet alchemy itself was subject to an elastic interpretation, especially within the secrets tradition. The vast majority of Sforza's recipes indexed under the heading 'Alchemy' were not secrets for what was referred to then as 'true' or

49 [Rusio,] *La mascalcia di Lorenzo Rusio.*

50 BNCF, Magl. XV 14, fols. 14v, 15r-v, 16r.

51 Principe, *Secrets of Alchemy.*

transmutational alchemy, but rather for the more pedestrian, result-oriented recipes often referred to as 'household alchemy'.[52] Both the recipes in the B volume and those referenced in the Palatino index affirm a broad understanding of alchemy: it could be applied to a set of methods, techniques, and processes in addition to secrets requiring chemical ingredients and those that delved into arcana. For instance, the Palatino index lists four recipes for dyeing the hair and beard under the letter T, heading alchemy.[53] While such recipes might just as easily be grouped with cosmetics ('lisci'), clearly the chemical ingredients as well as the corrosive processes they involved led to their classification as 'alchemy'.

A substantial portion of Caterina's secrets relied on distillation, which as a production method spanned both traditional Galenic and alchemical practices. Indeed, her recipe for making a 'marvellous' ointment for healing wounds was followed immediately by one for giving base metals a golden lustre and yet another for dissolving iron chains – all utilizing similar distillation methods.[54] After 1500, the knowledge and practice of distillation became increasingly commonplace within both aristocratic and artisan households across Europe, particularly since it was necessary for making certain Galenic medicines of great repute.[55] The Sienese physician Pietro Andrea Mattioli mistakenly claimed that distillation had been 'invented' in the sixteenth century, ignoring both its Arabic roots and John of Rupecissa's important treatise on distilling written in the fourteenth century. But Mattioli was certainly correct in observing its tremendous growth in popularity, in part due to the commercial success of printed vernacular handbooks – including his own – on distilling herbs for making perfumes and medicines.[56] The German surgeon Hieronymus Brunschwig published two widely disseminated books on distilling in 1500 and 1512. Both were how-to manuals instructing readers how to operate a still and make distillates: the first was intended for an unlearned audience, the second for a more learned group.[57]

Sforza's extensive use of distilling techniques points to broader trends in household medicine that are poorly understood for fifteenth-century Italy.

52 Moran, *Distilling Knowledge*. Eamon discusses the elastic interpretation of the term 'alchemy' in books of secrets in 'How to Read a Book of Secrets', 44, where he introduces the useful concept of 'result-oriented alchemy'. On the historical opposition of 'true alchemy' and 'false alchemy', see Nummedal, *Alchemy and Authority*.

53 BNCF, Palatino 1021, fol. 55r-v.

54 BNCF, Magl. XV 14, fols. 49r-50v (nos. 229, 230, 231).

55 Voights and Payne, 'Medicine for a Great Household'.

56 Franchi, 'Apparecchi e metodi'.

57 Rankin, 'How to Cure the Golden Vein'.

To date the enthusiasm for distilling remedies of all kinds has been studied mainly as it pertained to well-born German and English women from the sixteenth century onward.[58] Distillation required specialized equipment, such as lead distilling bells and glass alembics, as well as a concentrated heat source and other paraphernalia such as caps, connectors, and tubes. Still, these devices could be relatively simple from a technological standpoint, and high heat was not necessary to distill most plant materials, in contrast to the extreme temperatures required to melt gold. Evidence that Italian women of the mercantile classes had begun to install small-scale distilling equipment in their own homes by the mid-fifteenth century suggests that these practices penetrated normative models of female domesticity at an early date. In 1451, for instance, the well-connected Florentine widow Alessandra Macinghi Strozzi listed a distilling apparatus ('una chanpana da stillare') among the essential kitchen utensils included in the rental agreement for a house she leased to a kinsman.[59] This technology appeared in other Italian merchant households as well. A 'distilling bell made of lead' featured among the household goods recorded in the 1497 inventory of the Tornabuoni family villa located north of Florence.[60] Although Caterina can be considered an expert practitioner, it is clear that Italian city women of her day worked along a 'continuum of skills and knowledge' when engaging in the healing arts.[61]

Magic and the Censorship of Caterina's Recipes

Magic, whether symbolic, ritual, natural, or demonic, was the operative principle for a sizable portion of Caterina's collection of recipes. In her day, spirits and invisible properties called 'occult' (for instance, the attractive force of magnets) were widely believed to play a role in observable natural phenomena. The manipulation of invisible forces and properties through magic was regarded by a large cross-segment of the population as an effective enterprise for operating in the natural world.[62] While late medieval and

58 Rankin, *Panaceia's Daughters*; Leong, 'Making Medicines'.

59 Florence, Archivio di Stato, Carte Strozziane, ser. 5, vol. 15, fol. 80v.

60 DePrano, *Art Patronage, Family and Gender*, 225.

61 Klein and Spary, 'Introduction: Why Materials?', 2.

62 Copenhaver, 'Natural Magic'; and Park, 'Medicine and Magic', 138-39. Caterina herself partially cloaked a few of her recipes by using a substitution cipher (nos. 5, 6, 25), and Latin (nos. 41, 79, 164). Some of these were for maleficent ends (e.g. invisibility); others were for indecorous ones (e.g. laxatives). She did not systematically encipher her magic recipes.

early modern Europeans recognized that some forms of magic were licit while others were not, the boundaries between these two categories were widely debated.[63] Highly regarded Christian practitioners of magic such as William of Auvergne, Arnald of Villanova, Albertus Magnus, and Marsilio Ficino all believed that their magic was above reproach because it was carried out by means of occult properties in natural things rather than by means of demons.[64]

Attempting to distinguish between 'magic' and 'science', or 'magic' and 'medicine', in the age in which Caterina lived would be anachronistic, especially because the term 'magic' did not come to be defined consistently until long after her death.[65] Greater uniformity in the use of this term was forced by the intensification of disputes within the Counter-Reformation church over issues regarding demonology and other forms of occultism.[66] At the height of efforts to define the church's position on demonology, Paul IV updated the Index of Prohibited Books in 1559 to officially condemn all printed or manuscript writings dealing with 'magic'. Importantly, the Roman Inquisition, which was responsible for enforcing the new Index, began to define 'magic' in the broadest sense possible.[67]

The resulting seismic shift in the boundaries between orthodox and forbidden knowledge bears a direct connection to the removal of recipes in the category of 'incanti' from the B volume. This strategic campaign of expurgation was carried out principally by means of excision (cutting out the pages both partially and in their entirety) and obliteration (covering the text with meaningless forms to render it illegible).[68] Whereas the first method had the unintentional effect of sometimes damaging harmless recipes in the process, the second method was time-consuming and incomplete. The parameters of this campaign of destruction aimed at the B volume can be reconstructed rather precisely due to two circumstances. First, the B volume's index records the descriptive names of excised recipes; second, enough remains of some of the obliterated recipes to deduce their

63 Henry, 'Fragmentation of Renaissance Occultism', 16; Tarrant, 'Giambattista Della Porta', 612-13. For case studies, see Collins, 'Albertus, Magnus or Magus', and Herzig, 'Demons and the Friars'.

64 Thorndike, *History of Magic*, 2: 342-43, 546.

65 Henry, 'Fragmentation of Renaissance Occultism'.

66 See Kieckhefer, *European Witch Trials*, esp. chs. 1, 3, and 4; Clark, *Thinking with Demons*, esp. pt. 2, 'Science'; and Tarrant, 'Giambattista Della Porta', 605-6.

67 Tarrant, 'Giambattista Della Porta', 617-20.

68 Similarly expurgated recipe collections in Florentine libraries show that three kinds of secrets were targeted: recipes involving demonic magic; recipes meant for immoral ends (or involving ingredients obtained through immoral acts); and recipes that were potentially toxic.

operative principles. What is clear from all of this textual evidence is that the intentionally targeted recipes share certain verbal elements of ceremonial magic, specifically the recitation or writing of performative phrases.

Although this concern with verbal charms could be demonstrated by citing many examples such as the excised recipe 63 entitled 'Pain: heal it with words', the censor's exacting criteria are best understood by comparing recipes that did and did not escape destruction.[69] Whereas recipe 35 for inducing miscarriages and abortions was excised because it included an incantation, recipe 66, which used a potion of lichwort (*Parietaria officinalis*) for the same purpose, was left alone. Recipe 74 offering protection from ghosts was excised, but recipe 71 for overcoming witchcraft and breaking spells was judged licit because it used naturalia (a squash root worn on the neck) rather than words. Quelling a fever with incantations offered in recipes 45 and 108 was forbidden, whereas it was permitted to do so by wearing the words 'be cured of fever' based on the apocryphal story in recipe 43 about Christ healing St. Peter of fever in this way. In a similar case of what could be termed Christian magic, recipe 27 used the permissible incantation, 'Iob vermes habuit per gratiam Christi liberatus est' as an anthelmintic, while the words recited with the similar intention of eliminating parasites in recipes 32 and 33 were condemned to oblivion.

More evidence is needed to securely establish when the B volume was expurgated; however, circumstantial factors suggest that it occurred in the late sixteenth century. Duke Cosimo de' Medici, who possibly owned one or more volumes of Cuppano's transcriptions or perhaps even the original collection, was particularly vulnerable to politically motivated charges of heresy. This was especially true when his opponents sat on the papal throne. Under Paul III – a bitter enemy of the Medici duke – the powers of the Roman Inquisition were greatly enhanced beginning in 1543 and Inquisition officials gained the authority to bypass local bishops when searching for heretical writings, not only pushing their way into institutional libraries and commercial printing presses, but also prying into private houses and monasteries.[70] The Florentine court was caught in the snares of intolerance in the second half of the sixteenth century with the zealous persecution of a high-profile Medici favourite, the Valdesian adherent Pietro Carnesecchi (1508-1567). Initiated under Paul IV, the Inquisition's pursuit of this Florentine

69 'Dolori guarire con parole'. The censored recipes are nos. 15, 30-38, 40, 42, 45, 62-65, 70, 72, 74-79, 89-95, 98, 99, 102, 108, 122, 132-39, 142, 145-49, 163-64, 166, 279-82, 300-24, and 357.
70 On the Inquisition under Paul III, see Tarrant, 'Giambattista Della Porta', 613. On Paul III and the Medici, see Spini, *Cosimo I*, ch. 5; and Lupo Gentile, *La politica di Paolo III*.

nobleman was brought to its dreadful conclusion during Pius V's papacy when he was taken to Rome, decapitated, and burnt at the stake, despite the pleas of Cosimo's ambassadors.[71]

In this tense atmosphere, the aspects of Caterina's experimental knowledge that were increasingly viewed as demonic began to represent a threat to Medici fortunes. Despite the fact that the Medici court fostered experimentation, the Medici may have voluntarily expunged Caterina's text of illicit secrets in the late sixteenth century in order to protect themselves from charges of heresy (that is, if this purging was not carried out by an agent of the Roman Inquisition). Soon this censoring mentality was internalized by experimenters throughout Florence, and beginning in the 1590s, new recipe collections created within Medici court circles almost never involved magic of any kind.[72]

Conclusion

The newly recovered materials discussed here shed important light on Caterina Sforza's creative praxis as well as the contours of household medicine practised in a Renaissance court setting. As a careful steward of scant resources, Caterina showed an unmistakable practical bent and clear predilection for result-oriented recipes. Undoubtedly, her status as a highborn woman put her in a privileged position for acquiring the knowledge that was circulating within and among Renaissance courts and for trying it out. However, the encyclopedic nature of the B volume and Palatino index also demonstrates her capacity to transcend the boundaries of both class and gender in gathering know-how from diverse contexts and along a continuum of skills and knowledge. In doing so, Caterina aggregated to her recipe collection many secrets involving verbal charms capable of harnessing occult forces. While perfectly acceptable in her own era and considered part of the standard repertory of domestic medicine, such operations that worked by means of intelligible verbal communications rather than natural phenomena were later condemned by the Catholic Church. The painstaking censorship of her text destroyed a portion of her intellectual legacy, but it still allowed for the continued use of the rest of her vast store of knowledge for the care and cure of bodies amidst shifting epistemological boundaries.

71 Ortolani, *Pietro Carnesecchi*.

72 Such collections include Torresi, *Il ricettario Medici*; Torresi, *Il ricettario Bardi*; and Rosselli, *Mes secrets à Florence*.

Works Cited

Manuscripts

Florence, Archivio di Stato, Carte Strozziane, ser. 5, vol. 15.
Florence, BNCF, Magl. XV 14.
Florence, BNCF, Magl. XV 58.
Florence, BNCF, Palatino 1021.

Printed Works

Baker, Nicholas Scott. '*Dux ludens:* Eleonora of Toledo, Cosimo I de' Medici, and Games of Chance in the Ducal Household of Mid-Sixteenth-Century Florence', *European History Quarterly*, 46 (2016), 595-617.

Barker, Sheila. 'Christine of Lorraine and Medicine at the Medici Court', in *Medici Women: The Making of a Dynasty in Grand Ducal Tuscany,* ed. Giovanna Benadusi and Judith C. Brown (Toronto: Centre for Reformation and Renaissance Studies, 2015), 155-81.

—. 'The Contributions of Medici Women to Medicine in Grand Ducal Tuscany and Beyond', in *The Grand Ducal Medici and their Archive (1537-1743)*, ed. Alessio Assonitis and Brian Sandberg (Turnhout: Brepols, 2016), 101-16.

Blumenthal, Debra. 'Domestic Medicine: Slaves, Servants and Female Medical Expertise in Late Medieval Valencia', *Renaissance Studies*, 28 (2014), 515-32.

Cabré, Montserrat. 'Beautiful Bodies', in *A Cultural History of the Human Body in the Middle Ages*, ed. Linda Kalof (Oxford: Berg, 2010), 121-39.

—. 'Women or Healers? Household Practices and the Categories of Health Care in Late Medieval Iberia', *Bulletin of the History of Medicine*, 82 (2008), 18-51.

Clark, Stuart. *Thinking with Demons: The Idea of Witchcraft in Early Modern Europe* (Oxford: Oxford University Press, 1997).

Collins, David J. 'Albertus, Magnus or Magus? Magic, Natural Philosophy, and Religious Reform in the Middle Ages', *Renaissance Quarterly*, 63 (2010), 1-44.

Copenhaver, Brian. 'Natural Magic, Hermeticism and Occultism in Early Modern Science', in *Reappraisals of the Scientific Revolution*, ed. D.C. Lindberg and R.S. Westman (Cambridge: Cambridge University Press, 1990), 261-301.

Coppi da Gorzano, Carlo. 'Il conte Lucantonio Coppi detto Cuppano, ultimo condottiere delle Bande Nere e dimenticato Governatore Generale di Piombino (1507-1557)', *Rivista del Collegio araldico*, 3 (1960), 87-105.

Covini, Nadia. 'Tra patronage e ruolo politico: Bianca Maria Visconti (1450-1468)', in *Donne di potere nel Rinascimento*, ed. Letizia Arcangeli and Susanna Peyronel (Rome: Viella, 2008), 247-80.

Dean, Trevor. 'Court and Household in Ferrara, 1494', in *The French Descent into Renaissance Italy, 1494-95*, ed. David Abulafia (Aldershot: Ashgate, 1995), 165-87.
DePrano, Maria. *Art Patronage, Family and Gender in Renaissance Florence: The Tornabuoni* (Cambridge: Cambridge University Press, 2018).
Eamon, William. 'Appearance, Artifice, and Reality: Collecting Secrets in a Courtly Culture', in *The Gentleman, the Virtuoso, the Inquirer: Vicencio Juan de Lastanosa and the Art of Collecting in Early Modern Spain*, ed. Mar Rey-Bueno and Miguel López-Pérez (Newcastle upon Tyne: Cambridge Scholars, 2008), 127-43.
—. 'How to Read a Book of Secrets', in *Secrets and Knowledge in Medicine and Science, 1500-1800*, ed. Elaine Leong and Alisha Rankin (Aldershot: Ashgate, 2011), 23-46.
Fiumi, Fabrizia and Giovanna Tempesta. 'Gli "experimenti" di Caterina Sforza', in *Caterina Sforza: Una Donna del Cinquecento* (Imola: La mandragora, 2000), 139-46.
Franchi, Giuseppe. 'Apparecchi e metodi per "lambiccare" secondo Mattioli', in *I Giardini dei Semplici e gli Orti Botanici della Toscana*, ed. Sara Ferri and Francesca Vannozzi (Perugia: Quattroemme, 1993), 201-4.
Goethals, Jessica. 'The Patronage Politics of Equestrian Ballet: Allegory, Allusion, and Satire in the Courts of Seventeenth-Century Italy and France', *Renaissance Quarterly*, 70 (2017), 1397-1448.
Goldthwaite, Richard. 'The Practice and Culture of Accounting in Renaissance Florence', *Enterprise & Society*, 16 (2015), 611-47.
Graziani, Natale and Gabriella Venturelli. *Caterina Sforza* (Milan: Mondadori, 2001).
Henry, John. 'The Fragmentation of Renaissance Occultism and the Decline of Magic', *History of Science*, 46 (2008), 1-48.
Herzig, Tamar. 'The Demons and the Friars: Illicit Magic and Mendicant Rivalry in Renaissance Bologna', *Renaissance Quarterly*, 64 (2011), 1025-58.
Kieckhefer, Richard. *European Witch Trials: Their Foundations in Popular and Learned Culture, 1300-1500* (London: Routledge and Kegan Paul, 1976).
Klein, Ursula and E.C. Spary, 'Introduction: Why Materials?', in *Materials and Expertise in Early Modern Europe: Between Market and Laboratory*, ed. Ursula Klein and E.C. Spary (Chicago: University of Chicago Press, 2010), 1-23.
Laroche, Rebecca. *Medical Authority and Englishwomen's Herbal Texts, 1550-1650* (Aldershot: Ashgate, 2009).
LeJacq, Seth Stein. 'The Bounds of Domestic Healing: Medical Recipes, Storytelling, and Surgery in Early Modern England', *Social History of Medicine*, 26 (2013), 451-68.
Leong, Elaine. '"Herbals she peruseth": Reading Medicine in Early Modern England', *Renaissance Studies*, 28 (2014), 556-78.
—. 'Making Medicines in the Early Modern Household', *Bulletin of the History of Medicine*, 82 (2008), 145-68.
Leong, Elaine and Sara Pennell. 'Recipe Collections and the Currency of Medical Knowledge in the Early Modern "Medical Marketplace"', in *Medicine and the*

Marketplace in England and its Colonies, c.1450-c.1850, ed. Mark S.R. Jenner and Patrick Wallis (Houndsmills: Palgrave Macmillan, 2007), 133-52.

Leong, Elaine and Alisha Rankin. 'Testing Drugs and Trying Cures: Experiment and Medicine in Medieval and Early Modern Europe', *Bulletin of the History of Medicine*, 91 (2017), 157-82.

'Lettere di Giovanni de' Medici detto delle Bande Nere', *Archivio Storico Italiano*, n.s., 9.2a (1859), 109-47.

Long, Pamela O. *Artisan/Practitioners and the Rise of the New Sciences, 1400-1600* (Corvallis, OR: Oregon State University Press, 2011).

Lubkin, Gregory. *A Renaissance Court: Milan under Galeazzo Maria Sforza* (Berkeley/Los Angeles: University of California Press, 1994).

Lupo Gentile, Michele. *La politica di Paolo III nelle sue relazioni con la corte medicea* (Sarzana: Tipografia Lunense, 1906).

Martins, Julia Gruman. 'Understanding/Controlling the Female Body in Ten Recipes: Print and the Dissemination of Medical Knowledge about Women in the Early Sixteenth Century', in *Gender, Health, and Healing, 1250-1550*, ed. Sara Ritchey and Sharon Strocchia (Amsterdam: Amsterdam University Press, 2020), 167-88.

Moran, Bruce T. *Distilling Knowledge: Alchemy, Chemistry, and the Scientific Revolution* (Cambridge, MA: Harvard University Press, 2005).

Nolte, Cordula. 'Domestic Care in the Sixteenth Century: Expectations, Experiences, and Practices from a Gendered Perspective', in *Gender, Health, and Healing, 1250-1550*, ed. Sara Ritchey and Sharon Strocchia (Amsterdam: Amsterdam University Press, 2020), 215-43.

Nummedal, Tara. *Alchemy and Authority in the Holy Roman Empire* (Chicago: University of Chicago Press, 2007).

Ortolani, Oddone. *Pietro Carnesecchi: per la storia della vita religiosa italiana nel Cinquecento; con estratti dagli Atti del Processo del Santo Ufficio* (Florence: Le Monnier, 1963).

Park, Katharine. 'Medicine and Magic: The Healing Arts', in *Gender and Society in Renaissance Italy*, ed. Judith C. Brown and Robert C. Davis (London/New York: Longman, 1998), 129-49.

Pelling, Margaret. '"Thoroughly Resented?" Older Women and their Medical Role in Early Modern London', in *Women, Science and Medicine, 1500-1700: Mothers and Sisters of the Royal Society*, ed. Lynette Hunter and Sarah Hutton (Stroud: Sutton, 1997), 63-88.

Principe, Lawrence M. *The Secrets of Alchemy* (Chicago: University of Chicago Press, 2012).

Rankin, Alisha. 'Exotic Materials and Treasured Knowledge: The Valuable Legacy of Noblewomen's Remedies in Early Modern Germany', *Renaissance Studies*, 28 (2014), 533-55.

—. 'How to Cure the Golden Vein: Medical Remedies as *Wissenschaft* in Early Modern Germany', in *Ways of Making and Knowing: The Material Culture of Empirical Knowledge*, ed. Pamela H. Smith, Amy R.W. Meyers, and Harold J. Cook (Ann Arbor, MI: University of Michigan Press, 2014), 113-37.

—. *Panaceia's Daughters: Noblewomen as Healers in Early Modern Germany* (Chicago: University of Chicago Press, 2013).

Ray, Meredith K. *Daughters of Alchemy: Women and Scientific Culture in Early Modern Italy* (Cambridge, MA: Harvard University Press, 2015).

Rosselli, Stefano Francesco di Romolo. *Mes secrets à Florence au temps des Médicis, 1593: pâtisserie, parfumerie, médecine*, transcribed, ed. and trans. Rodrigo de Zayas (Paris: Jean-Michel Place, 1996).

[Rusio, Lorenzo.] *La mascalcia di Lorenzo Rusio, volgarizzamente del secolo XIV messo per la prima volta in luce*, ed. Luigi Barbieri (Bologna: Romagnoli, 1867-70).

Sforza, Caterina. *Experimenti de la Ex.ma S.r Caterina da Furlj Matre de lo Illux. mo S.r Giovanni de Medici*, ed. Pier Desiderio Pasolini, 3 vols. (Imola: Ignazio Galeati e Figlio, 1894).

Smith, Pamela H. *The Body of the Artisan: Art and Experience in the Scientific Revolution* (Chicago: University of Chicago Press, 2004).

Snook, Edith. 'English Women's Writing and Indigenous Medical Knowledge in the Early Modern Atlantic World', in *A History of Early Modern Women's Writing*, ed. Patricia Phillippy (Cambridge: Cambridge University Press, 2018), 382-97.

Spini, Giorgio. *Cosimo I e l'indipendenza dello stato mediceo* (Florence: Vallecchi, 1980).

Strocchia, Sharon T. *Forgotten Healers: Women and the Pursuit of Health in Late Renaissance Italy* (Cambridge, MA: Harvard University Press, 2019).

Strozzi, Alessandra Macinghi. *Letters to her Sons (1447-1470)*, ed. and trans. Judith Bryce (Toronto: Iter Academic Press, 2016).

Tarrant, Neil. 'Giambattista Della Porta and the Roman Inquisition: Censorship and the Definition of Nature's Limits in Sixteenth-Century Italy', *British Journal for the History of Science*, 46 (2013), 601-25.

Thorndike, Lynn. *A History of Magic and Experimental Science*, 8 vols. (New York: Columbia University Press, 1923-58).

Torresi, Antonio P. *Il ricettario Bardi: cosmesi e tecnica atistica nella Firenze medicea* (Ferrara: Liberty House, 2004).

—. *Il ricettario Medici: alchimia, farmacopea, cosmesi e tecnica artistica nella Firenze del Seicento* (Ferrara: Liberty House, 2004).

Trivellato, Francesca. 'Guilds, Technology and Economic Change in Early Modern Venice', in *Guilds, Innovation and the European Economy, 1400-1800*, ed. Stephen R. Epstein and Maarten Prak (Cambridge: Cambridge University Press, 2010), 199-231.

Tuten, Belle S. 'Care of the Breast in the Late Middle Ages: The *Tractatus de passionibus mamillarum*', in *Gender, Health, and Healing, 1250-1550*, ed. Sara Ritchey and Sharon Strocchia (Amsterdam: Amsterdam University Press, 2020), 119-37.
Viroli, Marco. *Caterina Sforza, Leonessa di Romagna* (Cesena: Il Ponte Vecchio, 2008).
Voights, Linda Ehrsam and Ann Payne, 'Medicine for a Great Household (ca. 1500): Berkeley Castle Muniments Select Book 89', *Studies in Medieval and Renaissance History*, ser. 3, 12 (2016), 87-269.
Welch, Evelyn. 'Women as Patrons and Clients in the Courts of Quattrocento Italy', in *Women in Italian Renaissance Culture and Society*, ed. Letizia Panizza (Oxford: Legenda, 2000), 18-34.

About the Authors

Sheila Barker directs the Jane Fortune Research Program on Women Artists at the Medici Archive Project (Florence). Her publications include 'Artemisia Gentileschi in a Changing Light' (2017) and 'Cosimo I de' Medici and the Renaissance Sciences: "To Measure and to See"', in *The Brill Companion to Cosimo I de' Medici* (2019).

Sharon Strocchia is Professor of History at Emory University in Atlanta. A social and cultural historian of Renaissance Italy, she has published widely on women, religion, and health-related topics. Her most recent book is *Forgotten Healers: Women and the Pursuit of Health in Late Renaissance Italy* (2019).

6 Understanding/Controlling the Female Body in Ten Recipes

Print and the Dissemination of Medical Knowledge about Women in the Early Sixteenth Century

Julia Gruman Martins

Abstract

In 1529, a book called *Dificio di ricette* was published in Venice. It included ten recipes concerned with the female body, which aimed to instruct readers but also allowed them to control the female body, especially where reproduction was concerned. This book initiated a new trend of vernacular medical texts directed to a broad audience; it described practices, prescribed models, and served as a tool for readers to create their own experiments. When translated into other vernaculars, recipes were adapted to new readerships, with publishers and translators closely engaging and transforming their texts, reshaping the knowledge they diffused. By encouraging the discussion of these matters more openly in the vernacular, recipes potentially allowed female readers to actively regulate their own bodies.

Keywords: books of secrets, medical recipes, translation, vernacular medicine, reproduction

In 1529, an anonymous book called *Opera nuova intitolata Dificio di ricette*, or 'New Work called House of Recipes', was published in Venice.[1] It was a cheaply printed in-octavo booklet, containing miscellaneous recipes to aid and amuse the reader in his or her everyday life. It addressed the readership in an informal tone, and its preface underscored its utility, since it had been

1 Anon., *Opera nuova intitolata Dificio di ricette.*

Ritchey, Sara & Sharon Strocchia (eds), *Gender, Health, and Healing, 1250-1550*. Amsterdam, Amsterdam University Press 2020
DOI: 10.5117/9789463724517_CH06

published for the 'benefit of all people' ('beneficio universale'). The *Dificio di ricette* was the first printed book of secrets in Italy, inaugurating more than a century of best-selling print compilations of recipes in Europe, and deeply influencing subsequent works by Alessio Piemontese, Leonardo Fioravanti, Giambattista Della Porta, and others. The *Dificio* promised to reveal 'secrets' to its readers in the form of straightforward recipes illustrated by woodcuts. Among the dozens of magic tricks, cosmetic, culinary, and medical recipes contained in the collection, the reader was presented with ten practical secrets about women's bodies. These recipes aimed to instruct, but also allowed the reader to control the female body, especially where fertility and reproduction were concerned. Thanks to this book, the periodicity, quality, and quantity of menstruation could be regulated, conception assured, and questions about future children answered.

Having served as an inspiration for most books of secrets that followed it, the *Dificio* continued to be printed well into the nineteenth century. It was particularly successful in France, even more so than in Italy, arguably thanks to its clever translation. The publication of the *Dificio* can also be considered a turning point toward broader dissemination of knowledge about the female body, which was made available to a general readership. In their orientation toward practical knowledge of the body, vernacular books of secrets were closely connected to regimens and other health texts that became popular in the period.[2] These materials broke away from medieval writings on the subject, which were usually written in Latin and aimed at a specialized readership. Hybrid versions of medical texts, such as the treatise on breast care explored by Belle Tuten earlier in this volume, sometimes bridged both Latin and Italian materials and learned and household medicine.[3] By and large, printed books of secrets fulfilled a demand for vernacular medical texts addressed to lay readers in a time of growing vernacular literacy. Scholars have argued that 'secrets of women' started to be broadly disseminated in print in the sixteenth century through two genres: midwifery manuals and recipe books.[4] While the former exhibited important continuities with their medieval predecessors, the latter arguably constituted the first genre of medical writing produced for (and often by) women.

In the sixteenth century, medical print was defined by what Mary Fissell calls the three R's: regimens, recipes, and religious medical texts.

2 Cavallo and Storey, *Healthy Living*; Cavallo and Storey, eds., *Conserving Health in Early Modern Culture*; Hobby, 'Secrets of the Female Sex'.

3 Tuten, 'Care of the Breast'.

4 Green, ed., *Trotula*; Lemay, ed., *Women's Secrets*; Davis, *Society and Culture.*

Regimens and recipes can be understood as opposite sides of a coin. The first advised readers how to stay healthy while the second counselled what to do when they fell ill.[5] While these genres varied from one country to another, recipe books were ubiquitous throughout early modern Europe, becoming virtual best-sellers. Many of them, such as the *Dificio di ricette*, had an Italian origin, and were often known as 'books of secrets', with 'secret' and 'recipe' becoming synonymous over time.[6] As Sheila Barker and Sharon Strocchia show elsewhere in this volume, recipe books often assumed that readers had experiential knowledge of both the ingredients and procedures to be followed.[7] The exact quantity of ingredients is often omitted, as are specifics about what part of the plant should be used; moreover, therapeutic instructions could be vague, such as 'make an ointment'. Printed books of secrets were a genre rooted in practical use, one that was deeply connected to the Italian urban middle classes from which the genre emerged and which constituted the books' expected readers.

When books of secrets were translated into other vernaculars, several changes were made to enhance their appeal to new readers, which helps account for their success. The French version of the *Dificio*, for instance, included many synonyms and alternatives to ingredients; it was more open to the reader's context and was incorporated into the Bibliothèque bleue, a collection of popular books sold by itinerant pedlers in cities and countryside. Books of secrets were often 'rebranded' in translation, with one type of recipe becoming more prominent in the new version by the addition of other similar recipes. French versions of the *Dificio* gave new prominence to 'secrets of women', transforming the original, shorter domestic guide into a more explicitly medical text. The broad vernacular tradition surrounding 'secrets of women' was not without contradictions. Even though women figured among expected readers, these materials often reinforced women's dependence on male physicians, much like most midwifery texts; recipe books, on the other hand, arguably encouraged more female agency, as did the *Dificio di ricette*.[8]

In this essay, I analyse how the process of translating recipes about the female body from Italian into French altered and adapted them for new

5 Fissell, 'Popular Medical Writing'.

6 Eamon, *Science and the Secrets of Nature*.

7 Barker and Strocchia, 'Household Medicine for a Renaissance Court'.

8 For a more detailed analysis, see Green, *Making Women's Medicine Masculine*, and Green, 'From "Diseases of Women" to "Secrets of Women"'.

readers. By focusing on one book, I show how the translation of individual recipes helped to 'rebrand' the book and even the genre of secrets itself by reshaping the content as well as the goal of the text for new readers. The translator demonstrated remarkable flexibility in offering synonyms and alternatives for the materia medica involved in each recipe and he often simplified recipes to facilitate memorization. This flexibility and simplification suggests an interest in transmitting body knowledge to a broad readership that included both women and men, residents of the city and countryside, and more as well as less literate individuals. In the ten recipes that offered handy solutions to 'conditions of women' (ranging from reproduction to venereal disease), the reader was confronted with the possibility of not only better understanding the female body but also acting upon it, thereby potentially giving female readers, in particular, more agency over their own bodies.

The *Dificio di ricette* was addressed to a broad readership and did not presume any specialized or theoretical knowledge about the body. It is unclear how and by whom these recipes were used, but there is no reason to believe that laywomen could not access this information. Still, more research is needed to fully understand the reception of recipes by analysing marginalia and reader's annotations.[9] Regardless of reading practices, printed recipe compilations made it possible for midwives, surgeons, and laywomen to access a corpus of medical knowledge that could have daily application in the household and the local community. Here I focus on the role of publishers and translators in both reshaping and diffusing 'secrets of women', demonstrating how closely they engaged with their texts.

The original Italian edition of the *Dificio di ricette* published in Venice consisted of 187 recipes, most of them simple and easy to follow. Reflecting its Venetian context, the *Dificio* was directed at urban elites and the middle classes, who were often more literate than their counterparts in other European cities.[10] The *Dificio* was meant to be both useful and amusing. It was a household manual that addressed domestic needs, but its imagined reader was someone sophisticated enough to entertain at home who was also interested in cosmetics and general hygiene practices.

9 While recent scholars have focused on manuscript recipes, the relationship between print and manuscript secrets has yet to be fully understood. Efforts at bridging that gap include Pennell, 'Perfecting Practice?'; Shanahan, *Manuscript Recipe Books as Archaeological Objects*; Leong, 'Collecting Knowledge for the Family'; Leong, '"Herbals she peruseth"'; DiMeo and Pennell, eds., *Reading Writing Recipe Books*.

10 Deblock, ed., *Le Bâtiment des recettes*.

The recipes contained in the *Dificio* therefore can be divided into two categories: those meant to entertain and those that were useful in a practical sense. The first group included magic tricks such as 'how to make a candle burn underwater' or 'how to cook an egg without fire'. Other 'fun' recipes might be used in popular festivities or to play pranks, such as 'how to dye a horse green' or 'how to paint a man's beard blue'.[11] When the *Dificio* was translated into French, these recipes lost some of their relevance, especially since new medical treatises were added to the original text, indicating that publishers anticipated a shift in readership. Indeed, the newly imagined reader seemed to be more concerned with domestic medicine and the care of the body, and less so with magic tricks for guests.

By contrast with the first group of recipes geared toward amusement, the second group was composed of 'useful recipes' that could be used in the household in a myriad of ways. These included recipes for 'how to make fruit preserves', 'how to make ink to write', and 'how to produce cosmetics'. Most of the recipes in this category, however, concerned medicaments that could be made and used by family members, especially female householders. Of the 187 recipes in the *Dificio di ricette*, the 10 concerning the female body account for roughly 6 per cent of the total.

The *Dificio di ricette* was enormously successful in Italy, being reprinted twenty-eight times by the end of the eighteenth century, but it reached an even broader readership in France.[12] Translated as the *Bâtiment des recettes*, it was reprinted sixty times, the last known edition dating from 1830.[13] The French edition also acted as a 'cultural mediator', to use Geneviève Deblock's expression; in 1545 the Dutch translation was made using the French version, and subsequently reprinted six times.[14] This kind of indirect translation was not unusual in the early years of print, nor was it considered to be inferior to direct translation from the original language; for instance, Alessio Piemontese's book of secrets was translated into English from the French edition, rather than the Italian original.[15] Indeed, publishers, translators,

11 Deblock, 'Astuces, farces, magie'.

12 Deblock, ed., *Le Bâtiment des recettes*.

13 *Le Bâtiment des recettes, traduit de l'italien, et augmenté d'une infinité de beaux secrets, avec un autre traité de recettes intitulé Le Grand jardin.*

14 Deblock, 'Le Bâtiment des recettes'; Van Heurck, *Les livres populaires flamands*, 144-45. The 'Pleasant garden' was also translated from French into Dutch and printed independently from the other parts of the *Bâtiment* in 1657.

15 Piemontese, *Secrets of the Reverend Maister Alexis of Piedmont*; Ferguson, 'Secrets of Alexis'; Demetriou and Tomlinson, '"Abroad in Mens Hands"'.

and booksellers formed an international network in which books circulated widely from one country and language to another. The famous Antwerp printer Christophe Plantin (1520-1589) undertook translations of Italian books into Latin, French, and Dutch, capitalizing on the market potential for books of secrets.[16]

Because the *Dificio* enjoyed an international circulation, one of the main questions arising from its study must concern translation. The first French edition was made in 1539 and published by Jean III Du Pre, a printer from Lyon. Another, possibly earlier, translation, entitled *Difficile des receptes*, was probably printed between 1529 and 1560 in Lyon.[17] As the title indicates, however, it is a very poor translation and was not reprinted elsewhere, to the best of my knowledge. In the long history of the *Dificio*, every publisher changed something, leaving the mark of his workshop in the book. However, Jean Du Pre dramatically transformed the nature of the *Dificio*, making it more focused on the 'secrets of women'. He added to it a compilation of obstetric recipes called 'other medical secrets, besides those proposed by the Italian compilation, specifically for women'. This addition, comprised of twenty-six recipes, brought the complement of 'secrets of women' to 17 per cent of the total recipes in the book. It was usual for publishers to add compilations to translations, but it happened more frequently with books of secrets, which were often printed with other works, including recipes by the translator himself.[18] In this case, however, the author of the compilation was anonymous, as was the translator. Nevertheless, the fact that the publisher decided to add these recipes 'specifically for women' indicates that he saw the 'secrets of women' already present as being important or useful enough to justify adding a whole new section on the subject. These additions undoubtedly made the text more marketable to female readers.

In 1551, another compilation was added to the *Bâtiment des recettes*, called the 'Pleasant garden' ('Le plaisant jardin'). It too was a translation of Italian recipes that had been printed elsewhere in France.[19] Unfortunately, the original Italian compilation has never been identified. The 'Pleasant garden'

16 Voet, *Golden Compasses*, vol. 1, ch. 1, 1-138.

17 Anon., *Difficile des receptes*.

18 Examples include Fioravanti, *Short Discours of the Excellent Doctour and Knight, Maister Leonardo Phioravanti Bolognese upon Chirurgerie*; Pantin, 'John Hester's Translations of Leonardo Fioravanti'; Piemontese, *De secretis libri septem*; Piemontese, *Kunstbuch des wolerfarnen Herren Alexii Pedemontani*.

19 This version was edited by the father-in-law of Jean Ruelle, who became the most important printer of the *Bâtiment* in France; Deblock, ed., *Le Bâtiment des recettes*.

was a mixed compilation of medical recipes, with only one concerning the female body, namely 'how to treat sore nipples'. The translator's name is mentioned as 'Quiller or Quilleri de Passebreve', who seems to have been a French physician known for his alchemical and astrological interests.[20] No translator is named for the other two parts of the book. From this point forward, these two recipe collections were always printed with the translation of the *Dificio di ricette*, making the French *Bâtiment des recettes* more than twice the size of the original book. To the 187 recipes from the original *Dificio*, another 26 recipes 'concerning women' were added, along with 202 recipes culled from the 'Pleasant garden'. These additions meant that about 9 per cent of the *Bâtiment des recettes* concerned 'secrets of women'.

By adding these materials, French publishers changed the nature of the *Dificio di ricette*. From a general household guide focused on entertaining and household tasks, it became oriented more specifically towards care of the body and 'self-medicine', with recipes about the female body becoming central to the book. This transformation included many actors involved in the printing world, ranging from compilers and publishers to correctors, collaborators, and especially translators. Their shared project adapted the empirical knowledge contained in the *Dificio* for French readers.

Once the *Bâtiment* became part of the famous collection of popular books known as the Bibliothèque bleue from the mid-seventeenth century, it started to be sold in the countryside by itinerant pedlers as well as in cities, reaching an even more diverse readership.[21] Some scholars suggest that Parisian readers alone represented half the potential readership for these books, since roughly half of literate French adults lived there. However, rural areas should not be forgotten as a part of the vibrant world of early modern print.[22] Since reading and writing were often learned separately, using the ability to sign one's name – the traditional indicator of literacy – may prove misleading.[23] Most likely, far more readers existed than is usually thought, both in cities and in the countryside, especially since collective reading was a customary practice in early modern Europe. Moreover, medical books were often collectively owned as well.[24]

The *Bâtiment* was one of the most popular books sold in rural areas as part of the Bibliothèque bleue, probably because of its practical nature.

20 Hoefer, *Nouvelle Biographie générale*.

21 Chartier, 'Stratégies éditoriales et lectures populaires'.

22 Mellot, 'La capitale et l'imprimé a l'apogée de l'absolutisme'.

23 Davis, *Society and Culture*, 194-95.

24 Chartier, 'Loisir et sociabilité'; Jones, 'Book Ownership and the Lay Culture of Medicine'.

The *Bâtiment* itself claimed that it was directed to 'men and women who could read and were refined', implying that it targeted urban social elites. However, intended and real readers often diverged, and in this case the readership was so diversified that generalizations may be unwise. In her survey of the sixty French reprints of the *Bâtiment*, for instance, Geneviève Deblock argues that the annotations in the books indicate readers who knew how to write poorly or not at all.[25] Still, the gap between reading and writing abilities, on the one hand, and collective reading practices, on the other, must be kept in mind in assessing the projected audience for these texts.

The *Bâtiment* attained its definitive version in the 1560 edition by Jean Ruelle. That edition included the greatest number of recipes concerned with medicine, particularly 'secrets of women'. In the following comparison, I use the original Italian *Dificio* of 1529 and the French translation of 1560, since most successive versions were reprinted from this definitive edition.[26] However, I do not include in this analysis the twenty-six recipes regarding the female body added by French printers, since the original Italian text has not been identified.

The first recipe of the 'secrets of women' is titled 'To know whose fault it is that a couple cannot have children, the man's or the woman's' ('A voler saper per chi mancha a ingravedare o per lhuomo o per la donna', D, 1v/'Pour savoir à qui il tient que la conception ne se face, ou s'il tient à la femme, ou s'il tient à l'homme, en cas qu'ils ayent longtemps este mariez ensemble', B, 2; see Appendix 6.1 for comparison). The first thing one notices about this recipe is that the duration of marriage is emphasized in the French title, perhaps suggesting that readers need to be patient and consult this recipe only after several years of childless marriage. This emphasis is absent from the original Italian title. The concern with infertility, the perpetuation of the lineage, and the 'precarious nature of fatherhood', to use Katharine Park's phrase, hinged to a large degree on the womb and its mysterious nature.[27] Important questions such as paternity and inheritance were therefore deeply connected to 'secrets of women'. While much attention has been given to abortifacients in early modern recipes, infertility – especially in relation to gender and masculinity – remains a

25 Deblock, ed., *Le Bâtiment des recettes*, 33.

26 Anon., *Opera nuova intitolata Dificio di ricette*; Anon., *Bastiment de receptes*. All further comparisons are drawn from these books and indicated by D (for *Dificio di ricette*) or B (for *Bâtiment des recettes*) and the page number.

27 Park, *Secrets of Women*.

subject that is only beginning to be explored, as seen in Catherine Rider's essay elsewhere in this volume.[28]

From a translation standpoint, the most intriguing aspect of this recipe is that the main ingredient in Italian, semolina ('semola'), appears in the French text as 'froment ou seigle ou orge', meaning respectively wheat, rye, or barley. Three grains are offered to the French reader, whereas only one was given in Italian. Interestingly, their order seems to be decrescent in price.[29] The translator probably had a diverse readership in mind; he considered readers with different budgets or living in different areas of the country, where access to grains might vary. Consequently, the translator created options for new readers. In this recipe, both the man and the woman were instructed to urinate in the grain. If worms appeared in one of the samples after three days, that person was responsible for the couple's infertility, thus offering the possibility of displacing feminine blame for infertility, often regarded as a woman's responsibility. Whether the same result could be obtained with alternative grains does not seem to have worried the translator.

The next recipe, 'to know whether one is a virgin, meaning if seed has been expelled' ('A conoscer se uno o una e verzene dico se lha sparso il seme', D, 2r/'A cognoistre si une personne est vierge, soit malle ou femelle, j'entens si elle est corrompue, ou de soy ou autrement', B, 9), is another example of how the titles are rendered more complex in French. The translator adds that the loss of virginity could happen through one's own action or that of someone else. This alteration may indicate a stronger concern in France about self-corruption through masturbation, or it may be that the Italian version is more pragmatic, only dealing with corruption that might jeopardize the marriage, such as a woman who is already pregnant with another man's child. Most likely, the French text indicates a greater concern with the health-promoting aspects of releasing seed. If so, the French translation transcends the context in which the seed was expelled to privilege instead the physiological aspect of the action. Medically speaking, these actions had the same result, even though masturbation and 'corruption' through intercourse were socially very different.[30] In any case, the focus shifts from expelled seed in Italian to the corruption of the body in French, with 'seed' being omitted from the translation. This could indicate that medical debates of the time about whether women as well as men released seed were more controversial in France.

28 Rider, 'Gender, Old Age, and the Infertile Body'.

29 Appleby, 'Grain Prices and Subsistence Crises'.

30 Cadden, *Meanings of Sex Difference*; Laqueur, *Making Sex*.

The third translated recipe is an emmenagogue designed to stimulate menstruation ('A far produr el suo tempo a una donna che lo variasse o perdesse', D, 7r/'Pour faire avoir les fleurs a une femme qui les eust perdues, ou qui en fust desreiglee', B, 64). Several herbs were known to provoke contractions of the womb, which regulated menstruation and treated amenorrhea.[31] Recipes to provoke menstruation were particularly common in this period, since purging the womb was understood to be central to women's health. A 'clean' womb was considered a more favourable environment for conception and essential to female health.[32] In this recipe, 'flower' and 'time' or 'terms' are used as synonyms, as was often the case in early modern Europe. The herb feverfew ('madrigale') is translated as 'espargoutte ou madrigal', indicating the translator's awareness that readers might know the plant by different names, depending on their level of instruction or geographical region. Hence the Latin-derived *madrigal* is complemented by the popular term *espargoutte*.[33] This practice of translating one word with two or more synonyms occurs often in books of secrets, indicating their practical function and the need to identify the herb correctly to a diverse readership.

Given the variety of local names for herbs, it is not surprising that some of them could not be translated. The usual solution was to leave the word in the original language, which rendered the recipe less useful but retained the secret's mystery. This is the case in the fourth recipe concerning menorrhagia (excessive menstruation), which aims 'to contain the natural flux of a woman who has it abundantly' ('A far restrenzer el corso natural de una donna se li abondasse', D, 7r/'Pour faire restraind[r]e le cours n[a]turel a une femme qui l'eust trop abondant et oultre mesure', B, 65). Women were instructed to make an ointment using something called *linardo* and to spread it around their vagina and pubic area. Although it has not been possible to definitively identify the untranslated ingredient in either language, it must have been common enough in early modern Venice. A seventeenth-century Spanish-Italian dictionary renders *linardo* as a synonym for *asarabacca*, our modern wild ginger or hazelwort.[34] If this identification is correct, *linardo* would be a diuretic, laxative, and emetic. It is not clear why it would be used to stop menstruation. Regardless, had

31 McClive, 'Bleeding Flowers and Waning Moons'; Hindson, 'Attitudes towards Menstruation and Menstrual Blood'.

32 Stolberg, 'Menstruation and Sexual Difference'.

33 *Espargoutte* could be used in baths as well as drunk in solutions; Renou, *Les Œuvres pharmaceutiques*, esp. ch. 14.

34 Franciosini, *Vocabulario Espanol e Italiano*.

the French translator understood the word, he might have opted for one of many available synonyms, such as *asaret, cabaret, oreille-d'homme*, or a more regional name such as *oreillette* or *rondelle*.[35] The point is that, instead of suppressing the recipe, the translator kept it despite the untranslatable word so as not to diminish the collection's overall value. It demonstrates the translator's effort to preserve and transmit useful remedies even in instances when certain ingredients remained mysterious or unavailable on a local level.

The fifth recipe, 'to make women pregnant' ('A far ingravedar le donne', D, 10v/'Pour trouver moyen de faire engrossir une femme qui ne peut avoir enfans de son mary', B, 107) further exemplifies the era's preoccupation with conception. While some recipes concentrate on one treatment, this one suggests several ways of enhancing fertility, including a pessary, eating eggs, drinking herbal mixtures, and taking medicinal baths. Readers could make a pessary of lemon and honey, using the juice of wormwood ('ascenzo'). In French, two synonyms are again offered to the reader, 'aluine' and 'absinthe', and ingredients absent from the original text are added, such as balm leaves and lily of the valley. The French version emphasizes that, when using a medicinal bath to enhance fertility, the reader should 'use odorant herbs *appropriate to her case*'. This inflection is missing in the Italian original; a fragrant bath is mentioned, but not that specific herbs should be picked with the woman's condition in mind. Underlining the importance of tacit and experiential knowledge, it is assumed that the reader will be sufficiently familiar with herbs to forego specific instructions. Similarly, mead or wine is substituted in the French version for the unfamiliar Moscato wine as the liquid base for herb mixtures. This adjustment illustrates how cultural translation often accompanied linguistic changes. Later editions also modernized the title of the recipe to stress its value in treating female infertility ('pour la stérilité des femmes'). This attention to issues of translation demonstrates an effort to localize body knowledge and to disseminate recipes to a broad audience, one that aimed to establish some amount of greater agency over their bodies.

Recipe no. 6 displayed similar concerns with issues of fertility: 'how to know if a woman can have children or not' ('A sapere se la donna pol haver figlioli overo no', D, 11r/'Pour savoir si la femme pourra concevoir ou non', B, 108). Again, the translator seems concerned with issues of access to ingredients, considering varied budgets and geography. At the

35 *Dictionnaire Larousse*, Les Editions Larousse, s.v. 'asaret', www.larousse.fr/dictionnaires/francais/asaret/5613.

same time, this recipe highlights some of the complexities underlying vernacular instructions for assuring fertility and reproductive health. Since the womb was invisible and largely inaccessible, it invited different ways of knowing that combined oral and written knowledge as well as manuscript and print information. 'Secrets of women' provided an 'open interpretative space', as Mary Fissell calls it, in which readers' practice and written instructions coexisted.[36] Recipes did not merely offer prescriptive models for what the reader should do. Rather, they offered a 'toolkit' from which people could select in developing their own empirical healthcare practices.[37] When the French translator rendered common mallow ('malba salvatica') as 'mauve sauvage ou guimauve' in this recipe, he simultaneously identified local ingredients while offering the reader additional tools with which to work.

The seventh recipe was eventually transformed into a new recipe in French reprints. Its subject concerned 'how to know how many children a woman will have by looking at her first' ('A saper quanti figlioli die haver una veduto il primo parto', D, 11r/'Pour savoir combien d'enfans doit avoir une femme en voyant son premier', B, 109). The first difference between Italian and French concerns the title. In Italian, the first labour indicates the number of children the woman may have; in French it is the first baby. It is significant that the French version specifically places the midwife in the birth scene, whereas in Italian that word (*levatrice* or *ostetrica*) is not used. Instead, the Italian recipe references a 'matron' ('comare'), an older woman who already had children and who would help with the childbirth, but who was not a specialized practitioner. The French version appears more open to childbirths attended by a midwife, a matron, or both, while in Italian the midwife is not as central. The relation of these terms to actual practice warrants further investigation, but regardless of the identity of the practitioner, the translation practice reveals an interest in localizing knowledge oriented around women's bodies.

This recipe also exemplifies another trend in publishing early modern books of secrets: rearranging recipes. Printers often would cut a recipe that was considered too long into two or more segments, making them more accessible to readers with limited reading skills; this division was important because recipes often had to be learned by memory. In Italian, this recipe ends with a section on how to figure the number of future male offspring. By contrast, in French this part is transformed into a

36 Fissell, *Vernacular Bodies*.

37 Gentilcore makes a similar point concerning vernacular regimens in *Food and Health*.

new recipe, 'how to know how many male children a woman can have' ('Pour savoir combien d'enfans masles pourra avoir une femme', B, 110). The reader was advised to count the number of 'crowns of hair' on the first baby's head. Regardless, both recipe books point to the importance of male progeny for sustaining familial property and reputation. Such knowledge could be incredibly useful to a woman negotiating status in filial relationships.

The final two recipes (nos. 8 and 9 in the *Dificio* and 9 and 10 in the *Bâtiment*) are very broad in scope. They deal with venereal diseases, specifically syphilis, as well as leprosy (in the first case) and gout (in the second). The first recipe is intended 'to purify the blood'. The recipe title goes on to state that 'the purification [is good] against most illnesses and especially against the French disease and leprous sores' ('A purificar el sangue la qual purification e contra la magior parte di ogni infirmita e massime contra li mal franzosi et rogne leurose', D, 17r/'Pour purifier le sang, qui est chose propre à la plus grand' partie de toutes les maladies, mesmement a la maladie de Naples, et toute rognes lepreuses qui pour onction quelconque ne se veulent partir', B, 147). This recipe aims to treat syphilis and leprosy indirectly by balancing the humors. It reminds us of the reach of the Hippocratic and Galenic humoral understanding of the body in early modern Europe, and how restoring the balance of the humors and their qualities would serve several purposes, including the cure of venereal ailments.[38]

This recipe is also noteworthy because it showcases the importance of cultural adaptations, or 'cultural translation', as Peter Burke puts it.[39] Indeed, expressions are often 'negotiated' from one language to another, according to Burke. In cultural exchanges such as translation, two languages can mutually influence one another, without a 'perfect translation' ever being reached. The arrangement reached in this process is not a definite translation, but still renders the circulation of ideas possible while adapting expressions to their new context.[40] In this case, syphilis was known by many names in the period, but was usually called the 'French evil' or 'French disease' ('mal francese') in Italian. When the text was translated into French, the expression was transformed into the 'Naples evil' or 'Neapolitan disease'. Each area associated the illness with its neighbour, giving the ailment several

38 King, *Hippocrates' Woman*; Keller, '"That Sublimest Juyce in Our Body"'; Fissell, *Vernacular Bodies*.

39 Burke, 'Cultures of Translation in Early Modern Europe'; Boutcher, 'From Cultural Translation to Cultures of Translation?'.

40 Burke, 'Cultures of Translation in Early Modern Europe', 9.

different names. Translators were attentive enough to replace the name of the disease in order to associate its stigma with a different geographical origin.

While the previous recipe treated syphilis through purification of the blood, the final recipe treated its symptoms specifically. This recipe, 'for every pain, whether from the French disease or from gout, or any other sort' ('Ad ogni dolia o si adel mal franzioso over delle gotte e de ogni altra sorte', D, 17v/'Contre toutes gouttes de quelque sorte qu'elles soient, ou de la verole ou autrement', B, 148), should be used in painful or uncomfortable stages of the disease. One of the ingredients in the remedy, worms ('vermi'), is translated by two synonyms, 'vers ou lombriz', reminding us that the translator carefully rendered the translation as complete as possible by choosing two synonyms for something as commonplace as earthworms.

In conclusion, these ten recipes tell us many things about the circulation of knowledge about the female body in early modern Europe. First, serious work went into its translation, despite its low-quality print, small format, and inexpensive paper and binding. Cheap print is often associated with mispagination and careless work by publishers and translators, but whoever translated the *Dificio* into French tried to do a thorough job, thereby blurring the lines between 'learned' and 'popular' print cultures. Second, the nature of this book suggests that positing too sharp a divide between 'elite' and 'popular' readers may prove fruitless when studying early modern vernacular books of secrets. Because most recipes offer synonyms for ingredients, it seems that translators and publishers carefully considered varied readerships. Synonyms appealed to readers with different skills, different budgets, and different access to local plants. In any case, these recipes represent a major departure from medieval writings about the female body that required a reading knowledge of Latin, as well as specialized, theoretical knowledge about the properties of herbs. Instead, printed books of secrets offered readers simple recipes to solve everyday problems.

Furthermore, the translation indicates the tension between the more prescriptive quality of the Italian recipes and their French version, which were necessarily adapted to a new context. It would be a mistake to suggest that Italian readers were prompted to follow recipes to the letter, while French readers were actively encouraged to experiment with them. Nevertheless, tensions between the two models are perceptible throughout books of secrets, which probably stem more from their print context and target audience than from different medical understandings. The dynamic, highly competitive Venetian print market shaped the *Dificio* into a short book composed of 187 straightforward recipes that could be retailed easily; by contrast, subsequent French editions offered a more comprehensive medical handbook containing more than 400 recipes. The Italian version targeted urban, middle-class readers, while its French counterpart aimed to be peddled in both city and countryside.[41] To be marketable in French rural areas, popular books like recipe collections needed to take geographical context, class differences, and levels of literacy into account.

The fact that the main modifications to these recipes concerned ingredients is also telling, rendering these books of secrets closer to herbals. There is little difference in the production processes indicated in the two recipe collections; in fact, sometimes these basic techniques are not even mentioned, implying that most readers would already be familiar with them. The rearrangement of recipes into shorter ones in the French translations also indicates a preference for short, simple texts, illustrating how perception of the intended audience took people with different literacy skills into account. Furthermore, by adding greater precision to the recipes, French translators expected that readers would actively try them out and wanted to help them achieve their goal.

The *Dificio di ricette* was one of the first printed books of secrets of a genre that flourished in early modern Europe. It inspired its successors as well as influenced other genres, such as herbals and medical manuals. Its success in France was partly due to the addition of original recipes, and partly due to the work of publishers and translators whose adaptations transformed it into a more comprehensive medical handbook. 'Secrets of women' held a significant place in that compendium. By adapting and reshaping recipes for the female body, translators and publishers tried to make those secrets as useful and understandable as possible. Despite their name, books of secrets aimed to reveal knowledge to a general readership, breaking with the tradition of secrecy in areas such as reproductive health. These books allow us to imagine, as Sara Verskin does in her essay in this volume, the ways in which medical information described as restricted might actually point to women's participation in the production and transmission of medical knowledge.[42] The commercial success of the *Dificio* in France is particularly intriguing, since its focus on self-care may have appealed

41 Andries and Bollème, *La Bibliothèque bleue*; Fontaine, *Histoire du Colportage en Europe*.

42 Verskin, 'Gender Segregation and the Possibility of Arabo-Galenic Gynecological Practice'.

especially to female readers eager to acquire more effective ways of caring for their health.[43]

Recipes about female reproductive issues offered readers a vernacular 'toolkit' from which they could pick and choose, creating their own arsenal of medical knowledge by adding to their recipe collections.[44] While it could be argued that these books present male readers with ways of controlling the female body as well, a closer reading indicates that the nature of these recipes focuses on self-care; that is, these medical recipes were meant to be prepared and used on one's own body, or perhaps by friends and family. Books of secrets seem to have been more of a resource for female readers than a way for male readers to 'manage' women's bodies, unlike many contemporary midwifery manuals written mainly by and for male practitioners. The assumption that the reader of these 'secrets of women' would be familiar with the appropriate herbs, quantities, and procedures to follow not only indicates a high level of tacit knowledge, it could also point to a likely female readership, since manuals about the subject addressed to men tended to follow a distinctive style.[45]

Using the female body as a category of analysis for translation offers unique insight into early modern perceptions of women and women's role in healthcare, especially in the universe of print. Translation is a key aspect of the study of vernacular texts because it shows how recipes could be adapted from one context to another, providing readers with different degrees of agency and autonomy. The translation of vernacular medical texts also raises important questions about how new markets for this kind of knowledge were developed, and how these markets influenced perceptions of the female body, especially in matters of reproduction. What I hope to have shown here is that translators rendered knowledge about the female body available to a myriad of new readers, including women who were potentially empowered by these 'secrets'.

43 Pennell, 'Perfecting Practice?'

44 Leong, '"Herbals she peruseth"'.

45 A famous example of this trend is Raynalde's 1540 translation of Rösslin's *Der Rosengarten*. A modern version is published as *When Midwifery Became the Male Physician's Province*.

Appendix

Table 6.1 Recipe ingredients compared

Title in Italian	Title in French	Ingredients (Italian)	Ingredients (French)
A voler saper per chi mancha a ingravedare o per lhuomo o per la donna (D. 1v)	Pour savoir à qui tient que la conception ne se face, ou s'il tient à la femme, ou s'il tient à l'homme, en cas qu'ils ayent longtemps este mariez ensemble (B. 2)	Semola	Froment ou Seigle ou Orge
A conoscer se uno o una e verzene dico se lha sparso il seme (D. 2r)	A cognoistre si une personne est vierge, soit masle ou femelle, j'entens si elle est corrom-pue ou de soy ou autrement (B. 9)	Ace over spago	Fillet ou Fisselle
A far produr el suo tempo a una donna che lo variasse o perdesse (D. 7r)	Pour faire avoir les fleurs à une femme qui les eust perdues ou qui en fust des reiglee (B. 64)	Madrigale	Espargoutte ou madrigal
A far restrenzer el corso natural de una donna se li abondasse (D. 7r)	Pour faire restrain-dre le cours naturel a une femme qui l'eust trop abondant et oultre mesure (B. 65)	Incenso Linardo Gala Bon vino caldo Ascenzo verde	Encens Linardo Noix de galle Bon vin vermeil Aluine verde
A far ingravedar le donne (D. 10v)	Pour trouver moyen de faire engrossir une femme qui ne peult avoir enfans de son mary (B. 107)	Citrone Mele Ascenzo Herbe odorifere Ovo fresco Bon vino Moscato	Citrons secs Miel Absynthe ou Aluine Herbes odorantes et propices Œuf frais Bon vin ou hydromel Citron Melisse Muguette
A sapere se la donna pol haver figlioli overo no (D. 11r)	Pour savoir si la femme pourra concevoir, ou non (B. 108)	Malba salvatica	Mauve sauvage ou guimauve

Title in Italian	Title in French	Ingredients (Italian)	Ingredients (French)
A saper quanti figlioli die haver una veduto il primo parto (D. 11r)	Pour vouloir savoir combien d'enfans doit avoir une femme, en voyant son premier (B. 109)	No ingredients – Guardar i nodi del boligolo	No ingredients – Regarder combien de neuds au nombril de la creature
(Part of the previous recipe)	Pour savoir combien d'enfans masles pourra avoir une femme (B. 110)	Second part of the previous recipe: No ingredients – Guardare le coronelle dei capelli	No ingredients – Prendre garde aux cercles ou chappelets de cheveux
A purificar el sangue laqual purification e contra la magior parte di ogni infirmita e massime contra li mal franzosi et rogne leurose (D. 17r)	Pour purifier le sang, qui est chose propre à la plus grand' partie de toutes les maladies, mesmement a la maladie de Naples, et toute rognes lepreuses qui pour onction quelconque ne se veulent partir (B. 147)	Sene Polipodi Epitimi Mirabolani citrini Sebeste Iua artice Acqua di lupuli Siropo di lupuli Fiori di boragine Bugolose Fiori di basilico Siropo di fumo Oximellis Siropo violato Zaffrayan scropulo Ambra Muschio	Fueilles de sené mundees Polipode Eptime Mirabolans citrins Sebesten Reglisse Germansree ou yua arthretica Fleurs de buglosse Bourroche Baselic Syrop de houbelon Oximel Syrop violat Scrupule de saffran Ambre Musc
Ad ogni dolia o si adel mal franzioso over delle gotte e de ogni altra sorte (D. 17v)	Contre toutes gouttes de quelque sorte qu'elles soient, ou de la verole ou autrement (B. 148)	Canuzole Vermi	Cannes d'hyebles Vers ou lombriz

N.B *Batiment* recipes are B + number, in which number is not the page number, but the number of the recipe in the book, while for the *Dificio* recipes the number is for the page.

Works Cited

Printed Works

Andries, Lise and Geneviève Bollème. *La Bibliothèque bleue: littérature de colportage* (Paris: Robert Laffont, 2003).

Anon. *Bastiment de receptes* (Paris: Jean Ruelle, 1560).

—. *Difficile des receptes* (Lyon: Jacques Moderne, *s.a.*).

—. *Opera nuova intitolata Dificio di ricette* (Venice: Giovannantonio e fratelli da Sabbio, 1529).

Appleby, Andrew B. 'Grain Prices and Subsistence Crises in England and France, 1590-1740', *Journal of Economic History*, 39.4 (1979), 865-87.

Barker, Sheila and Sharon Strocchia. 'Household Medicine for a Renaissance Court: Caterina Sforza's *Ricettario* Reconsidered', in *Gender, Health, and Healing, 1250-1550*, ed. Sara Ritchey and Sharon Strocchia (Amsterdam: Amsterdam University Press, 2020), 139-65.

Boutcher, Warren. 'From Cultural Translation to Cultures of Translation? Early Modern Readers, Sellers and Patrons', in *The Culture of Translation in Early Modern England and France (1500-1660)*, ed. Tania Demetriou and Rowan Tomlinson (Hampshire: Palgrave Macmillan, 2015), 22-40.

Burke, Peter. 'Cultures of Translation in Early Modern Europe', in *Cultural Translation in Early Modern Europe*, ed. Peter Burke and Ronnie Po-chia Hsia (Cambridge: Cambridge University Press, 2007), 7-38.

Cadden, Joan. *Meanings of Sex Difference in the Middle Ages: Medicine, Science, and Culture* (Cambridge: Cambridge University Press, 1993).

Cavallo, Sandra and Tessa Storey. *Healthy Living in Late Renaissance Italy* (Oxford: Oxford University Press, 2013).

—, eds. *Conserving Health in Early Modern Culture: Bodies and Environments in Italy and England* (Manchester: Manchester University Press, 2017).

Chartier, Roger. 'Loisir et sociabilité: lire à haute voix dans l'Europe moderne', ed. Patrick Dandrey, *Littératures Classiques*, 12 (1980), 127-47.

—. 'Stratégies éditoriales et lectures populaires, 1530-1660', in *Histoire de l'édition française*, vol. 1: *Le livre conquérant, du moyen age au milieu du XVII*[e] *siècle*, ed. Roger Chartier and Henri-Jean Martin (Paris: Fayard, 1989), 698-721.

Davis, Natalie Z. *Society and Culture in Early Modern France* (Malden: Polity Press, 1975).

Deblock, Geneviève. 'Astuces, farces, magie: les recettes de divertissements du "Bâtiment des recettes" (XVIe-XIXe siècles)', *Techniques & Culture*, 59 (2012), 25-39.

—. 'Le Bâtiment des recettes: un livre de secrets réédité du XVIe au XIXe siècle', MA diss., L'École Pratique des Hautes Études, 2012.

—, ed. *Le Bâtiment des recettes: présentation et annotation de l'édition Jean Ruelle, 1560* (Rennes: Presses universitaires de Rennes, 2015).

Demetriou, Tania and Rowan Tomlinson. '"Abroad in Mens Hands": The Culture of Translation in Early Modern England and France', in *The Culture of Translation in Early Modern England and France, 1500-1660*, ed. Tania Demetriou and Rowan Tomlinson (Basingstoke: Palgrave Macmillan, 2015), 1-21.

DiMeo, Michele and Sara Pennell, eds. *Reading Writing Recipe Books 1550-1800* (Manchester: Manchester University Press, 2013).

Eamon, William. *Science and the Secrets of Nature: Books of Secrets in Medieval and Early Modern Culture* (Princeton, NJ: Princeton University Press, 1994).

Ferguson, John. 'The Secrets of Alexis: A Sixteenth Century Collection of Medical and Technical Receipts', *Proceedings of the Royal Society of Medicine* 24.2 (1930), 225-46.

Fioravanti, Leonardo. *A Short Discours of the Excellent Doctour and Knight, Maister Leonardo Phioravanti Bolognese upon Chirurgerie, with a Declaration of Many Thinges, Necessarie to Be Knowne, Never Written before in This Order; Wherunto Is Added a Number of Notable Secrets* (London: Thomas East, 1580).

Fissell, Mary. 'Popular Medical Writing', in *The Oxford History of Popular Print Culture: Cheap Print in Britain and Ireland to 1660*, ed. Joad Raymond (Oxford: Oxford University Press, 2011), 417-30.

—. *Vernacular Bodies: The Politics of Reproduction in Early Modern England* (Oxford: Oxford University Press, 2004).

Fontaine, Laurence. *Histoire du Colportage en Europe: XVe-XIXe siècle* (Paris: Albin Michel, 1993).

Franciosini, Lorenzo. *Vocabulario Espanol e Italiano* (Rome: Camera Apostolica, 1638).

Gentilcore, David. *Food and Health in Early Modern Europe: Diet, Medicine and Society, 1450-1800* (London: Bloomsbury, 2015).

Green, Monica. 'From "Diseases of Women" to "Secrets of Women": The Transformation of Gynaecological Literature in the Later Middle Ages', *Journal of Medieval and Early Modern Studies*, 30.1 (2000), 5-40.

—. *Making Women's Medicine Masculine: The Rise of Pre-modern Gynaecology* (Oxford: Oxford University Press, 2008).

—, ed. *The Trotula* (Philadelphia: University of Pennsylvania Press, 2001).

Heurck, Émile H. van. *Les livres populaires flamands* (Antwerp: J.E. Buschmann, 1931).

Hindson, Bethan. 'Attitudes towards Menstruation and Menstrual Blood in Elizabethan England', *Journal of Social History*, 43.1 (2009), 89-114.

Hobby, Elaine. 'Secrets of the Female Sex: Jane Sharp, the Reproductive Female Body, and Early Modern Midwifery Manuals', *Women's Writing*, 8 (2001), 201-12.

Hoefer, Jean Chrétien Ferdinand. *Nouvelle Biographie générale, depuis les temps les plus reculés jusqu'à nos jours* (Paris: Firmin Didot, 1863).

Jones, Peter Murray. 'Book Ownership and the Lay Culture of Medicine in Tudor Cambridge', in *The Task of Healing: Medicine, Religion and Gender in England and the Netherlands 1450-1800*, ed. Hilary Marland and Margaret Pelling (Rotterdam: Erasmus, 1996), 49-68.

Keller, Eve. '"That Sublimest Juyce in our Body": Bloodletting and Ideas of the Individual in Early Modern England', *Philological Quarterly*, 86.1-2 (2007), 97-122.

King, Helen. *Hippocrates' Woman: Reading the Female Body in Ancient Greece* (New York: Routledge, 1998).

Laqueur, Thomas. *Making Sex: Body and Gender from the Greeks to Freud* (Cambridge, MA: Harvard University Press, 1990).

Le Batiment des recettes, traduit de l'italien, et augmenté d'une infinité de beaux secrets, avec un autre traité de recettes intitulé Le Grand jardin (Troyes: Jean-Antoine Garnier et Baudot, 1830).

Lemay, Helen Rodnite, ed. *Women's Secrets: A Translation of Pseudo-Albertus Magnus' De Secretis Mulierum with Commentaries* (Albany, NY: State University of New York Press, 1992).

Leong, Elaine. 'Collecting Knowledge for the Family: Recipes, Gender and Practical Knowledge in the Early Modern English Household', *Centaurus*, 55.2 (2013), 81-103.

—. '"Herbals she peruseth": Reading Medicine in Early Modern England', *Renaissance Studies*, 28.4 (2014), 556-78.

McClive, Cathy. 'Bleeding Flowers and Waning Moons: A History of Menstruation in France c. 1495-1761', PhD diss., University of Warwick, London, 2004.

Mellot, Jean-Dominique. 'La capitale et l'imprimé a l'apogée de l'absolutisme (1618-1723)', *Histoire et Civilisation du Livre*, 5 (2009), 17-44.

Pantin, Isabelle. 'John Hester's Translations of Leonardo Fioravanti: The Literary Career of a London Distiller', in *Renaissance Cultural Crossroads: Translation, Print and Culture in Britain, 1473-1640*, ed. Andrew Pettegree, S.K. Barker, and Brenda M. Hosington (Leiden/Boston: Brill, 2013), 159-83.

Park, Katharine. *Secrets of Women: Gender, Generation, and the Origins of Human Dissection* (New York: Zone Books, 2006).

Pennell, Sara. 'Perfecting Practice? Women, Manuscript Recipes and Knowledge in Early Modern England', in *Early Modern Women's Manuscript Writing: Selected Papers from the Trinity/Trent Colloquium*, ed. Victoria Burke and Jonathan Gibson (Aldershot: Ashgate, 2004), 237-58.

Piemontese, Alessio. *De secretis libri septem, a Ioan Iacobo Veckero Doctore Medico, ex Italico sermone in Latinum conversi, & multis bonis secretis aucti; accessit hae editione eiusdem Weckeri opera, octavus de artificiosis vinis liber* (Basel: Petrum Pernam, 1563).

—. *Kunstbuch des wolerfarnen Herren Alexii Pedemontani, von mancherleyen nutzlichen unnd bewerten Secreten oder Künsten, jetzt newlich auß welscher und lateinischer Sprach in Teutsch Gebracht, durch Doctor Hanß Jacob Wecker* (Basel: König, 1616).

—. *The Secrets of the Reverend Maister Alexis of Piedmont* (London: Thomas Wight, 1595).

Renou, Jean. *Les Œuvres pharmaceutiques de Jean Renou* (Lyon: A. Chard, 1626).

Rider, Catherine. 'Gender, Old Age, and the Infertile Body in Medieval Medicine', in *Gender, Health, and Healing, 1250-1550*, ed. Sara Ritchey and Sharon Strocchia (Amsterdam: Amsterdam University Press, 2020), 267-89.

Rösslin, Eucharius. *When Midwifery Became the Male Physician's Province: The Sixteenth-Century Handbook, The Rose Garden for Pregnant Women and Midwives, Newly Englished* (Jefferson, NC: McFarland & Co., 1994).

Shanahan, Madeline. *Manuscript Recipe Books as Archaeological Objects* (London: Lexington Books, 2015).

Stolberg, Michael. 'Menstruation and Sexual Difference in Early Modern Medicine', in *Menstruation: A Cultural History*, ed. Andrew Shail and Gillian Howe (Basingstoke: Palgrave Macmillan, 2005), 90-101.

Tuten, Belle S. 'Care of the Breast in the Late Middle Ages: The *Tractatus de passionibus mamillarum*', in *Gender, Health, and Healing, 1250-1550*, ed. Sara Ritchey and Sharon Strocchia (Amsterdam: Amsterdam University Press, 2020), 119-37.

Verskin, Sara. 'Gender Segregation and the Possibility of Arabo-Galenic Gynecological Practice in the Medieval Islamic World', in *Gender, Health, and Healing, 1250-1550*, ed. Sara Ritchey and Sharon Strocchia (Amsterdam: Amsterdam University Press, 2020), 291-313.

Voet, Leon. *The Golden Compasses: The History of the House of Plantin-Moretus*, 2 vols. (London: Routledge, 1969-72).

About the Author

Julia Gruman Martins is a PhD candidate at King's College London. Her thesis focuses on the translation of 'secrets of women' in early modern Europe, especially from Italian into French and English. She holds a joint Master's (honours) degree from the University of Bologna and the University of Paris VII.

Part 3

Infirmity and Care

7 *Ubi non est mulier, ingemiscit egens?*

Gendered Perceptions of Care from the Thirteenth to Sixteenth Centuries

*Eva-Maria Cersovsky**

Abstract

This essay studies the feminization of different caring practices by examining the cultural meanings attached to the biblical proverb Sirach 36:27. Touching on diverse sources, it investigates three interrelated contexts of use. In particular, I explore discourses on wifely responsibilities towards the needy husband; on charitable care for the sick and poor; and on the nature and social status of women. I suggest that by using the proverb as an argument, learned men subsumed a wide variety of caring practices under received notions of essentially female duties and innate qualities, connected above all to gendered ideas of compassion. However, the essay also highlights ambivalent attitudes towards female caregivers, as well as their agency and power, that surface within these complex discourses.

Keywords: healthcare, nursing, charity, women, medieval, early modern

The title of this essay is taken from verse 36:27 of the biblical book of Sirach as handed down through the Latin Vulgate: 'Where there is no woman, the needy groans'.[1] This short proverb appeared in conduct manuals, hospital

* My thanks to Letha Böhringer for drawing my attention to the proverb explored in this chapter, and to the volume editors as well as Isabelle Cochelin for their helpful comments on earlier versions of the essay.

1 Note that Weber and Gryson, *Biblia sacra iuxta vulgatam*, 1075, use 'gemescit' in their critical edition, giving 'ingemiscit' as a variant reading. Here I do not aim to provide a history of manuscript or textual transmission, but I have chosen to use 'ingemiscit' because it is the dominant form used in the Latin texts examined in this essay. There seems to be no significant difference in meaning between the two forms; both verbs denote the act of groaning or sighing.

Ritchey, Sara & Sharon Strocchia (eds), *Gender, Health, and Healing, 1250-1550*. Amsterdam, Amsterdam University Press 2020
DOI: 10.5117/9789463724517_CH07

ordinances, works of literature, and rhetorical tracts throughout the medieval and early modern period. With translations of the Latin into English, French, Spanish, or German, learned men of varying backgrounds related the biblical reference and its renditions to women and caring for those in need, the sick in particular. Broadening its original context of use, which centred on wifely duties towards a needy husband, they brought a range of interpretations and layers to the phrase in order to assert, parody, or call into question the suitability of women as caregivers.

Thus far, no study has been devoted to an analysis of the societal views encapsulated in the proverb.[2] In this essay I consider these meanings and cultural assumptions attached to Sirach 36:27 during the thirteenth to sixteenth centuries. Exploring the proverb's history, I suggest, offers a useful point of entry into long-standing patterns of thinking about women in relation to those in need of care. This approach allows us to examine documented moments when women, as *women*, were discussed as the most effective caregivers, and to ask what it was about their gender that made them particularly suitable. Through my reading of this biblical passage, I intend to demonstrate how a broad spectrum of caring activities, such as care for the husband in need, charity to the poor, or hospital nursing, could be explicitly feminized, while at the same time illuminating the complexities, ambiguities, and tensions that subtended such discourses.

In investigating ideas about women as caregivers, this essay builds on the burgeoning scholarship over the past decade that has given us a fuller, more nuanced picture of women's engagement in palliative and therapeutic care throughout the medieval and early modern period.[3] Anglo-American scholars in particular have adopted an inclusive approach focused more broadly on providers of care and 'bodywork', thereby revealing the broad

On the shift from 'egens' to '(a)eger' which only occurred within the exegetical tradition and prompted more substantial semantic change, see my comments throughout this chapter.

2 Here I follow the broad definition of proverbs provided by Mieder and Röhrich, *Sprichwort*, 3: 'Proverbs are generally well known, firmly established sentences, which express a maxim or wisdom in striking, short form' (translated from German in Morewedge, 'Proverbs', 2027). My argument is also premised on the assumption that proverbs are both stable and adaptable sayings. As research on medieval literary texts has shown, they could occur in variant or abbreviated form while still remaining highly recognizable, and they could vary in meaning depending on their use and context when embedded in longer texts. For a concise overview of definitions, characteristics, and scholarship, see Morewedge, 'Proverbs'.

3 See especially the essays compiled in Green, ed., *Women's Healthcare*; and the articles in Fissell, ed., *Women, Health, and Healing*, and in Strocchia, ed., *Women and Healthcare*. Additionally, see the synthetic monographic studies by Whaley, *Women and the Practice of Medical Care*, and Broomhall, *Women's Medical Work*.

spectrum of activities women from different social strata performed in their capacities as wives, mothers, kin, neighbours, or hospital nurses. These activities ranged from providing bedside care, making and administering foods and medicaments, dressing wounds, interpreting bodily signs, and generating and consuming medical knowledge.[4] While recent studies have focused mainly on social practices, some historians have also pointed to the equally wide variety of perceptions towards women and caregiving. They have put into perspective the negative stereotypes presented in the writings of learned men, in particular medical practitioners, about 'old women' and women engaging in paid medical care.[5] It has also been attested that women often were perceived to be particularly suited for providing bedside care, especially in the domestic setting, and that notions of charity played an important role in constructing their relationship to a variety of caring practices.[6]

Interestingly, renditions of Sirach 36:27 have made repeated appearances within twentieth-century historiography that argues for a central, respected role of women as caregivers. Muriel Hughes, for example, alluded to quotes taken from Albertano da Brescia (d. 1251) and Geoffrey Chaucer (d. *c.*1400) to support her broad claim that women were widely acknowledged as both nurses and healers and 'sufficiently successful to win them the gratitude, the devotion, and the respect of their contemporaries' throughout the Middle Ages.[7] Similarly, Conrad Brunner and Robert Jütte referred to the proverb in relation to medieval hospital nurses and sixteenth-century domestic care respectively; the latter author specifically cites the French humanist physician François Rabelais (d. 1553) as a point of reference.[8] However, none of these scholars provides information about the specific premodern contexts of use and the meanings associated with the phrase.

4 On new interpretative frameworks that move beyond the focus on official work identities, see Green, 'Bodies, Gender, Health, Disease'; Cabré, 'Women or Healers?'; and Fissell, 'Introduction', where the concept of 'bodywork' is introduced.

5 Agrimi and Crisciani, 'Immagini e ruoli'; Rawcliffe, *Medicine and Society*, 170-215; Kinzelbach, 'Wahnsinnige Weyber'; Harkness, 'View from the Streets'.

6 On the provision of bedside care, see Pelling, 'Compromised by Gender'; Riddy, 'Authority and Intimacy'; Cabré, 'Women or Healers?'. On notions of charity see Rawcliffe, *Medicine and Society*, 170-215, and Kinzelbach, 'Konstruktion und konkretes Handeln'. Both topics are discussed in Broomhall, *Women's Medical Work*, 81-82, 98-101, and Rankin, *Panaceia's Daughters*, 10-14, 113.

7 Hughes, *Women Healers*, 137-38, as well as the page following the table of contents where she prominently placed the two renderings of the proverb.

8 See Brunner, *Medizin und Krankenpflege*, 112 ('Ubi non est mulier, ingemiscit aeger'), who does not even identify the original source text; and Jütte, 'Familie und Krankheit', 21, n. 1, as well as his title which features a modern German translation of the proverb.

The present essay sets out to show that this neglect disguises the manifold assumptions behind the use of the proverb. By providing a more detailed inquiry into the interpretations, renderings, and layers connected to Sirach 36:27, it enlarges our understanding of the argumentative strategies and tropes that coexisted within the varied discussions of female caregiving in Europe from roughly 1200 to 1600. The choice of time period, however, is to some extent a pragmatic one, since an exploration into the interpretations of Sirach could certainly start earlier or be extended well into the nineteenth-century discourse on poor relief, or twentieth-century scholarship as just mentioned.[9] The chronological focus is justified by the new layers of interpretation Sirach 36:27 received when incorporated into discourses of charity and compassion emerging in the thirteenth century, as well as in the *querelle des femmes* taking shape in the early sixteenth century. Nevertheless, my intention is neither to propose a full picture of the proverb's exegetical tradition nor a definite trajectory for the period under consideration. Rather, I offer a preliminary survey of small-scale case studies in an attempt to historicize their social, cultural, and discursive contexts and to reconstruct three different traditions of use. In so doing, I contrast different source types, each of which embodies specific characteristics, audiences, and functions that must be considered. However, all three traditions of use share a normative quality that, while not necessarily indicative of actual practices, nevertheless sheds important light on expectations and idealized social roles.

Caring Wives and Needy Husbands

Neither the association with care for the sick nor the wider array of caregiving environments later referenced are evident from the proverb's biblical origins, the book of Sirach, also known as the book of Ecclesiasticus. The Hebrew text dates to the second century BCE and provides instructions on various aspects of life within an idealized faith community of Jews living in the diaspora of Ptolemaic-Hellenistic Egypt.[10] In the Latin Vulgate, chapter 36 (verses 21 to 27) focuses on the commendable characteristics of wives. Here verse 27 does not refer to *(a)eger*, sick, specifically, but more

9 See for instance the nineteenth-century example cited in Sohn-Kronthaler, which in its interpretation of Sirach 36:27 in relation to compassion, charity, and feminine healing powers strongly resembles the discourses explored in this essay; 'Armutsdiskurse und Gender(-frage)', 330.

10 On the book of Sirach see Marböck, 'Sirach/Sirachbuch'.

generally to *egens*, needy. In this context, it is related to the wife as a helper to her husband and to her responsibilities within marriage and household, not to caregiving in general.[11] Furthermore, the first part of the biblical verse links her to safeguarding domestic possessions ('Where there is no fence, the property will be plundered'), a notion that is lost in some of the later contexts of use.

A closer examination of the examples cited in twentieth-century scholarship – Albertano da Brescia, Geoffrey Chaucer, and François Rabelais – indicates that these were part of an interpretative tradition that remained close to the biblical context. Albertano da Brescia, a Lombard jurist, magistrate, and writer of several sermons and social treatises, addressed his first work *Liber de amore et dilectione Dei et proximi* to his eldest son Vicenzio in 1238. His widely read treatise imparts counsel about Christian life and social behaviour, promoting values associated with a lay urban elite to which Albertano himself belonged.[12] Albertano referred to Sirach 36:27 in Book 2, chapter 16 ('De uxore diligenda'), which discusses the values of marriage and underscores why a husband should love his wife through a combination of citations from biblical and ancient authorities. His first argument centred on the fact that a wife was a helper to her husband. Taking a customary approach, Albertano used creation to explain both sex and gender roles: formed from Adam's side, a woman was deemed man's helpmate by divine creation.[13] Further, Albertano explained that, whereas houses and wealth were inherited from parents, a prudent wife was God's gift; his explanation was based on Proverbs 19:14, which he wrongly attributed to Sirach. According to him, this relationship also held true because the wife was a helper to man and the neediest ('adiutorium hominis et maxime egeni'). Albertano supported his argument by citing Sirach 36:27 ('Ubi non est sepis, dirunpitur possessio; et ubi non est mulier, ingemiscit egens').[14] Significant for this essay, the extant manuscripts of the *Liber de amore* seem to vary

11 Sirach 36:25-28 (Biblia Sacra Vulgata): '25 Si est lingua curationis et mitigationis misericordiae, non est vir illius contra filios hominum. 26 Qui possidet mulierem inchoat possessionem, adiutorium contra illum est et columna ut requies. 27 Ubi non est sepis diripietur possessio, et ubi non est mulier gemescit egens. 28 Cui credit qui non habet nidum, et deflectens ubicumque obscuraverit, quasi succinctus latro exiliens de civitate in civitatem'. On the variant readings of 'gemescit' see note 1.

12 On Albertano and his work see Powell, *Albertanus of Brescia*.

13 Albertano da Brescia, *De amore*, 119-20.

14 Ibid., 120: 'Dixit enim Ihesus filius Syrac, "Domus et divitie dantur a parentibus, a Domino autem proprie uxor bona vel prudens." Est enim ut dixit adiutorium hominis et maxime egeni, unde idem dixit, "Ubi non est sepis, dirunpitur [possessio]; et ubi non est mulier, ingemiscit egens"'.

in regard to the exact words used within the quotation of the proverb. While the fourteenth-century Italian manuscript that Sharon Hiltz used as the basis of her critical edition appears to use 'egens', other manuscripts apparently note the word 'eger'.[15] Therefore, translations of the book or texts that drew upon it as a source not only referred to a husband in need, but specifically to a sick husband. This becomes apparent, for instance, in a fifteenth-century German translation by the Carthusian Heinrich Haller or in Chaucer's *Merchant's Tale*, which I discuss below.[16]

While Albertano did not elaborate on exactly how a wife would help a needy or sick husband – and thus cannot be interpreted in Hughes' sweeping manner with regard to medical care – other medieval authors were more specific. Gabriela Signori has pointed out that most medieval jurists interpreted *adiutorium* within marriage as the wifely duty to nurse an older, infirm husband and that late medieval didactic works on marriage, too, routinely emphasized assistance in the case of old age and sickness.[17] Similarly, historians of medieval and early modern medicine have highlighted the fact that guides to proper conduct of well-bred women expected the noble or bourgeois housewife to be responsible for the health and wellbeing of both her husband and larger family.[18] Some of the most familiar examples include the instructions written by the French provincial knight Geoffroy, Chevalier de la Tour Landry, for his daughters (1371-72) or the popular *De institutione feminae christianae* which the Spanish humanist Juan Luis Vives dedicated to Catherine of Aragon in 1523. Both conduct manuals relate tales of wives who devoted themselves to nursing their sick spouses, encouraging their audience to do the same.[19] Still, scholars such as Monica Green and Alisha Rankin have suggested that such instructions varied in outlining the nature of the expected health-related tasks, as well as in the degree of autonomy a housewife was supposed to show in caring for sick

15 Hiltz used University of Pennsylvania, Latin MS 107, Albertanus Causidicus Brixiensis, which originated in late fourteenth-century northern Italy (ibid., xvii). By contrast, Koeppel cites from Bayerische Staatsbibliothek, Cod. Lat. 14230, which has 'eger' ('Chaucer und Albertanus Brixiensis', 41).

16 For Haller see Bauer, *Albertanus von Brescia*, 110: 'Vnd darum spricht Salomon: "Wo nicht ain czaun ist, da würt zerstört die pesiczung, vnd wo das weib nicht ist, da ist seüfften der dürfftig oder der kchrankch mensch"' ('[...], and where there is no woman, the needy or the sick person groans').

17 Signori, *Paradiesehe*, 26.

18 Rawcliffe, *Medicine and Society*, 170-215; Broomhall, *Women's Medical Work*, 81-82, 98-101; Rankin, *Panaceia's Daughters*, 10-14.

19 See the English translations by Wright, ed., *Book of the Knight of la Tour-Landry*, 155; and Vives, *Education of a Christian Woman*, 199-204.

family members throughout this period.[20] The essay by Cordula Nolte in this volume provides further insight into how spousal caregiving was practised in urban homes in sixteenth-century Germany.[21]

Returning to our proverb, the literary works of Chaucer and Rabelais likewise underscore the complexities and ambiguities that subtend the discourse on wifehood and marriage. These texts also point to the importance of considering the genre and functions of texts alluding to the biblical phrase.[22] Both Chaucer and Rabelais appeal to Sirach 36:27, but call into question the notion of the caring wife in a paradoxical and ironic way. Chaucer's *The Merchant's Tale* centres on January, a 60-year-old knight, his decision to take a wife, and his subsequent marriage to the young May. A translation of Sirach 36:27 is included in the marriage encomium at the very beginning of the tale.[23] This section of the story in particular is concerned with contrasting the positive and negative aspects of marriage, or rather wives themselves, in an argumentative and exhortative style. It explicitly references Theophrastus, Aristotle's successor at the Athenian lyceum and the supposed author of the misogynist *Liber de nuptiis* – a work that sparked debate on the question of whether a (wise) man should marry. This controversy was picked up by various authors in the twelfth century across a number of genres to refute marriage and denounce wives, or to praise them.[24]

Like Albertano's *Liber de amore*, which is assumed to be one of Chaucer's sources for the encomium, the *Merchant's Tale* counts among the arguments in favour of marriage the notion that a wife is God's gift and a faithful helper to her husband.[25] Chaucer's rendering of Sirach 36:27, too, is believed to be taken from Albertano: 'A wyfe is kepere of thyn housbondrye;/ Wel may the sike man biwaille and wepe,/ Ther as ther nys no wyf the hous to

20 Green, 'Possibilities of Literacy', 21-23, 32-34; Rankin, 'Housewife's Apothecary'. Similarly, some of the examples given by Signori suggest that both husband and wife were expected to care for each other in old age or sickness; Signori, *Paradiesehe*, 26.

21 Nolte, 'Domestic Care in the Sixteenth Century'.

22 Schnell has pointed out that the qualities and responsibilities of spouses put forward in medieval and early modern texts on marriage can differ tremendously not only with regard to genre but also depending on whether a text addresses the topic from the perspective of either only one sex or of both; Schnell, 'Discourse on Marriage', esp. 776-79, 784-86.

23 See Benson, *Riverside Chaucer*, 154-56, verses 1267-1392. On the encomium see Benson, 'Marriage "Encomium"'; and more recently Pugh, 'Gender, Vulgarity, and the Phantom Debates'.

24 See Roth, *'An uxor ducenda'*.

25 Benson, *Riverside Chaucer*, 155, verse 1311 ('A wyf is Goddes yifte verraily'), and verse 1324 ('That womman is for mannes helpe ywroght'). For a compilation of Chaucer's sources see ibid., 884. On Albertano specifically see Koeppel, 'Chaucer und Albertanus Brixiensis', 40-44.

kepe'.[26] Here the husband is not only needy but sick. However, Chaucer relates the absence of a wife more to the first part of the biblical verse about domestic government, and less to tending to the sick husband, which he had already discussed in earlier verses.[27] Ultimately, Chaucer's tale invites an ironic reading of both sentiments. Within the encomium, he not only recounts Theophrastus' arguments that servants and friends constituted better caregivers than wives, but the whole story speaks to the anxieties about women taking advantage of their old, infirm husbands.[28] Thus, May neither takes good care of the blind January nor his household, but betrays her husband with a young lover and then convinces him to stay morally blind to her adultery, despite the restoration of his physical sight.[29]

Like Chaucer, the French humanist and physician François Rabelais also integrated his translation of Sirach 36:27 into a literary discussion of the advantages and disadvantages of marriage. In the third book of his five-part series *La vie de Gargantua et de Pantagruel*, published in 1546, the young giant Pantagruel and his friend Panurge seek advice on the issue of taking a wife, visiting a variety of different people who present them with contradictory opinions.[30] The second part of the biblical verse is applied in chapter 9 headed 'How Panurge asks counsel of Pantagruel whether he should marry'. Here the proverb constitutes one of the arguments seemingly put forward in favour of marriage by Panurge himself: 'The wise man says, where there is no woman – I mean the mother of a family and wife in the union of a lawful wedlock – the sick is in great strife, as by clear experience has been made apparent in the persons of popes, legates, cardinals, bishops, abbots, priors, priests, and monks'.[31] However, in view of the substantial medical care such clergymen could receive at courts or in monasteries, this statement appears highly ambivalent. Perpetuating an established topos, Panurge counters his own argument by explicitly voicing the suspicion that if a wife became upset with a sick and impotent husband, she could

26 Benson, *Riverside Chaucer*, 156, verses 1380-82. Also see Koeppel, 'Chaucer und Albertanus Brixiensis', 41.

27 Benson, *Riverside Chaucer*, 154, verses 1286-92.

28 For Theophrastus' argument see ibid., 155, verses 1301-4.

29 Ibid., 154-68. For an exploration of May's pregnancy as disability, see Vanderveter Pearman, who also argues that 'May's excessively physical body usurps January's sight'; *Women and Disability*, 35-44, quote at 35.

30 On the *Tiers livre* see Duval, *Design of Rabelais's Tiers Livre*.

31 Rabelais, *Le Tiers livre*, 78-79: 'Et si par cas tombois en maladie, traicté ne serois qu'au rebours. Le saige dict: là où n'est femme, j'entends merefamiles, et en mariage legitime, le malade est en grand estrif. J'en ay veu claire experience en papes, legatz, cardinaulx, evesques, abbez, prieurs, prieurs, presbtres et moines'.

cease to help him, embezzle his goods, or even prostitute herself to another man. He even asserts to have seen this happen to many other men.[32] Like Chaucer, Rabelais's use of the proverb therefore cannot be read as praise of female caring abilities, but indicates conflicted attitudes towards wifely caregiving and an underlying unease with the power women might wield over their weakened husbands and their economic possessions.

Charitable and Compassionate Care for the Poor and Sick

Having examined some of the meanings that could be attached to Sirach 36:27 with regard to the husband in need, we turn now to another tradition of use, which associated the proverb with female charity, compassion, and help to the poor. Again, I start by examining a thirteenth-century conduct book, which enjoined the practice of charity upon noblewomen as part of their household duties and social role as wives. In the widely disseminated princely instruction *De eruditione principum* written by the French Dominican Guillaume Peyraut *c.*1265, Sirach 36:27 makes an appearance in the fifth book, which purports to discuss the virtues of young princes and princesses.[33] Here chapter 57 is concerned with the merciful and charitable deeds expected from a married *puella nobilis*.[34] After exalting the value of mercy as a virtue particularly loved by God, Peyraut explained that married princesses in particular should be a refuge for the poor. They were particularly apt to perform charity, since women by nature possessed a soft heart; by contrast, men's hearts were harder. It was thus women's responsibility to soften their husbands' hearts and convince them to give alms. According to Peyraut, if a woman was not at home, the poor did not receive refreshment; for this reason Sirach had said: 'Ubi non est mulier, ingemiscit egens'. Girls having a noble heart should therefore strive to be merciful, feed the needy, and fulfil the five other works of corporal mercy

32 Ibid., 79.

33 On Guillaume Peyraut and his work see Dondaine, 'Guillaume Peyraut'; and more recently Verweij, 'Princely Virtues'.

34 Peraldus, *De eruditione principum*, 116: 'Puella nobilis cum nupserit, pauperum refugium esse debet, habent naturaliter mulieres corda tenera, cum viri habeant corda dura; earum est emollire viros; [...]. Si mulier in domo non fuerit, pauper ad domum veniens refrigerium non invenit, juxta illud Eccl. 39: ubi non est mulier, ingemiscit egens. Debent puellae nobiles, quae habent nobilitatem carnis, habere magnum desiderium veri honoris, qui pietate acquiritur, juxta illud Matth. 25: accipite regnum quod vobis est paratum ab origine mundi. Esurivi enim et dedistis mihi manducare etc.'

laid out in Matthew 25:35-36 (providing drink, shelter, and clothing, visiting the sick and the imprisoned). For Peyraut, these wifely charitable practices complemented the husband's social role and entailed a political dimension. While her husband ventured from home to fight enemies with weapons, a noble wife should fight adversaries by giving charity, thus providing a stabilizing power within the religious realm.[35]

In his discussion of female mercy, Peyraut adopted an established theme. As Sharon Farmer has shown, portrayals of the pious wife softening her husband's heart to perform charitable economic actions can be traced back to eleventh-century monastic authors and became even more prominent at the beginning of the thirteenth century, when scholars like Thomas Chobham encouraged women to give charity even against their husband's wishes.[36] Unlike Chobham's *Manual for Confessors* (*c.*1215), Peyraut neither paired this notion with the persuasive power of a wife's speech; nor did he emphasize the redemptive effect charity would have on a husband's soul. Instead, he placed greater emphasis on feminine nature and social responsibilities, an approach that was continued by subsequent authors of conduct manuals. Although charitable behaviour was certainly regarded as important for all Christians, both male and female, asserting women's innate affectivity and particular aptness to perform works of mercy benefitting the poor remained a widespread tradition in conduct books and marriage tracts up to the sixteenth century.[37] For example, the fourteenth-century instructions of the Chevalier de Tour Landry labelled a lack of pity 'mannish'. In contrast, he presented the tale of the Countess of Anjou, who visited the poor, the sick, and women in childbed, dispensed alms and food, and obligated her physicians and surgeons to provide healing care, as a 'womanly' way of expressing compassion and charity.[38]

These invigorated discussions of mercy and charity directed at a lay audience disseminated ideals of charitable service and a larger 'culture of compassion', as Adam Davis recently put it, which took root in the twelfth and thirteenth centuries.[39] Sirach 36:27 seems to have gained new layers

35 Ibid. Reinle, 'Was bedeutet Macht', 70-71, focuses on medieval concepts of power and offers a similar interpretation.

36 Farmer, 'Persuasive Voices'.

37 Rawcliffe, *Medicine and Society*, 170-215. On gendered understandings and practices of charity see also Cullum, 'And hir Name was Charite'.

38 Wright, *Book of the Knight of la Tour-Landry*, 136-37. In the sixteenth century, the production of medicines and their distribution to the local poor by German noblewomen was equally couched in terms of charity; Rankin, *Panaceia's Daughters*, 113.

39 Davis, 'Hospitals, Charity, and the Culture of Compassion'. See his concise overview of the relevant historiography in 'Social and Religious Meanings of Charity'.

of meaning that did not refer solely to wifely duties towards the husband. Scholars have demonstrated that the promotion of piety and compassion as modes of feeling directed toward suffering in general and toward the suffering Christ in particular, could take on a decidedly female face in a variety of contemporary texts and contexts.[40] For example, affectivity, charity, and care of the poor were also increasingly and intimately connected with female religious and saints.[41] In contrast to the noblewomen addressed in conduct books, these religious women were more readily associated with hands-on bodily care in *vitae* or miracles which, among other things, portrayed them as both founding and visiting hospitals, and actually nursing their inmates.[42] Sara Ritchey's essay in this volume, for example, illuminates the intricate links between the beguines of thirteenth-century Liège, hospital staff, and modes of oral, performative, and affective bedside care.[43] Indeed, renderings of Sirach 36:27 can also be found in statutes regulating the hospital life of *mulieres religiosae* and the sick poor for whom they were perceived to be particularly suited as caregivers. Although such hospital ordinances certainly had a pragmatic function, they still present a normative, idealized picture of hospital life, roles, and tasks, and lend themselves to an analysis of their rhetoric and semantic strategies.[44]

An early Italian example can be situated within the complex institutional responses to new groups of religious women emerging in the thirteenth century.[45] In 1254, the bishop of Spoleto, Bartolomeo Accoramboni, institutionalized part of a female *bizzoche* community that followed an unregulated apostolic life in a hermitage close to the city. Bartolomeo – who had conducted the canonization process for Clare of Assisi the previous year – assigned them the Augustinian rule and obligated them to care for the inmates of the newly built urban hospital, the Ospedale Nuovo or della Stella, which he had founded himself.[46] In the short constitutions he drafted for the institution, he employed a rendering of Sirach 36:27, without citing its origins, to reason for a new spirituality and way of life for the female community. The bishop promoted a combination of a contemplative, cloistered life and the active performance of works of mercy within the

40 McNamer, *Affective Meditation*.
41 Ritchey, 'Affective Medicine'.
42 On this point see also Rawcliffe, *Medicine and Society*, 205-6; Rankin, *Panaceia's Daughters*, 10.
43 Ritchey, 'Caring by the Hours'.
44 On the characteristics of medieval hospital ordinances see Drossbach, 'Hospitalstatuten'.
45 On these developments in relation to the example discussed here, see Sensi, 'Anchoresses and Penitents'.
46 For a history of the hospital see Ceccaroni, *La storia millenariana degli ospedali*.

hospital.[47] While in his view observing enclosure was necessary to fully enjoy the effects of contemplation, the assistance to the sick poor of the hospital was similarly important because, the statutes tell us, it was women who were particularly apt to provide care: 'ubi non est mulier/ ingemiscit eger'. Therefore, two sisters should alternately see to the inmates' needs, while being careful to cover head and face, to neither leave the hospital nor linger within, and to perform their pious works speedily. In an effort to institutionalize female piety, an appeal to the proverb thus married spiritual ideals with social needs.

Some 300 years later, in 1535, the statutes of the Paris Hôtel-Dieu made similar if more elaborate use of the proverb when changes occurred in the life of the hospital community. The existence of Paris's main hospital is attested since the ninth century. According to the earliest surviving statutes composed *c.*1220, its staff was comprised of both male and female religious who followed an Augustinian rule adapted to the hospital's needs.[48] Whereas the number of female religious grew to about eighty in the sixteenth century, the number of priests and lay brothers decreased to about twenty.[49] Work within the Hôtel-Dieu was divided along gendered lines. Female religious performed most of the health-related tasks, ranging from the provision of a clean environment and nursing care to diagnosing and treating illnesses; the men were responsible mainly for inmates' spiritual wellbeing. Male medical practitioners, physicians, surgeons, and apothecaries are occasionally mentioned throughout the fifteenth century and, after 1536, they were supposed to visit the hospital weekly. Nevertheless, the bulk of medical care remained in the hands of the Augustinian sisters.[50]

During the late fifteenth and sixteenth centuries the hospital saw repeated conflicts about its governance, administration, and the conduct of personnel. After a number of failed attempts at reform, it received a new and lengthy set

47 Fausti, 'Degli antichi ospedali di Spoleto', 104-6: 'ab arce contemplationis ad opera misericordia aliquando descendendo. [...][T]amen quia ubi non est mulier/ ingemiscit eger, ad mandatum magistre, que pro tempore fuerit, due sorores, velato capite et facie ut solummodo videre possint, per vices suas simul egrediantur pro necessitatibus infirmorum/ pauperum hospitalis [...]'. ('finally descending from the summit of contemplation to the works of mercy. [...] Yet since where there is no woman, the sick groans, on the order of the mistress who will have been there for the time being, two sisters, with their heads and faces veiled so that they could just see, should go out together in turns to see to the needs of the sick paupers of the hospital.')

48 Coyecque, *L'Hôtel-Dieu*, 27-53, discusses the history of the hospital.

49 On the number of male and female religious see Jéhanno, 'Sustener les povres malades', 150-57, 661-707 (append. 3 for sisters, 4 for brothers). Names and numbers were collected for the period 1392 to 1535 according to available documents.

50 Coyecque, *L'Hôtel-Dieu*, 27-53, 97-100; Broomhall, *Women's Medical Work*, 72-76.

of rules in 1535 intended to renew the institution 'en chefz et en members'.[51] The longest section within this ordinance is devoted to the nursing sisters and begins by presenting arguments about why these women were especially suited for their tasks. Aristotle, it asserted, testified that women were naturally more inclined toward pity and compassion than men. Accordingly, this would match what the wise man said in Ecclesiasticus chapter 36: 'Where there is no woman, the sick groans'.[52] Here the ordinance referred to Aristotle's *Historia animalium* 9.1, which described females as softer than males in disposition and overall less spirited. This notion was connected to the inability of the female body to produce semen due to its cold nature, as well as to a more general aura of incapacity.[53] While these characteristics were not regarded as necessarily beneficial in an Aristotelian context, women's supposedly soft, compassionate nature was interpreted more positively in relation to charity, and had been connected to Sirach 36:27 since at least the thirteenth century, as discussed above. In explaining its rationale, the ordinance rendered yet another of Sirach's proverbs to feminize attributes of kindness, faithfulness, and diligence, and to indicate their importance in nourishing the sick back to health (Sirach 26:16, 'The kindness of the faithful and diligent woman pleases the man, and shall fatten his bones').[54] Therefore, the ordinance continued, the hospital should follow former custom and continue to assign religious women to serve the sick poor, including forty professed sisters and forty novices who adhered to the Augustinian rule.[55]

Why did the statutes place such emphasis on the sisters' suitability before presenting the actual hospital rules they were expected to follow? Thomas Frank has suggested that, although the ordinance was declared a reform text, it tried to reconcile continuity and change while also concealing unresolved tensions.[56] Naturalizing the nursing work of female religious seems to have served both intentions. Highlighting the women's supposed 'natural' qualities and duties concealed the fact that the sisters themselves had not only

51 Jéhanno, 'L'Alimentation hospitalière', 131-32. On these reforms see also Broomhall, *Women's Medical Work*, 76-90, who does not analyse the statutes; and Frank, *Heilsame Wortgefechte*, 163-212.
52 Jéhanno, 'L'Alimentation hospitalière', 147: 'Le prince de philosophes Aristote tesmoigne et enseigne que la nature de la femme est plus incline et plus prompte a pitié et compassion que n'est la nature de l'home, et a icelle sentence convient et acorde le saige disant an ung sixiesme chappitre de l'*Ecclesiastique*: "Ou il n'y a poinct de femme le mallade se plainct" […]'.
53 Aristotle, *History of Animals* 9.1, 608a22-27, 608b1-3; Maclean, *Renaissance Notion of Woman*, 41-42, 89-90; Cadden, *Meanings of Sex Difference*, 172, 183-88, 204.
54 Jéhanno, 'L'Alimentation hospitalière', 147: 'et au vingt sixiesme chappitre d'icelluy: "La doulceur de la femme fidelle et dilligente faict plaisir a l'homme et engressera les os d'icelluy"'.
55 Ibid.
56 Frank, *Heilsame Wortgefechte*, 201, 204.

complained about the lack of support for their work in interviews with the reform committee – for instance, in the form of heating, food, and medical resources – but also had shown hostility towards earlier reform efforts. In 1505, the introduction of female tertiaries to help reform religious life within the institution had met with disapproval, anger, and even violent behaviour by the Augustinian sisters.[57] This was probably why the reform committee was adamant about ensuring continuity in their choice of caregivers, even though it once again tried to impose a stricter religious life on the community.[58] Furthermore, the following chapters of the statutes encoded several concerns about the sisters' behaviour that had been raised repeatedly by the governors in previous years. For example, the ordinance restricted the sisters' freedom to leave the hospital and visit patients in their own homes – a practice which the governors confounded with sexual licentiousness, neglect of hospital patients, and inobservance of the religious rule.[59] The reformers' praise of female caregiving must therefore be understood as part of a complex process of negotiating, defining, and ultimately controlling the sisters' agency as both nurses and *mulieres religiosae.*

Caring and the Nurturing Qualities of the Female Body

The last line of inquiry I pursue in exploring the meanings attached to Sirach 36:21 leads us back to a more literary if no less complex context of use. In the *querelle des femmes*, the debate about the nature and values of women that unfolded in Europe from the fourteenth century into the early modern period, the proverb could be used as an argument in favour of women's social worth and superiority to men. The *querelle* can be considered a continuation of the debate on marriage and wives discussed above.[60] However, *querelle* texts do not figure Sirach in relation to the husband in need, but instead continue the tradition of associating the proverb with compassion and caregiving in more general terms. While the proverb already appeared in

57 Ibid., 181-85; Broomhall, *Women's Medical Work*, 76-80, 87-88.

58 Another group of religious, the canons regular and 'religieuses reformees' of the congregation of St. Victor who followed a reformed Augustinian rule, were supposed to assist in implementing reform; Frank, *Heilsame Wortgefechte*, 192-208.

59 Jéhanno, 'L'Alimentation hospitalière', 155. On the concerns raised by the governors see Frank, *Heilsame Wortgefechte*, 189-204; Broomhall, *Women's Medical Work*, 81-86.

60 Bock and Zimmermann, 'Die *Querelle des Femmes* in Europa', 16. Campbell, 'Querelle des Femmes', offers a concise introduction to the state of scholarship on the French, Italian, and English contexts.

the fifteenth-century debate by way of short enumeration, it gained more elaborate interpretative dimensions in one of the *querelle*'s seminal texts written at the beginning of the sixteenth century.[61]

In 1529, the German humanist theologian and physician Henricus Cornelius Agrippa von Nettesheim published his declamation *De nobilitate et praecellentia foeminae sexus* (*Declamation on the Nobility and Preeminence of the Female Sex*) in Antwerp. The text was reprinted several times and translated almost immediately into French, English, Italian, German, and Polish. It exerted enormous influence throughout the sixteenth century, with the bulk of the literature for and against women written during the following century referencing Agrippa as an immediate source. *De nobilitate* rejected traditional misogyny on a number of grounds, claiming for instance that it was not women's intellectual inferiority but rather social custom based on male tyranny that had prevented them from taking on public offices and responsibilities.[62] In his chapter on women's superior virtue, Agrippa alluded to Sirach 36:27 in relation to arguments about female compassion, caregiving, and the healing powers of their bodies.

Like the Paris hospital ordinance written six years later, Agrippa explicitly drew on Aristotle and combined his feminized notion of mercy with our proverb, which he however attributed to Solomon. In the absence of women, the sick groaned, he elaborated, because women also showed a specific adeptness and good humour when serving the sick. Further, Agrippa argued, their breast milk provided a powerful healing remedy for the infirm and dying. Similarly, the heat of the female breast when placed on an old man's chest displayed rejuvenating capacities, as exemplified by Abishag and King David (1 Kings 1:4).[63] Agrippa had already mentioned the efficaciousness of breast

61 For example, in his *Triunfo de las doñas* written in the mid-fifteenth century, the Galician Franciscan and court poet Juan Rodriguez de la Cámara (or del Padrón) asserted that women were more compassionate than men and then offered a translation of Sirach 36:27. See Paz y Meliá, ed., *Obras de Juan Rodríguez de la Cámara*, 97: 'La decima sesta razon es, por ser mas misericordiosa. De la cual el fijo de Sirac dize: Onde non ay mugger, comiença fuerte mente gemir el enfermo; e donde non ay seto, la possession se destruye'. ('The sixteenth reason is that she is more compassionate. This is why the son of Sirach says: Where there is no woman, the sick starts to groan loudly; and where there is no hedge, the possession is destroyed.')

62 For an overview of Agrippa and his work, see Rabil's introduction to *Declamation on the Nobility*, 3-32.

63 Agrippa, *De nobilitate et praecellentia*, 46: 'Constat autem semper fere mulierem maioris esse pietatis et misericordiae quam virum, quod et Aristoteles ipse foemineo sexui proprium tribuit. Quamobrem arbitror dixisse Salomonem: Ubi non est mulier, ingemiscit aeger, vel quod in inserviendo et adsistendo valetudinariis mirae est dexteritatis et alacritatis, vel quod lac muliebre potissimum aegris debilibus etiam morti vicinis praesentaneum remedium est, quo ad vitam restituantur. Hinc, ut ferunt medici, calor earundem papillarum virorum nimio senio confectorum

milk in the previous paragraph. Here he related the widely known ancient story of the unnamed Roman daughter whose milk nourished her imprisoned mother, thereby preventing her death by starvation. In keeping with a well-established tradition, he interpreted this milk relationship as manifestation of maternal-filial bonds and female piety.[64] Combining the tale with Aristotle, Sirach, and Solomon, Agrippa thus presented an elaborate argument regarding women's piety, compassion, and caregiving to (adult) patients of both sexes.

However, he not only drew on literary or biblical sources, but also alluded to medical arguments regarding the therapeutic value of breast milk for both male and female patients, which he appropriated from Pliny the Elder's *Natural History* (23-79 BCE). These healing qualities were also discussed in contemporary medical treatises, in particular with regard to the cure of gout.[65] In a similar vein and again drawing on Pliny, Agrippa also argued for the healing powers of menstrual blood, which in his view had the power to cure a number of illnesses, both physical and psychological.[66] Furthermore, he attested that women also had 'the power of healing themselves of all sorts of illnesses by their own means, without recourse to some foreign or external aid'.[67]

pectori applicatus, calorem vitalem in illis excitat, adauget et conservat [...]'. (Agrippa, *Declamation on the Nobility*, 58: 'It is, moreover, recognized that the woman nearly always manifests more piety and mercy than the man, and even Aristotle himself asserts that these qualities are characteristics of the female sex. For this reason, I think, Solomon said: "Where there is no woman, a sick man groans," doubtless because the woman has an adroitness and an astonishing good humor when she aids and assists the sick, or because her milk is the most powerful remedy that can be found at the immediate disposition of the feeble, the sick, and even the dying, for restoring them to life'.)

64 Agrippa, *De nobilitate et praecellentia*, 44, 46. Jutta Sperling has shown that this story, which originated in Valerius Maximus's *Memorable Doings and Sayings* (*c.*31 BCE), was widely known among learned and illiterate audiences throughout the medieval and early modern period. In the context of the *querelle*, both Giovanni Boccaccio and Christine de Pizan had already included retellings of it in their respective works, *On Famous Women* (1361) and *Book of the City of Ladies* (1404); Sperling, *Roman Charity*, 231-68.

65 See Agrippa, *Declamation on the Nobility*, 58; Sperling, *Roman Charity*, 269-306.

66 Agrippa, *De nobilitate et praecellentia*, 46: 'Quanta etiam propter haec ipsa in mulieribus natura producere gaudeat miracula, nemo mirabitur, qui philosophorum medicorumque volumina perlegerit; quorum exemplum [...] praesto est et ad manum in menstruo qui sanguis propter quod a quartanis [...] et multis id generis perniciosissimis aegritudinibus liberat [...]'. (Agrippa, *Declamation on the Nobility*, 59: 'No one will be astonished at the number of prodigious phenomena – beyond those I have cited – that nature is pleased to create among women, if he has read the works of philosophers and doctors, of which an example [...] is ready to hand: menstruation. Menstrual blood, in addition to the fact that it cures some quartan fevers [...] and many other similar pernicious illnesses [...]'.)

67 Agrippa, *Declamation on the Nobility*, 59. For the Latin original see Agrippa, *De nobilitate et praecellentia*, 46: 'quo ipsaemet suis propriis dotibus in omni morborum genere sibi ex seipsis mederi possint, nullo etiam exotico aut aliunde accersito adminisculo accedente'.

As many scholars have attested, Agrippa's tract remains ambivalent. On the one hand, as a *declamatio*, it presents itself as an exercise in rhetoric, offering all probable arguments to prove its point, which might not reflect a serious intent, but rather an interest in paradox or exaggerated tongue-in-cheek for its own sake. On the other hand, this format also allowed heterodox ideas to travel and some of Agrippa's arguments regarding theological topics were taken seriously by contemporaries.[68] The medical layers that the argument regarding female caregiving received in this text certainly can be viewed as a response to concerns of Agrippa's time. Gianna Pomata has convincingly argued that the pro-woman medical arguments of the sixteenth-century *querelle* were related to changing attitudes toward the female body on the part of humanist physicians, who rejected the negative presentations that dominated scholastic thought.[69] In *De nobilitate*, too, we see Agrippa reversing misogynistic views of Aristotelian scholasticism about women's anatomy. Contrary to Aristotle, Agrippa presented the female body not as a defective male but as a wonder of nature, which also relates to the healing powers he ascribed to it.[70] Furthermore, when referencing the heat of Abishag's breast, he addressed Aristotle's notion that cold and moist humors predominated in women, arguing instead that woman's heat was efficacious.[71] With regard to the powerful capacities of menstrual blood, he again went against a popular medical tradition that emphasized its dangerous, destructive qualities, such as preventing seeds from germinating, rusting iron, giving dogs rabies, and so forth.[72] Moreover, Agrippa had referred to the medical care provided by women in a positive light before. In *De incertitudine et vanitate scientiarum* (1527), he pointed out not only that leading physicians learned excellent remedies from women but that the simple medicines of 'an old wife of the country' could prove more efficacious than the elaborate mixtures of physicians.[73]

Ultimately, Agrippa's arguments regarding female caregiving testify to the complexity and ambiguities of gendered ideas about women and

68 Agrippa, *Declamation on the Nobility*, quote at 59. See also Brinker-von der Heyde, 'Der Frauenpreis'; Maclean, *Renaissance Notion of Woman*, 91.

69 Pomata, 'Was There a *Querelle des Femmes*'.

70 Agrippa, *Declamation on the Nobility*, 59-61.

71 Ibid., 16.

72 Ibid. On traditions highlighting the venomous capacities of menstrual blood see Cabré and Salmon, 'Blood, Milk, and Breastbleeding', this volume.

73 Agrippa, *Declamation on the Nobility*, 58, n. 71. This argument serves less to assert the superiority of women over physicians than it does the advantages of simple over compound drugs, but it nevertheless presents a favourable view of women as providers of medical care.

care. They also demonstrate the range of possible interpretations that late medieval and early modern writers could bring to Sirach 36:27. Moreover, the relations Agrippa established between compassion, the aptitude to heal the sick, and the almost thaumaturgic powers of the female body, travelled into several later texts of the *querelle* tradition, continuing into the seventeenth century.[74]

Conclusion

This essay has offered a preliminary exploration of premodern patterns of thought that feminized the connections between women and caregiving in complex ways. The history of Sirach 36:27 has provided important insights into discourses, at once stable and permeable, which furnished the vocabulary and conceptual tools for understanding a variety of caring practices as extensions of duties and qualities perceived to be specifically and naturally feminine, across different genres, countries, and languages. These discourses were far from being entirely uniform, but the biblical reference and its renditions seem to have provided a stable platform for naturalizing feminine compassion and women's practices of care: wifely duties towards the husband in need and of charitable care for the poor growing out of household responsibilities; care for the sick poor in hospitals by female religious; and medical care provided by the physical presence and the supposed medicinal powers of the female body, which turned into a potent proof of women's innate caregiving capacities. These findings complement what Montserrat Cabré has argued regarding female practices of healthcare being associated with the context of the home and the 'semantic domain of "woman" and "mother," as well as to other categories that designate women at certain life stages'.[75]

This theme could also be elaborated, however, in more ambivalent directions that called into question the notion of a 'natural' feminine aptness for care that lay at the core of interpretations of the proverb. Situated in the context of marriage or hospital reform, the use of Sirach 36:27 points to tensions regarding the dynamics of agency and authority between women, their patients, and their expected social roles as wives, hospital nurses, or female religious. These complexities and ambiguities prompt intriguing questions for further research. More exhaustive studies, whether focusing

74 Angenot, *Champions des Femmes*, 114-17.

75 Cabré, 'Women or Healers?', 23.

on Sirach 36:27 or not, would have to be more rigorous both in regard to the issues of continuity and change and those of source type. Systematic and comparative explorations of the same genre – for example, the large corpus of didactic works on marriage or hospital ordinances – over a longer period of time might yield fruitful results. While we are clearly just beginning to establish a full picture of both women's caregiving practices and their perceptions, the varied evidence provided here also raises the question of how men were perceived in relation to care in medieval and early modern times. In order to fully understand ideas of femininity and care, we should more rigorously explore parallel constructions of masculinity.

Works Cited

Printed Works

Agrimi, Joel and Chiara Crisciani. 'Immagini e ruoli della vetula tra sapere medico e antropologia religiosa (secoli XIII-XV)', in *Poteri carismatici e informali: chiesa e società medioevali*, ed. Agostino Paravicini Bagliani and André Vauchez (Palermo: Sellerio, 1992), 224-61.

Agrippa, Henricus Cornelius. *Declamation on the Nobility and Preeminence of the Female Sex*, ed. and trans. Albert Rabil, Jr. (Chicago: University of Chicago Press, 2007).

—. *De nobilitate et praecellentia foeminei sexus: von Adel und Vorrang des weiblichen Geschlechts*, ed. and trans. Otto Schönberger (Würzburg: Königshausen & Neumann, 1997).

Albertano da Brescia. *De amore et dilectione Dei et proximi et aliarum rerum et de forma vite*, ed. Sharon Lynne Hiltz, PhD diss., University of Philadelphia, 1980.

Angenot, Marc. *Les champions des femmes: examen du discours sur la supériorité des femmes 1400-1800* (Montréal: Presses de l'Université du Québec, 1977).

Aristotle. *History of Animals, Volume III: Books 7-10*, ed. and trans. D.M. Balme, Loeb Classical Library 439 (Cambridge, MA: Harvard University Press, 1991).

Bauer, Erika, ed. *Albertanus von Brescia: 'De amore Dei et proximi' in der Übersetzung Heinrich Hallers* (Salzburg: Analecta Cartusiana, 2001).

Benson, Larry D. 'The Marriage "Encomium" in the "Merchant's Tale": A Chaucerian Crux', *Chaucer Review*, 14.1 (1979), 48-60.

—, ed. *The Riverside Chaucer*, 3rd ed., with a new foreword by Christopher Cannon (Oxford: Oxford University Press, 1987).

Bock, Gisela and Margarete Zimmermann. 'Die Querelle des Femmes in Europa: eine begriffs- und forschungsgeschichtliche Einführung', in *Die europäische*

Querelle des Femmes: Geschlechterdebatten seit dem 15. Jahrhundert, ed. Gisela Bock and Margarete Zimmermann (Stuttgart: Metzler, 1997), 9-38.

Brinker-von der Heyde, Claudia. 'Der Frauenpreis des Agrippa von Nettesheim: persönliche Strategie, politische Invektive, rhetorisches Spiel?', in *Text im Kontext: Anleitung zur Lektüre deutscher Texte der frühen Neuzeit*, ed. Alexander Schwarz and Laure Abplanalp (Bern: Peter Lang, 1997), 31-48.

Broomhall, Susan. *Women's Medical Work in Early Modern France* (Manchester: Manchester University Press, 2004).

Brunner, Conrad. *Über Medizin und Krankenpflege im Mittelalter in schweizerischen Landen* (Zurich: Seldwyla Zürich, 1922).

Cabré, Montserrat. 'Women or Healers? Household Practices and the Categories of Health Care in Late Medieval Iberia', *Bulletin of the History of Medicine*, 82 (2008), 18-51.

Cabré, Montserrat and Fernando Salmón. 'Blood, Milk, and Breastbleeding: The Humoral Economy of Women's Bodies in Late Medieval Medicine', in *Gender, Health, and Healing, 1250-1550*, ed. Sara Ritchey and Sharon Strocchia (Amsterdam: Amsterdam University Press, 2020), 93-117.

Cadden, Joan. *Meanings of Sex Difference in the Middle Ages: Medicine, Science, and Culture* (Cambridge: Cambridge University Press, 1993).

Campbell, Julie D. 'The Querelle des Femmes', in *The Ashgate Research Companion to Women and Gender in Early Modern Europe*, ed. Allyson M. Poska, Jane Couchman, and Katherine A. McIver (Burlington, VT: Ashgate, 2013), 361-80.

Ceccaroni, Sandro. *La storia millenariana degli ospedali della città e della diocese di Spoleto* (Spoleto: Ente Rocca di Spoleto, 1978).

Coyecque, Ernest. *L'Hôtel-Dieu de Paris au Moyen Âge: histoire et documents*, vol. 1: *Histoire de l'Hôtel-Dieu: documents (1316-1552)* (Paris: H. Champion, 1891).

Cullum, Patricia Helena. '"And hir Name was Charite": Charitable Giving by and for Women in Late Medieval Yorkshire', in *Woman is a Worthy Wight: Women in English Society c. 1200-1500*, ed. Peter Jeremy Piers Goldberg (Stroud: Sutton, 1992), 182-211.

Davis, Adam J. 'Hospitals, Charity, and the Culture of Compassion in the Twelfth and Thirteenth Centuries', in *Approaches to Poverty in Medieval Europe: Complexities, Contradictions, Transformation, c. 1100-1500*, ed. Sharon Farmer (Turnhout: Brepols, 2016), 23-46.

—. 'The Social and Religious Meanings of Charity in Medieval Europe', *History Compass*, 12 (2014), 935-50.

Dondaine, Antoine. 'Guillaume Peyraut: vie et œuvres', *Archivum Fratrum Praedicatorum*, 18 (1948), 162-236.

Drossbach, Gisela. 'Hospitalstatuten im Spiegel von Norm und Wirklichkeit', in *Hospitäler in Mittelalter und Früher Neuzeit: Frankreich, Deutschland und Italien;*

eine vergleichende Geschichte, ed. Gisela Drossbach (Munich: Oldenbourg, 2007), 41-54.

Duval, Edwin M. *The Design of Rabelais's Tiers Livre de Pantagruel* (Genève: Librairie Droz, 1997).

Farmer, Sharon. 'Persuasive Voices: Clerical Images of Medieval Wives', *Speculum*, 61 (1986), 517-43.

Fausti, Luigi. 'Degli antichi ospedali di Spoleto', *Atti dell'Accademia Spoletina* (1920-22), 59-111.

Fissell, Mary E. 'Introduction: Women, Health, and Healing in Early Modern Europe', *Bulletin of the History of Medicine*, 82.1 (2008), 1-17.

—, ed. *Women, Health, and Healing in Early Modern Europe*, special issue of *Bulletin of the History of Medicine*, 82.1 (2008).

Frank, Thomas. *Heilsame Wortgefechte: Reformen europäischer Hospitäler vom 14. bis 16. Jahrhundert* (Göttingen: V&R Unipress, 2016).

Green, Monica. 'Bodies, Gender, Health, Disease: Recent Work on Medieval Women's Medicine', *Studies in Medieval and Renaissance History*, ser. 3, 2 (2005), 1-46.

—. 'The Possibilities of Literacy and the Limits of Reading: Women and the Gendering of Medical Literacy', in *Women's Healthcare in the Medieval West: Texts and Contexts* (Aldershot: Ashgate, 2000), 1-76.

—. *Women's Healthcare in the Medieval West: Texts and Contexts* (Aldershot: Ashgate, 2000).

Harkness, Deborah E. 'A View from the Streets: Women and Medical Work in Elizabethan London', *Bulletin of the History of Medicine*, 82.1 (2008), 52-85.

Hughes, Muriel Joy. *Women Healers in Medieval Life and Literature* (New York: Books for Libraries Press, 1968).

Jéhanno, Christine. 'L'Alimentation hospitalière à la fin du Moyen Âge: l'exemple de l'Hôtel-Dieu de Paris (avec édition de texte)', in *Hospitäler in Mittelalter und Früher Neuzeit: Frankreich, Deutschland und Italien; eine vergleichende Geschichte*, ed. Gisela Drossbach (Munich: Oldenbourg, 2007), 107-62.

—. '"Sustener les povres malades": alimentation et approvisionnement à la fin du Moyen Âge; l'exemple de l'Hôtel-Dieu de Paris', PhD diss., Université Paris I-Panthéon Sorbonne, 2000. Microfilm.

Jütte, Robert. '"Wo kein Weib ist, da seufzet der Kranke" – Familie und Krankheit im 16. Jahrhundert', *Jahrbuch des Instituts für Geschichte der Medizin der Robert-Bosch-Stiftung*, 7 (1988), 7-24.

Kinzelbach, Annemarie. 'Konstruktion und konkretes Handeln: Heilkundige Frauen im oberdeutschen Raum, 1450-1750', *Historische Anthropologie*, 7 (1999), 165-90.

—. '"Wahnsinnige Weyber betriegen den unverstendigen Poeffel": Anerkennung und Diffamierung heilkundiger Frauen und Männer 1450 bis 1700', *Medizinhistorisches Journal*, 32 (1997), 29-56.

Koeppel, Emil. 'Chaucer und Albertanus Brixiensis', *Archiv für das Studium der Neueren Sprachen und Litteraturen*, 86 (1891), 29-46.

Maclean, Ian. *The Renaissance Notion of Woman: A Study in the Fortunes of Scholasticism and Medical Science in European Intellectual Life* (Cambridge: Cambridge University Press, 1980).

Marböck, Johannes. 'Sirach/Sirachbuch', in *Theologische Realenzyklopädie*, ed. Horst Balz and others, vol. 31 (Berlin: De Gruyter, 2000), 307-17.

McNamer, Sarah. *Affective Meditation and the Invention of Medieval Compassion* (Philadelphia: University of Pennsylvania Press, 2010).

Mieder, Wolfgang and Lutz Röhrich. *Sprichwort* (Stuttgart: J.B. Metzler, 1977).

Morewedge, Rosmarie Thee. 'Proverbs', in *Handbook of Medieval Studies: Terms – Methods – Trends*, ed. Albrecht Classen, vol. 2 (Berlin: De Gruyter, 2010), 2026-55.

Nolte, Cordula. 'Domestic Care in the Sixteenth Century: Expectations, Experiences, and Practices from a Gendered Perspective', in *Gender, Health, and Healing, 1250-1550*, ed. Sara Ritchey and Sharon Strocchia (Amsterdam: Amsterdam University Press, 2020), 215-43.

Paz y Meliá, Antonio, ed. *Obras de Juan Rodríguez de la Cámara (o del Padrón)* (Madrid: Imprenta de Miguel Ginesta, 1884).

Pelling, Margaret. 'Compromised by Gender: The Role of the Male Medical Practitioner in Early Modern England', in *The Task of Healing: Medicine, Religion and Gender in England and the Netherlands 1450-1800*, ed. Hilary Marland and Margaret Pelling (Rotterdam: Erasmus, 1996), 101-34.

Peraldus, Guillelmus. *De eruditione principum*, ed. Roberto Busa, in *S. Thomae Aquinatis Opera Omnia ut sunt in indice thomistico additis 61 scriptis ex aliis medii aevi auctoribus*, vol. 7: *Aliorum medii aevi auctorum scripta 61* (Stuttgart/Bad Canstatt: Fromann-Holzboog, 1980), 89-121.

Pomata, Gianna. 'Was There a *Querelle des Femmes* in Early Modern Medicine?' *Arenal: Revista de Historia de las Mujeres*, 20.2 (2013), 313-41.

Powell, James Matthew. *Albertanus of Brescia: The Pursuit of Happiness in the Early Thirteenth Century* (Philadelphia: University of Pennsylvania Press, 1992).

Pugh, Tison. 'Gender, Vulgarity, and the Phantom Debates of Chaucer's *Merchant's Tale*', *Studies in Philology*, 114.3 (2017), 473-96.

Rabelais, François. *Le Tiers livre*, ed. Michael Screech (Paris: Droz, 1974).

Rankin, Alisha. 'The Housewife's Apothecary in Early Modern Austria: Wolfgang Helmhard von Hohberg's Georgica Curiosa (1682)', *Medicina & Storia*, 8.15 (2008), 55-76.

—. *Panaceia's Daughters: Noblewomen as Healers in Early Modern Germany* (Chicago: University of Chicago Press, 2013).

Rawcliffe, Carole. *Medicine and Society in Later Medieval England* (Stroud: Sutton, 1995).

Reinle, Christine. 'Was bedeutet Macht im Mittelalter?', in *Mächtige Frauen? Königinnen und Fürstinnen im europäischen Mittelalter*, ed. Claudia Zey (Ostfildern: Jan Thorbecke, 2015), 35-72.

Riddy, Felicity. 'Authority and Intimacy in the Late Medieval Urban Home', in *Gendering the Master Narrative: Women and Power in the Middle Ages*, ed. Mary Erler and Maryanne Kowaleski (Ithaca, NY: Cornell University Press, 2003), 212-28.

Ritchey, Sara. 'Affective Medicine: Late Medieval Healing Communities and the Feminization of Health Care Practices in the Thirteenth-Century Low Countries', *Journal of Medieval Religious Cultures*, 40.2 (2014), 113-43.

—. 'Caring by the Hours: The Psalter as a Gendered Healthcare Technology', in *Gender, Health, and Healing, 1250-1550*, ed. Sara Ritchey and Sharon Strocchia (Amsterdam: Amsterdam University Press, 2020), 41-66.

Roth, Detlef. '*An uxor ducenda*: zur Geschichte eines Topos von der Antike bis zur frühen Neuzeit', in *Geschlechterbeziehungen und Textfunktionen: Studien zu Eheschriften der frühen Neuzeit*, ed. Rüdiger Schnell (Tübingen: Max Niemeyer, 1998), 171-223.

Schnell, Rüdiger. 'The Discourse on Marriage in the Middle Ages', *Speculum*, 73.3 (1998), 771-86.

Sensi, Mario. 'Anchoresses and Penitents in Thirteenth- and Fourteenth-Century Umbria', in *Women and Religion in Medieval and Renaissance Italy*, ed. Daniel Bornstein and Roberto Rusconi, trans. Margary J. Schneider (Chicago: University of Chicago Press, 1996), 57-83.

Signori, Gabriela. *Von der Paradiesehe zur Gütergemeinschaft: die Ehe in der mittelalterlichen Lebens- und Vorstellungswelt* (Frankfurt: Campus, 2011).

Sohn-Kronthaler, Michaela, 'Armutsdiskurse und Gender(-frage) im deutschsprachigen Katholizismus des 19. Jahrhunderts', in *Konfessionen in den west- und mitteleuropäischen Sozialsystemen im langen 19. Jahrhundert: ein 'edler Wettkampf der Barmherzigkeit'?*, ed. Michaela Maurer and Bernhard Schneider (Berlin: LIT, 2013), 325-50.

Sperling, Jutta Gisela. *Roman Charity: Queer Lactations in Early Modern Visual Culture* (Bielefeld: transcript, 2016).

Strocchia, Sharon T., ed. *Women and Healthcare in Early Modern Europe*, special issue of *Renaissance Studies*, 28.4 (2014).

Vandeventer Pearman, Tory. *Women and Disability in Medieval Literature* (New York: Palgrave Macmillan, 2010).

Verweij, Michiel. 'Princely Virtues or Virtues for Princes? William Peraldus and his *De erudinione principum*', in *Princely Virtues in the Middle Ages, 1200-1500*, ed. István P. Bejczy and Cary J. Nederman (Turnhout: Brepols, 2007), 51-71.

Vives, Juan Luis. *The Education of a Christian Woman: A Sixteenth-Century Manual*, ed. and trans. Charles Fantazzi (Chicago: University of Chicago Press, 2000).

Weber, Robert, and Roger Gryson, ed. *Biblia sacra iuxta vulgatam versionem*, 5th ed. (Stuttgart: Deutsche Bibelgesellschaft, 2013).
Whaley, Leigh Ann. *Women and the Practice of Medical Care in Early Modern Europe, 1400-1800* (New York: Palgrave Macmillan, 2011).
Wright, Thomas, ed. *The Book of the Knight of La Tour-Landry*, Early English Text Society 33 (London: Trübner, 1868).

About the Author

Eva-Maria Cersovsky is completing her PhD dissertation on healthcare, charity, and gender in fifteenth- and sixteenth-century Strasbourg at the a.r.t.e.s. Graduate School for the Humanities, Cologne. She co-organized the international workshop, 'Gender(ed) Histories of Health, Healing and the Body, 1250-1550', held at the University of Cologne in January 2018 that forms the basis of this volume.

8 Domestic Care in the Sixteenth Century

Expectations, Experiences, and Practices from a Gendered Perspective

Cordula Nolte

Abstract
This essay combines a gendered approach with a perspective on the spatial, material, and performative dimensions of care practices within sixteenth-century German domestic environments. Terminological and semantic challenges of premodern and modern vocabularies are discussed first. The essay questions dichotomies between public, communal, and institutional care versus private, domestic care in light of the collaboration between internal and external experts and the collective nature of infirmity and caregiving. Using a case study of written and pictorial instructions in an illustrated surgeon's manual, the essay suggests the value of interdisciplinary approaches to the field of premodern care.

Keywords: spatial environment, material environment, performance of care, body, bed, terminology

Unlike institutional care, domestic care in the premodern era has only recently begun to emerge as a field of interdisciplinary research. New perspectives on social groups and networks, body history, dis/ability history, and other overlapping approaches have favoured a shift of focus towards caregiving within families, households, friendships, and neighbourhoods. Microhistorical and case studies have unearthed a number of formerly unknown or disregarded sources that shed light on the practices and spaces, organization, and financing of domestic or 'private' care for infirm persons.[1] Scholars using the lens of gender have added details and contours to formerly

1 Frohne, *Leben*, 188-281; Cabré, 'Women or Healers?'; Harkness, 'View from the Streets'.

Ritchey, Sara & Sharon Strocchia (eds), *Gender, Health, and Healing, 1250-1550*. Amsterdam, Amsterdam University Press 2020
DOI: 10.5117/9789463724517_CH08

general notions that in premodern societies both women and men actively engaged in caregiving and were cared for. Domestic caregiving was identified as an acknowledged field of female and male work within late medieval and early modern urban economies. Linking communal and private spheres, it created and shaped social nets between women and men of different social strata.[2]

Still, many aspects of domestic care have not yet been examined systematically. There are few studies that cross disciplinary borders or proceed comparatively. General assumptions that within households women were more often associated with active care than men, or that specific activities were performed in accordance with gender-related norms and expectations, have to be tested by scrutinizing written, visual, and material evidence. Also, some basic questions should be considered in order to assess the extent to which premodern domestic care was a gendered field of action. Above all, what is the meaning of 'domestic care' with regard to premodern societies?

It seems useful to start with reflections on premodern and modern terminologies before turning to the concrete, specific acts performed within the work of domestic care for infirm persons. Who performed them? Who is presented as a recipient of care in the role of patient? In which social and spatial environments did domestic care actually take place?[3] How were rooms of care organized? Which kinds of furnishing, equipment, and material objects were part of them and shaped the interaction of women and men in the field of care? These last questions are inspired by recent object-centred analyses of historical and modern care practices. Against a backdrop of spatial, material, and performative 'turns' in the humanities, they conceive of care as an interaction of humans and objects within spaces that follows a specific choreography.[4] Read alongside the essays by Iliana Kandzha on relics, Ayman Atat on bathtubs, and Sara Ritchey on books and images, my contribution underlines the performative and spatial dimensions of care, including therapeutic tools for transmitting medical knowledge and facilitating medical practice.[5] Due to the fragmentary and diverse character of source material, however, it may be difficult to grasp some kind of premodern 'care choreography'.[6] Yet, studying 'care things',

2 Frohne, 'Unterstützungsnetzwerke'; Munkhoff, 'Poor Women and Parish Public Health'.

3 The essay collection, Horden and Smith, eds., *Locus of Care*, departs from a broad concept of support, including care for infirm persons.

4 Kollewe et al., 'Pflegedinge'; see also Braunschweig, ed., *Pflege*.

5 Kandzha, 'Female Saints as Agents of Female Healing'; Atat, 'Bathtubs as a Healing Approach'; Ritchey, 'Caring by the Hours' – this volume.

6 The term 'care choreography' is used by Atzl and Depner, 'Home Care Home', 279.

material environments, and spatial arrangements of bodies seems to be a fresh, original approach.[7] Thus, this essay is an experiment.

This essay draws on a variety of written evidence: autobiographical narratives and family records, as well as urban administrative material and manuals. Since my observations are based on a selection of sources, they offer suggestive findings which may contribute to exploring the field in a systematic and comparative way. Due to the limited range of materials, however, my results may not be representative and generalization should be avoided. Beginning with some remarks on terminology, I will then comment on categories within the field of care before turning to care practised among household members in the environment of the *stube*, the heated centre of dwelling houses. Considering urban networks and social nets shifts the focus from wealthy households to poorer parts of the population. The final section presents a case study based on textual and pictorial evidence. I will analyse an illustrated manual for surgeons written by the German surgeon Caspar Stromayr. His *Practica copiosa von dem Rechten Grundt Deß Bruch Schnidts* (1559), a manual on herniotomy, offers instructive information regarding agents of domestic care and their collaboration within the spatial and material setting of a civic household.

Terminology

Writing an article in English based on sixteenth-century German records requires some remarks concerning vocabularies and semantics. Premodern written German was hardly standardized but instead reflected regional differences in speech. Due to changes of terminology and semantics in recent centuries, texts must be translated from premodern to modern German. Moreover, the semantic contents of the English word field 'care' and its German equivalent *Pflege* are far from being congruent. In addition, there is a multitude of definitions of care within different modern languages and disciplines which fuels current debates about how to use the modern German term *Pflege*.[8] In some discourses a double term or conjunction, linking the German and the English noun ('Pflege und Care'), is used. Thus the specific, limited meaning of *Pflege* as nursing infirm or needy persons is combined with the broader range of meaning conveyed by the English term 'care'. In some contexts the latter corresponds to the German term *Sorge*,

7 See also Ott, 'Disability Things'.

8 Kollewe et al., 'Pflegedinge', 19-26.

which is understood by some scholars as a set of attitudes and practices towards human beings that is both the basis for and a constituent part of the activities labelled as *Pflege*.

The medieval noun *pflege* and the corresponding verb *pflegen* originally referred to caring and guarding in administrative and juridical contexts. It was only at the end of the Middle Ages that they were regularly used as umbrella terms in the sense of caring for infirm persons. In sixteenth-century records the term 'pfleger', which previously had denoted administrators and supervisors with official or legal authority, is applied to male caregivers, and the female equivalent 'pflegerin' is introduced. At the time these terms only occasionally referred to professional care workers, whereas later they became modern professional titles. When Jacob Oetheus (d. 1586), a professor of medicine, published a manual on health and healing addressed to healthy and sick persons and to caregivers, he used the term 'pfleger' without indicating the gender of caregivers or defining an institutional or domestic context. He expected relatives as well as non-relatives to care for patients. The third part of his book is considered to be the first manual that provides instruction on the (professional) care of infirm persons.[9]

In addition to *pflegen*, the term *warten* was used until the nineteenth century. Implying attendance and service towards infirm persons, *warten* was a synonym for *pflegen*; however, it sometimes also included the meaning of watching and warding in the context of custody. This latter meaning is maintained in the modern German denomination *Wärter* for guards, keepers, and warders. Other terms frequently used in premodern documents such as 'cur' (from Latin *cura*), 'hailung' (healing), 'hilf' (help), and 'hantreichung' (assistance) summarized therapeutic and supportive measures in the domain of care and cure without specifying concrete activities. As may be expected, premodern rhetorics did not differentiate between care and cure, as this field characteristically was perceived as a continuum. In keeping with contemporary concepts of health based on the theoretical system of the six non-naturals, there was no need to categorize medical treatment as curative *stricto sensu* or to distinguish it from other ways of striving for health and healing. Of course, with regard to actual practices and practitioners, explicit distinctions were made in order to mark specific competencies, achievements, and responsibilities. In Nuremberg, for example, Marcella Praunbergerin, a 'bruchärztin' (female practitioner specializing in hernia),

9 Oetheus, *Gründtlicher Bericht*, 116-82. For a commentary see Hähner-Rombach, *Quellen*, 158-63.

received payment for her work as a surgeon ('artztlohn am bruchhailn'), as well as a separate wage called 'Wartgeld' for giving care to her patients and extra money for the bandages.[10] Further examples of pragmatic specifications within the conceptual entity of care and cure are mentioned below in the section on urban webs.

Fields of Action

When identifying the specific elements of domestic care, most autobiographical narratives and family histories are vague or fragmentary. Consequently, it is helpful to look at institutional documents such as hospital ordinances as supplements. Some of these normative texts contained detailed catalogues of duties assigned to different staff members, including those who nursed sick inmates. We may assume that the most basic activities were performed within domestic environments as well.

Nurses in hospitals were expected to organize the beds of infirm persons; arrange the bedding, cushions, and sheets; cook and administer food; lift and turn the infirm in bed; wash their bodies, clothing, and bedlinen; lead them to the commode chair or privy; empty and clean the chamber pot and other vessels; clean the room and its furniture; burn incense, sit up with the sick, comfort and admonish them and provide for all their needs.[11]

According to these lists, institutional care basically consisted of four fields of action. These are prominent in narratives on domestic settings as well, as discussed below. Centred on the body, the bed, housework, and emotional and spiritual support, these four fields overlapped.[12] Field 1: Caring for infirm persons meant being close to their bodies, performing such actions as touching and moving, nourishing and cleaning, dressing and covering them. It was bodily work in the double meaning of physical labour performed on another person's body. Field 2: The most important site and tool of care was the bed, which allowed nurses to perform their

10 Frohne, 'Unterstützungsnetzwerke', 216.

11 This list is compiled from several ordinances: Scheutz et al., *Quellen*, no. 1 (Spitalordnung des Wiener Hofspitals, 1551, with additions from 1568, pp. 306-21), at pp. 312-13. Winckelmann, *Das Fürsorgewesen*, no. 5 (Ordnung der Küsterin, fifteenth century, pp. 10-12), at p. 11; no. 10 (Ordnung des großen Spitals zu Straßburg [...], *c.*1540, pp. 20-27), at p. 27; no. 15 (Ordnung der Mägt im Spital [...], 1547), pp. 46-49; see also p. 182, n. 4, on communally employed female and male nurses who did ambulant service in private households. See Vanja, 'Aufwärterinnen', 14; Strocchia, 'Caring for the "Incurable"'.

12 Cabré, 'Women or Healers?', 25-26.

work on the body and required considerable attention in and of itself.[13] By washing and changing bedclothes, arranging cushions, sheets, and linen-covered bedspreads, nurses created an environment that was both hygienic and comfortable to body and mind. Field 3: Laundering the clothes of the infirm involved dealing with textiles which, like cooking and administering food, was part of basic household activities and daily-life routines. Field 4: Emotional support, or consolation, is often indicated in the context of round-the-clock care. In institutions as well as in private households, infirm persons were expected to be assisted at all times. Thus caregivers had to stay close to them, taking turns if necessary, and answer their needs. As Eva Cersovsky comments in her essay in this volume, the laborious nature of these tasks were compounded by the fact that they were often carried out in difficult conditions. The psychological dimension of this attendance was taken as seriously as bodily assistance.[14] All of these activities aiming at body, mind, and soul within the material environment were regarded as health-preserving and curative according to the theory of the non-naturals. Recent studies have underlined that this concept, which formed the base of premodern medicine and healthcare, oriented daily life practices.[15]

Household Members as Patients and Caregivers

Autobiographical narratives, family records, and letters present caring for sick, debilitated or aging family members, relatives, and servants as a normal part of household routines and a collective obligation, but they often do not mention who performs specific activities.[16] Their descriptions of care arrangements cannot be read as reports on concrete situations, since they did not intend to present complete information but were stylized according to literary traditions and moral ideals.[17] Thus narratives may have been shaped by intentions to show that husbands, wives, parents, daughters, and sons fulfilled the mutual obligations demanded by role models. Also, fragmentary details on the material and spatial environment only occasionally allow glimpses into rooms and their equipment.[18]

13 Heitmann-Möller and Remmers, 'Pflegebett'.

14 See below (on Stromayr), and Cersovsky, '*Ubi non est mulier*', this volume.

15 Frohne, *Leben*, 256-57; Nolte, '*der leib*', 53; Cabré, 'Women or Healers?', 23, 26.

16 Frohne, *Leben*, 262, on the description of care as a diffuse collective family effort.

17 Frohne, *Leben*, 257, n. 319.

18 The sites and utensils of caregiving in hospitals are more completely documented by texts, images, and archaeological findings. Some unearthed objects allow conclusions with regard to

An episode from Margery Kempe's 'Book' is illustrative here, even though her work was written in late medieval England and, in terms of genre, is an extraordinary hybrid of religious fiction and autobiography.[19] Margery Kempe (*c.*1373-after 1438) vividly describes how her alter ego, the creature, nursed her aging husband who had been injured when falling down the stairs. Social pressure from 'people' and the immediate command of Christ himself urged the wife to look after her husband, although at that time the couple lived separately after taking a vow of chastity:

> Then she took her husband home with her and looked after him for years afterwards, as long as he lived. She had very much trouble with him, for in his last days he turned childish and lacked reason, so that he could not go to a stool to relieve himself, or else he would not, but like a child discharged his excrement into his linen clothes as he sat there by the fire or at the table – wherever it was, he would spare no place. And therefore her labour was all the greater, in washing and wringing, and so were her expenses for keeping a fire going. All this hindered her a very great deal from her contemplation, so that many times she would have disliked her work, except that she thought to herself how she in her young days had had very many delectable thoughts, physical lust, and inordinate love for his body. And therefore she was glad to be punished by means of the same body, and took it much the more easily, and served him and helped him, she thought, as she would have done Christ himself.[20]

Caring for the old man with his progressing dementia is represented as hard labour and a burden, yet at the same time interpreted as an act of love from a spiritual perspective. Its religious message aside, the text points to the ambivalent attitude of the caregiver in an unusually outspoken way; it also evokes details of care in a specific material and spatial environment by mentioning concrete acts of service and help, aspects of diet and hygiene, the quality of clothes, pieces of furniture, and permanent heating. Apparently the infirm husband is accommodated in a well-equipped, heated central room. Special care devices such as a commode chair are available, and his underwear is changed frequently. It is unlikely that a wealthy household

the care choreography. See Egan, 'Material Culture', 68, on a reversible ash-wood bowl with a flange from a hospital site that 'could be a design specifically for a second person to hold steady by the foot while an infirm patient was fed'.

19 Staley, *Fictions*.

20 [Kempe,] *Book of Margery Kempe*, bk. 1, ch. 76, 219-21. For a commentary see Nolte, 'Häusliche Pflege'.

like this did not include servants who did the laundry. In order to focus attention on the wife's efforts, they may have been omitted in this scene.

Margery Kempe's narrative is representative by showing the heated centre of the house as the locus of care. Well into the sixteenth century the interior architecture of urban houses and the functional organization of rooms were characterized by medieval structures that basically differentiated between heated and unheated rooms (*stube* versus *cammer*) and between rooms having different access and publicity. In premodern urban houses of wealthy families, sleeping chambers used to be unheated or poorly heated at best. Located on an upper floor, they were less accessible than the *stube* or *dornse* which served as the main living room and was heated by a stove or a fireplace. The *stube* seems to have been the only place that maintained a comfortable temperature. Here all kinds of daily-life activities – meals, pastimes, reception of visitors, festivities – took place. Thus persons who had been infirm for long periods or were not expected to recover were moved into this multifunctional, public place in order to facilitate caregiving, company, and participation. They were seated in easy chairs, shared meals with the family, talked to visitors, and received therapy. Special beds were made up that could be easily moved and fitted to the room; these supported caregiving by being accessible from several sides.

In his family records Hermann Weinsberg (1518-1597), a member of the council of Cologne, describes several care situations in his own household and among relatives. In 1573 his wife Drutgin Barß, who had suffered from a 'terrible cough' for ten years, fell seriously ill. After sixteen days she left the marital sleeping chamber on the upper floor, had a small bed ('rutzbetgin') installed in the 'stoben' [sic], and 'stayed there day and night with her servant Else' for six weeks until her death.[21] Weinsberg also gives details about other smaller beds that were transported into the 'stobe' [sic] so that family members and guests could easily gather around.[22] Visual representations show beds of infirm persons with a tool (a cloth hanging down), which enabled the bedridden person to sit up and turn independently.[23] Obviously these beds provided maximum comfort for the patient and ensured that she or he was at the centre of attention. Whereas such comfortable places of care are well documented in cases of highly respected family members, such as heads of households or their fathers and mothers, it seems unlikely that household members of less prestige enjoyed such convenient arrangements.

21 [Weinsberg,] *Liber iuventutis*, fols. 629r, 630v-632v.

22 Jütte, 'Familie und Krankheit', 7; Frohne, *Leben*, 206.

23 Frohne, *Leben*, 206-7, 366. See below (on Stromayr).

However, Weinsberg's sister-in-law had such a bed installed in case she, her husband, or one of the handmaids fell ill.

Weinberg's narrations are instructive in several ways. They illustrate that in premodern households spatial arrangements were flexible and easily adapted to care exigencies.[24] They pay attention to environmental details that reflect familial cohesion, noting, for example, that during meals Druitgin sat at table or nearby on a low easy chair ('uff eim niddern raststoil'). They show the closeness of individual female servants to their mistresses and masters, which implied caregiving around the clock. Handmaids generally slept in close proximity to the marital couple and their children, sometimes sharing chambers with their daughters. They were readily available, well informed, and experienced about household needs.[25] Furthermore, Hermann's narrative on Drutgin's infirmity and death evokes material and spatial details of the scene that are loaded with emotional meaning. Druitgin's exit from the sleeping chamber implies the loss of marital intimacy.[26] When some years before his infirm wife had slept alone for eight weeks, he noted that 'she felt pity for me, sent away the servants, and I nursed her this once by myself as I wished to, but afterwards I had to sleep alone all the time until God would bring about recovery'.[27]

Records from Stralsund regarding the second marriage of mayor Bartholomäus Sastrow (1520-1603) allow glimpses into the interrelations between intimacy, bodily closeness, and care. According to Sastrow, his late wife Katharina Froböse had often helped him ('gedecket und geholfen') when he had severe fits at night due to a 'catarrhum suffocatum'.[28] When she died after forty-eight years of marriage, the widower was afraid of suffocating without 'jemand im Bette' ('someone in his bed').[29] Sastrow, a man of 78 years, now wished to marry Anna Haseneier, a servant in his household, just

24 Nolte, *Frauen*, 54, and Frohne, *Leben*, 205, on the dynamics of premodern families and households.

25 The accommodation of servants in urban households deserves further investigation with regard to social nets and daily life practices. See [Weinsberg,] *Liber iuventutis*, fol. 660r-v, on living as a widower with his servant ('min jong') Bochart Lintlar.

26 Druitgin 'did not return to the sleeping chamber; before we had slept on two separate beds in our sleeping chamber as she wished to lay alone due to her constant cough'; [Weinsberg,] *Liber iuventutis*, fol. 632r.

27 Ibid., fol. 539r: 'Und wie ich an 8 wochen nit bei ir gesclaiffen jamert sei meiner schickt daß gesindt auß, und ich wartet irer daß mail nach minem willen allein, malst aber darnach alleß allein sclaiffen biß es got besser foegen wirt'.

28 [Sastrow,] *Herkommen*, 217. On caring wives and needy husbands see Cersovsky, '*Ubi non est mulier*', this volume.

29 [Sastrow,] *Herkommen*, 212-13.

weeks after Katharina's death. This caused some scandal among council members. Sastrow justified this intention by his infirmity and the resulting inability to run the household.[30] In particular, he underlined his need for urgent assistance, especially at night: after his wife's death he tried in vain to wake the handmaids by calling out, and almost suffocated.[31] Apparently these servants were accommodated nearby, but in his opinion not close enough. Besides, he had observed that his new bride had loyally cared for his sick wife, reading to her, nursing her day and night and staying at her deathbed. As a long-term servant Anna was well-informed about the condition of his household and his body.[32] Her moral integrity, expertise, and faithfulness as a nurse, along with her knowledge of his domestic and personal needs, qualified her for marriage with him.

Compared to narratives on female household members, evidence that male servants performed intimate acts of care is rare.[33] When the shoemaker Sebastian Fischer (b. 1513) was infected by a sort of plague, he spent several weeks in bed and developed sores on his back. Having recently lost his wife, Fischer felt frail, painful, and deserted. Nevertheless, he was treated by physicians and his aunt cooked for him; moreover, his servant Jacob Ott not only kept his business running but cleaned his sores, laundered his underwear, emptied the chamber pot, 'and treated me as faithfully as if I were his father'.[34] By making this analogy, Fischer evoked the ideal of filial devotion as a model for a male caregiver's attitude towards his patient. Undoubtedly sons felt obliged to take in infirm parents and organize domestic care for them. Cyriacus Gottschalck, for example, repeatedly asked his mother to live with him and his wife, and promised to give her a chamber of her own. In case she fell ill, he would be able to provide better care than if she lived with strangers ('bei einem frömden').[35] The Hildesheim citizen Joachim Brandis (1553-1615) mentioned that 'someone' had to nurse his old, infirm, demented mother all the time and assist her in all matters ('einer stets up se warten und alle hantreikunge doin moiste').[36] He does

30 Ibid., 217. Sastrow was almost blind, could walk only with a guide, and could not access the kitchen or pantry.

31 Ibid., 217: 'könne seine Mägde mit Rufen nit aufwecken vnd habe oft ersticken wollen'.

32 Ibid., 218-19.

33 Frohne, *Leben*, 263.

34 *Sebastian Fischers Chronik*, 27-28, quote at 28: 'vnd mir trewlich gethon sam ich sein vatter sey'.

35 Letter to his mother, 28 January 1539; Hölscher, 'Handwerkerbriefe', 263, no. 13. Frohne, *Leben*, 301.

36 [Brandis,] *Diarium*, 257. See Prühlen, *Annäherung*, 250.

not say who actually performed this work and, like Cyriacus Gottschalck, does not mention his own contributions. However, Brandis notes that his sisters took turns spending the nights with his sick father.[37] When both of his parents fell ill, his sisters stayed with them and assisted them.[38] This is remarkable, since the brother was evacuated to a safe place due to a plague outbreak.[39] Other narratives confirm the role of daughters in performing various care activities. Josua Maler (1529-1599), a cleric from Zurich, lists shopping, cooking, washing the body and clothes, sitting up, 'and all other ways of befitting care' when he mentions his widowed sister's care for their old, infirm father.[40]

The important role played by wives and daughters in the field of domestic care has been underlined by scholars who have analysed autobiographical and familial records of the sixteenth century.[41] As Bianca Frohne has observed, these documents stem from the upper strata and their findings should not be generalized to less affluent households.[42] Interestingly, communal records on the distribution of alms indicate that – from the perspective of alms commissioners – husbands did not contribute sufficient support in some poor households with infirm housewives. In Luzern, for instance, lists of needy individuals and families indicate that some infirm women were permitted to receive domestic or institutional care on the grounds that they were not 'helped' by their husbands ('hatt kein hillff von ime').[43] 'Help' may refer here to caring in the sense of nursing (*pflägen*) as well as economic maintenance (*erhallten*). In many households men were absent due to mercenary service or foreign work.[44] Sometimes the records hint at a husband's disorderly conduct and careless behaviour. In the case of an epileptic woman who at times was mentally disturbed and unable to work, her husband was expected to assist her ('sol der mann ouch handreichung thůn'). Yet, in spite of being home he refused to be around her.[45] Eva Cersovsky has revealed similar findings with regard to the welfare system in Strasburg by identifying stereotypes

37 [Brandis,] *Diarium*, 403.

38 Ibid., 107.

39 Ibid.

40 *Ynkaufen, Kochen, Wüschen, Wäschen, Wachen und aller anderen gebührenden Pfleg.* quoted in Frohne, 'Häusliche Krankenversorgung', 469.

41 Prühlen, *Annäherung*, 250; Frohne, 'Häusliche Krankenversorgung', 469; Frohne, *Leben*, 263-64.

42 Frohne, 'Häusliche Krankenversorgung', 469.

43 Jäggi, *Arm sein in Luzern*, 188 (1591/12), 192 (1591/37).

44 Ibid., 38-39.

45 'Er ist heim, will aber nit zů ir'; ibid., 171 (1590/197).

of the 'absent husband' and the 'deserted woman'.[46] Whereas the records from Luzern name several daughters who nursed their mothers, they do not mention any caregiving sons.[47] Poor and infirm Anna Krämerin, for instance, had four robust sons who were in service and an 18-old daughter who nursed her. When the alms commissioners asked the sons whether they could help their mother, the answer was negative.[48] Even if a son was explicitly mentioned as living with his mother, he was not named as a caregiver.[49] Although in principle sons and daughters were guided by similar expectations and obligations, gendered practices prevailed in daily life.

Urban Webs of Care

Domestic care included outside personnel who collaborated with household members when necessary. In keeping with premodern medical pluralism, a wide range of external experts contributed to the work of care and cure: learned physicians, male and female empirically trained surgeons and other practitioners, specialists for conditions such as cataract and hernia, diverse sorts of healers and pharmaceutical empirics, apothecaries, beguines and so-called sisters of religious houses. In wealthy households, there seems to have been a constant traffic of experts coming and going. The family records of Hermann Weinsberg are particularly informative about the number and diversity of persons who participated in domestic care and cure, including friends who offered advice.[50]

In view of the 'overlapping and complementary' contexts and structures of services, researchers have argued that households should be regarded as 'open and receptive centers of care'. They also advocate looking at premodern urban healthcare systems as 'a web of multiple resources'.[51] Consequently,

46 Cersovsky, 'Blind Fraw'.

47 For example, Dorothea Sattlerin, a poor, bedridden, and infirm widow: 'Hatt ein tochter by iro, 18 järig, so iro pflägt' ('lives with an eighteen-year old daughter who nurses her'); Jäggi, *Arm sein in Luzern*, 106 (1590/50), 200 (1591/988), 209 (1591/146).

48 'sol man den sönen nachfragen, ob sy vermöchtend handreichung zthund. Sy sagen, die sön vermögent nüt'; Jäggi, *Arm sein in Luzern*, 140 (1590/139). There are further entries on the inability of sons to 'help' their infirm mothers; ibid., 184 (1590/230).

49 Elsbeth Hessin, a poor and infirm widow, lived with her son, an eighteen-year-old student; Jäggi, *Arm sein in Luzern*, 146 (1590/143), 209 (1591/147).

50 His home was 'half an inn' ('war ein half gasthus bei uns') when his wife and two sons were bedridden; [Weinsberg,] *Liber iuventutis*, fol. 535v. Jütte, *Ärzte*.

51 Cabré, 'Women or Healers?', 26, 50; Harkness, 'View from the Streets', 56, 65.

the assumption of clear-cut boundaries between private households and public institutions has become obsolete. Microhistorical studies with a regional focus create a complex, differentiated picture of care that shows the reciprocal nature of interaction across different socio-economic strata and the multitude of formal and informal arrangements.[52]

The city of Luzern exemplifies this connection between domestic and communal spheres. When the city council reorganized the welfare system in 1590, a new alms ordinance was introduced and protocols of the alms commission's decisions were drawn up. Needy persons were registered in catalogues (1590-92), which described their individual and familial situation in detail.[53] In many cases poverty went hand in hand with infirmity, impairment, and inability to work. Apart from food, clothes, and money, these persons were supported by various measures ranging from reception in the hospital to the provision of medical services by a surgeon and other male and female practitioners paid by the alms fund. The surgeon Hans Rublin had the double function of a paid hospital barber and a barber who was paid separately for each cure when treating alms recipients; he also earned an annual salary for further therapies and 'geng' (probably visits to his patients at home).[54] His therapeutic work is characterized by the verb 'artznen' and the noun 'Cůr' and his payment called 'Artzetlon' ('surgeon's salary').[55] This terminology is also applied to the work of an unnamed woman who, at the request of Hans Rublin, promised to medically treat ('ze artznen') an infirm woman in exchange for any wage the alms commissioners would pay.[56] Since she was given 2 florins for her own maintenance, she seems to have been a poor woman who offered therapy in tandem with master Rublin.[57] She both contributed to and benefitted from the welfare system. Dorothea an der Gant, an infirm widow, was another communally supported practitioner who got paid for assisting other poor persons. A specialist on

52 Frohne, *Leben* (on Nürnberg and Southern Germany); Munkhoff, 'Poor Women and Parish Public Health' (on London); McIntosh, 'Networks' (on Hadleigh); Dinges, 'Self-help' (on Bordeaux); Cersovsky, 'Pflege und Geschlecht' (on Strasburg). For a comparative approach see Van Steensel, 'Variations'.

53 Jäggi, *Arm sein in Luzern*, 9-19.

54 Staatsarchiv Luzern, COD 5145, fol. 172r.

55 Ibid., fols. 218r, 248r.

56 Ibid., fol. 258r: 'Begert nüt für die Cůr dann was den Allmůsnern gefellig'.

57 According to a different reading the money is given to the patient: Jäggi, *Arm sein in Luzern*, 237. However, paid caregiving by women as a way of subsistence ('narung') is mentioned frequently. Ibid., 82 (1590/1): The widow Anna Ärni subsisted from caregiving and journey work. *Sebastian Fischers Chronik*, 10: 'Ir narung [ist] gwesen das sy krancken leytten hat zugsehen vnd zugsprochen' ('she lived on looking after infirm persons').

dermatophytosis ('erbgrind'), she had children 'in der Cůr'.[58] This term probably implied that Dorothea treated children in her own household. Her work did not always include providing food and clothing, since this was organized by the alms commission or the hospital.[59]

Frequently poor and infirm individuals were granted trips to bathing resorts. In the case of Elsbeth Hessin, the alms commission even paid for her medicine and the female nurse ('pflägerin') who cared for her while travelling.[60] From a communal perspective, therapeutic bathing must have been perceived as an expensive but effective way of restoring the working ability of infirm individuals. Thus visits to curative spas were not exclusive to wealthy households but were also made available to the poor.[61]

The welfare system in other cities was based on similar structures. Bianca Frohne has explored links between 'private' and 'public' spheres in Nuremberg by examining networks of men and women drawn from different socio-economic milieus and their relevance for the urban economy.[62] In Nuremberg the above mentioned female surgeon Marcella Praunbergerin 'cured old and young persons from hernia' ('allte vnnd junge am bruch heilet'). She was paid from communal funds if her patients could not afford treatment. She was awarded an annual amount for nursing patients ('Wartgeld') plus a fixed sum per treatment, which differed according to gender and age. The accounts of the welfare office do not mention whether Marcella worked in her own household or visited patients. Other women in Nuremberg temporarily housed and fed infirm persons in their own households. One of the councilmen, for instance, paid a surgeon for removing a boy's kidney or bladder stones and gave the same amount to a woman who afterwards nursed the boy in her household for four weeks. From the perspective of these women, this was domestic care practised in their own spaces.[63] Widows of low economic status in particular benefitted from

58 Luzern, Staatsarchiv, COD 5145, fol. 258v; Jäggi, *Arm sein in Luzern*, 92.

59 Jäggi, *Arm sein in Luzern*, 239.

60 Luzern, Staatsarchiv, COD 5145, fol. 172v; Jäggi, *Arm sein in Luzern*, 158-59.

61 On Nürnberg see Mummenhoff, 'Gesundheits- und Krankenpflege', 64. Nolte, 'Arbeits(un)fähigkeit', on Lucas Rem (1481-1542), who visited therapeutic baths with large parts of his household; [Rem,] 'Tagebuch', 28. On 'therapeutic tourism' see Atat, 'Bathtubs as a Healing Approach', this volume.

62 Frohne, 'Unterstützungsnetzwerke', 216. In the following passage I draw on this article. See also Frohne, *Leben*.

63 Some surgeons also took in patients. For an example from Strasburg, see Winckelmann, *Das Fürsorgewesen*, no. 64 (Bestallung Lienhard Reinlins als Blatterarzt für die Armen, 3 November 1526), 111-13: A 'platerarzet' (specialist in treating smallpox) was given a house with six furnished beds that were reserved for poor sick persons sent by the leading health official.

boarding patients.[64] Whether paid communally or privately by councilmen, they participated in a welfare system that made extensive use of informal support networks. Thanks to cooperation between the council, wealthy citizens, and experienced practitioners, it was possible for poor and deserted persons to be treated, nursed and maintained, while providers of these services also obtained paid work.

The division of labour between diverse collaborators was just as typical in the organization of care as the interlacing of private households and public functions. Domestic and institutional spheres, even if spatially separate, were linked by persons who contributed specific services in different places like hospitals, their own dwellings, or their patients' houses. The surgeon Caspar Stromayr (1530-1567) was part of this system. When he obtained citizenship in Lindau, he offered to treat poor patients gratis and was granted the right of free residence in return.[65] In addition to this communal obligation, he worked independently as a specialist on hernias and cataracts. According to his manual *Practica copiosa* he may have performed surgery and follow-up care in his patients' households. This scenario deserves further investigation.

Pflegen / Wartten / vnnd Hailen: Care and Cure as Collective Labour

Stromayr's manual has been characterized as a pragmatically oriented work of medical prose, knowledge transfer, and an arcane book ('Geheimbuch') which instructed readers through both written and visual communication about the process of herniotomy.[66] The written text and pictorial programme explain and comment on each other without being identical.[67] They create an extraordinarily detailed picture of the surgical procedures involved and the performative, material, and spatial dimensions of cure and care.

The book opens with diagnostics that are represented by a series of male nudes, since the standard patient referenced in both text and image

According to the employment contract, the practitioner was obliged to cure them, house and supply them with food, drink, and medicine, and have them nursed. These tasks were to be performed by the man and his household members, probably his wife, relatives, and servants. In return, the physician was exempt from paying rent on the house. He also received a fixed weekly sum per patient to cover expenses, plus a wage for each cure and sufficient wood to heat his own and the patients' rooms.

64 McIntosh, 'Networks', 80, on a 'more varied pattern' in Hadleigh.

65 Stromayr, *Practica copiosa*, commentary by Kümmel, 4-5.

66 Stromayr, *Practica copiosa*, see the commentaries of Kümmel, and Keil and Proff.

67 Stromayr, *Practica copiosa*, commentary by Keil and Proff, 31.

is male. However, since Stromayr observed that women suffered hernia as well, he explains in a separate chapter how to perform surgery on them.[68] A single female patient is depicted fully dressed and is cited as feeling ashamed in a versed caption, which acknowledges the decency required when female bodies are represented visually. It does not imply that women actually feel or should feel ashamed when their bodies are examined by male practitioners. Also, a female nude is used when internal pathologies need to be shown.

The surgeon is instructed how to talk to a patient – female or male, young or old – and how to inform friends and family members of particular risks. Next the author explains each object and instrument needed for the operation and postsurgical care. Wound dressings, bandages, knives, and scissors are first shown in separate images as single objects and then as a symmetrically arranged collection on a table in front of the surgeon who explains them to another male figure, probably the addressee of the manual (Figure 8.1). These objects are thus assigned to male experts and symbolize, apart from their functionality, a gendered realm of professional work. The transfer of this realm into the domestic space is represented in an image showing the precise arrangement of utensils needed during the operation (fol. 75v). The bathtub and the plates and dishes in front of the patient also function as the surgeon's requisites because he is responsible for balneotherapy and diet.

After preparing everything for the herniotomy, the surgeon speaks with the patient's 'friends, father or mother, sisters or brothers and all persons standing around the infirm who take care of him'. They enter into a contract concerning his pay. In the corresponding picture (fol. 80r), women are absent, perhaps due to their limited legal capacity. The surgeon's 'Oration' in front of his audience refers to mutual obligations on both sides and to infirmity as a collective, public phenomenon. Therapeutic decisions, particularly about risky procedures such as herniotomy, were discussed among family members, neighbours, and friends.[69] Further, infirm individuals and practitioners usually communicated in the presence of a number of people 'standing around' ('vmbstender'), who as an audience gained knowledge and contributed to

68 Stromayr, *Practica copiosa*, ch. 14, fol. 110r-v; ch. 21, fols. 144r-149v, deals with uterine prolapse which, according to contemporary medicine, was a kind of hernia.

69 Hermann Weinsberg's nephew who suffered from hernia was examined by several physicians but his relatives could not decide whether to risk a herniotomy. Finally the boy's grandmother decided against surgery; [Weinsberg,] *Liber iuventutis*, fol. 541v. Weinsberg himself lived for decades with a hernia that caused him pain, impaired his mobility, and influenced his diet and dressing; fol. 723r.

Figure 8.1 'Die Jnstrumenta soltu han/ Ee dich deß schnidts solt vnderstan' ('You must have these instruments before performing herniotomy')

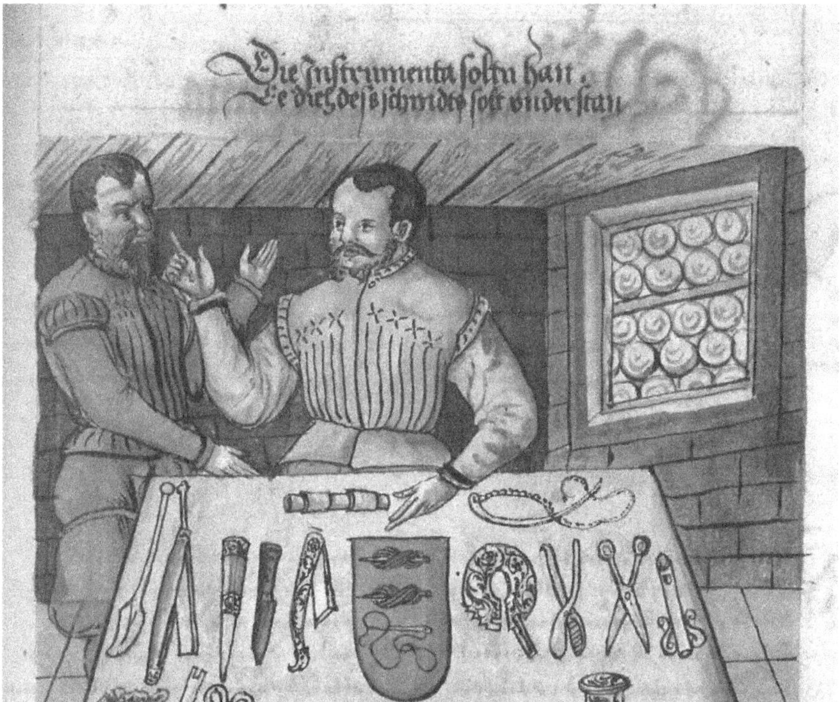

Caspar Stromayr, *Practica copiosa von dem Rechten Grundt Deß Bruch Schnidts*, 1559, fol. 63r. Lindau, Ehemals Reichsstädtische Bibliothek, P I 46.

caregiving.[70] Narrative and normative documents present household members as informed mediators between patients and practitioners. Stromayr, for instance, advises the surgeon to pass detailed knowledge about the festering wound to the *vmbstendern* in order to prevent them from panicking and running after him.[71] Persons who transported a person's urine to a physician had to relay details about the patient's condition in order to obtain a correct diagnosis.[72] Oetheus dedicates a chapter to this topic. If an ignorant person is sent, it is difficult to prescribe a useful therapy; moreover, prescriptions may be applied incorrectly. Thus messengers should be able to report accurately to the physician and communicate his orders to the patient in intelligible fashion.[73]

The surgical procedure is described step by step and demonstrated in a series of images. Both media are very detailed regarding the spatial positions of persons and objects, as well as individuals using specific tools. The architecture, configuration of persons, and display of objects are highly stylized, and the images stage an ideal environment. Nevertheless, the manual conveys a plausible notion of how teamwork was performed in a domestic frame. It describes and visualizes the care choreography based on experiences and practices.

The images show different patients and assistants in various versions of the *stube*, whereas the surgeon is portrayed as the same individual throughout.[74] Herniotomy is depicted as a concerted action of male figures. Three robust men are placed at the patient's head, side, and feet, with a stretcher serving as mobile surgical table. They assist the surgeon by binding and holding the patient. In one of these images a woman looks into the room through an open door in the background. Her coif indicates that she is a married woman. She appears at an advanced stage of the procedure when the cutting has been finished and the wound is closed by sewing. We may assume that her appearance alludes to imminent measures of care.

Such female engagement in postsurgical care is represented in an image found in a separate chapter on a specific kind of herniotomy caused by *hernia aquosa* ('Wasser Carniffel'). Here a woman enters the room at the moment when the surgeon finishes his work by affixing a drainage to the wound (Figure 8.2). Carrying a vessel shaped like a beer stein, she seems ready

70 Stolberg, *Praktiken*, ed. Brendecke, 112.

71 Stromayr, *Practica copiosa*, fol. 138v.

72 [Weinsberg,] *Liber iuventutis*, fol. 541v; *Sebastian Fischers Chronik*, 21.

73 Oetheus, *Gründtlicher Bericht*, pt. 3, ch. 5, 120-22.

74 Herniotomy is apparently performed in the patient's home. Stromayr also mentions places in the country and the surgeon's house when giving instructions concerning the mobile operating table; *Practica copiosa*, fols. 77r, 78r.

Figure 8.2 The surgeon applies a drainage while a woman provides the patient with a potion

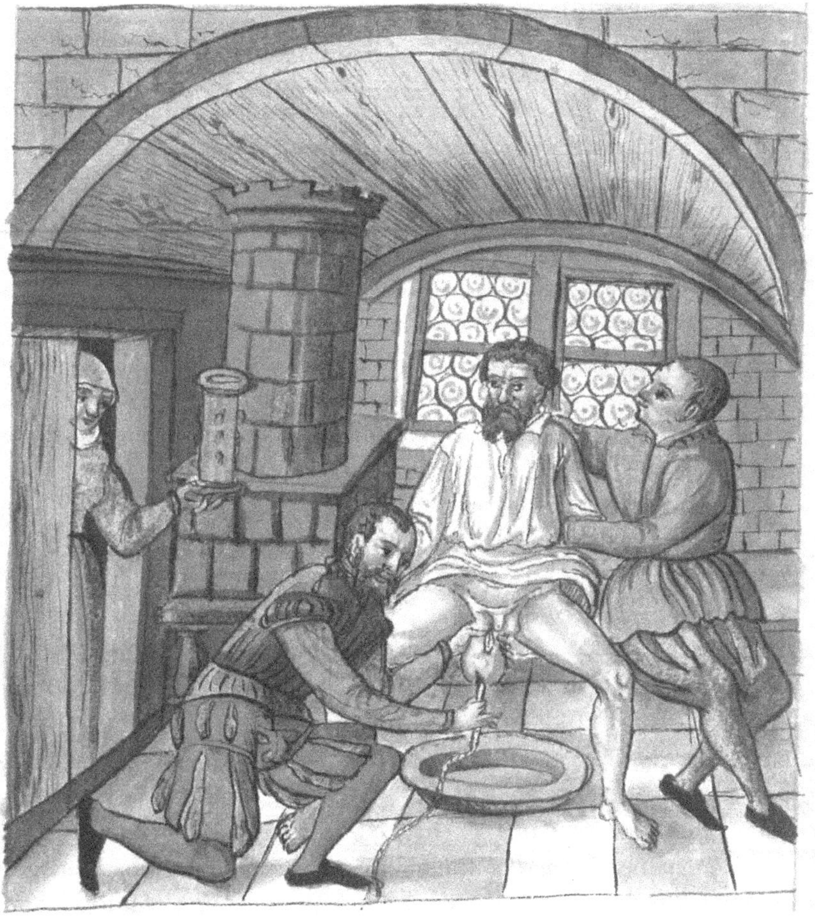

Caspar Stromayr, *Practica copiosa von dem Rechten Grundt Deß Bruch Schnidts*, 1559, fol. 129v. Lindau, Ehemals Reichsstädtische Bibliothek, P I 46.

to provide a drink. An important part of the diet prescribed by Stromayr was a potion based on boiled barley. With regard to gender the vessel may be interpreted as a counterpart to the collection of surgical instruments previously presented as the male practitioner's equipment. An iconic female attribute, the stein also implies gender-related practices in the field of care. Medieval visual representations of women presenting food and drink to the sick abound. They often propagandize saintly female charity but at the same time reflect women's responsibility to prepare and administer food in daily life as well as in specific care contexts.

Figure 8.4 The surgeon applies the warm, moist wound dressing (*Beefetzen*)

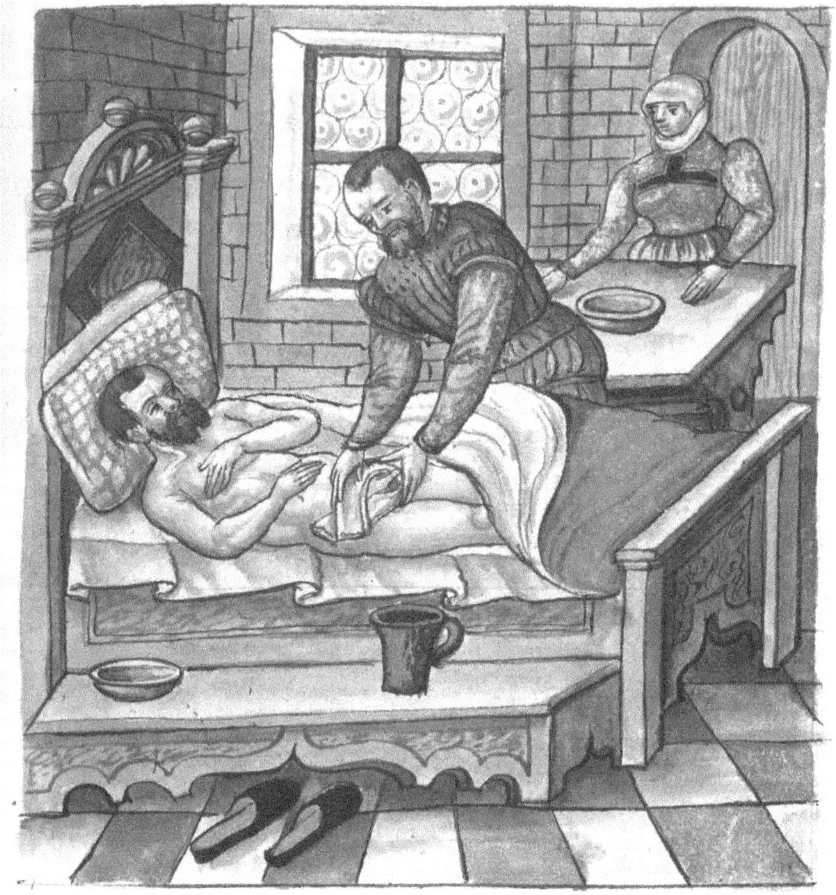

The vessel on the table probably contains the decoction of boiled herbs with which the *Beefetzen* is drenched. The presence of the female figure may indicate her learning how to change the wound dressing. Caspar Stromayr, *Practica copiosa von dem Rechten Grundt Deß Bruch Schnidts*, 1559, fol. 142r. Lindau, Ehemals Reichsstädtische Bibliothek, P I 46.

soon as the patient has been put to bed after surgery, the surgeon admonishes the assembled group ('alle die so jnn der stuben sein, vmb stender') to appoint a *reasonable* person – man or woman – to dedicate himself or herself exclusively to patient care.[80] Putting aside all other activities, he or she has to stay close to the patient for one or two days without interruption. This permanent attendance is not only deemed necessary to the patient's bodily needs, but since patients are often traumatized and have nightmares,

80 Ibid., fol. 132r-v.

they must be cared for psychologically as well. Caregivers are advised to gently wake and calm patients by touching them, calling their names, and talking to them.

Children and careless individuals ('Kinder oder sunst haillose Liederliche leüt') are excluded from this job. Also, young women should be avoided due to a potential lack of moral decency and to the danger of menstruation. According to contemporary medical theory, the flow of menstruation puts the male patient at risk of bleeding. Besides giving an *exemplum* on libido having killed a patient, Stromayr inserts a story about a man whom he had nursed together with the patient's wife ('dem jch vnnd sein aigne Hausfraw selbs gepflegen').[81] When the wife changed the wound dressing she began to menstruate and her husband died from gangrene.

Apart from these topoi Stromayr does not comment on gender in the field of care. He applies a combination of the male and the female term ('pfleger oder pflegerin') to the person delegated as nurse by the assembled group.[82] Above all he stresses that the surgeon has to initiate collective efforts. This is represented in a scene that shows the surgeon ordering the nurses and surrounding persons to care for the patient (fol. 136v). The image presents himself and three figures, two men and a woman, at the bedside of the patient, who holds on to the sling hanging from the ceiling. Obviously, as already underlined in the surgeon's remarks before the operation, care was understood as an obligation shared by social networks comprising women and men. This seems to be the main message of written and pictorial directions on the performance of care and of narrations on lived experiences.[83] However precisely this performance is represented, it conveys only fragmentary information on gendered practices within its choreography.

Conclusion

In this essay I combine a gendered lens with an approach that highlights spatial, material, and performative dimensions of care. Domestic care emerged as a field with various sectors that were gendered to different degrees. This investigation confirms previous research findings that female household members took the leading role in performing diverse acts, whereas

81 Ibid., fol. 133r-v.

82 Ibid., fol. 136v.

83 Weinsberg mentions collective efforts of household members who tried to lift his infirm wife's body; [Weinsberg,] *Liber iuventutis*, fol. 623r.

care practised by sons and husbands was rarely specified. Not surprisingly, Stromayr's images on wound care show only female figures next to the surgeon in order to represent specific practices.

Many questions remain about external providers of care and cure. Did male and female versions of the same occupational signifiers, such as *artzt* and *ärtztin*, refer to the same practices? Did female surgeons, such as the hernia specialist Marcella Praunbergerin, perform the same invasive operations as male surgeons as addressed by Stromayr's manual? Were women and men paid equally for identical services at the same time in the same town?[84] Due to ambiguous, inconsistent terminologies, it is difficult to assess which (gendered) practices are indicated by unspecific terms such as *helfen* or *hailen* ('help' and 'heal'). Questions like these must be dealt with systematically, in particular by scrutinizing archival repositories of administrative records, many of which have not been published.

The collaborative nature of domestic care and the participation of many individuals with diverse expertise required intense and constant communication, agreements, and exchange of knowledge. Care had to be organized in a concerted, interactive way with specific tasks being distributed. Grasping the choreography of this teamwork has proven difficult. Still, positing the spatial arrangements of bodies and objects within built and furnished domestic environments helps to recognize essential instruments such as the bed and to interpret care as a complex performance of female and male actors. An interdisciplinary approach that draws on written, visual, and material sources promises new ways of investigating the field of premodern care.

Works Cited

Manuscripts

Lindau, Ehemals Reichsstädtische Bibliothek, P I 46: Caspar Stromayr, *Practica copiosa von dem Rechten Grundt Deß Bruch Schnidts*, 1559.

Luzern, Staatsarchiv, COD 5145: Der Statt Lucern Allmuosen Ordnung Buoch vffgericht und erstmals angfangen anno 1590.

Nürnberg, Staatsarchiv, Rep. 54a II: Nürnberger Stadtrechnungsbelege, no. 74: Gesundheitswesen.

84 Bianca Frohne called my attention to a list of seventeen persons (fourteen women and three men) who were paid equally for giving care ('warten') to infirm persons in Nuremberg 1547; Nürnberg, Staatsarchiv, Rep. 54a II, no. 74. I thank her for sharing this finding with me.

Printed Works

Atat, Ayman Yasin. 'Bathtubs as a Healing Approach in Fifteenth-Century Ottoman Medicine', in *Gender, Health, and Healing, 1250-1550*, ed. Sara Ritchey and Sharon Strocchia (Amsterdam: Amsterdam University Press, 2020), 245-63.

Atzl, Isabel and Anamaria Depner. 'Home Care Home: Reflections on the Differentiation of Space in Living and Care Settings', in *Care Home Stories: Aging, Disability, and Long-Term Residential Care*, ed. Sally Chivers and Ulla Kriebernegg (Bielefeld: transcript, 2017), 265-81.

[Brandis, Joachim, des Jüngeren.] *Diarium* [...], ed. Max Buhlers (Hildesheim: Gerstenberg, 1902, repr. Hildesheim: Gerstenberg 1994).

Braunschweig, Sabine, ed. *Pflege – Räume, Macht und Alltag; Beiträge zur Geschichte der Pflege* (Zurich: Chronos, 2006).

Cabré, Montserrat. 'Women or Healers? Household Practices and the Categories of Health Care in Late Medieval Iberia', *Bulletin of the History of Medicine*, 82 (2008), 18-51.

Cersovsky, Eva. 'Blind Fraw – bresthaft Man: Überlegungen zu Beeinträchtigung, Versorgung und Geschlecht in Städten des 15. und 16. Jahrhunderts', paper given at the 52. Deutschen Historikertag, Münster, 25-28 September 2018.

—. 'Pflege und Geschlecht: Männer und Frauen im Straßburger Gesundheits- und Fürsorgewesen des späten Mittelalters', thesis, Universität zu Köln, in prep.

—. '*Ubi non est mulier, ingemiscit egens*? Gendered Perceptions of Care from the Thirteenth to Sixteenth Centuries', in *Gender, Health, and Healing, 1250-1550*, ed. Sara Ritchey and Sharon Strocchia (Amsterdam: Amsterdam University Press, 2020), 191-214.

Dinges, Martin. 'Self-help and Reciprocity in Parish Assistance: Bordeaux in the Sixteenth and Seventeenth Centuries', in *The Locus of Care: Families, Communities, Institutions, and the Provision of Welfare since Antiquity*, ed. Peregrine Horden and Richard Smith (London: Routledge, 1998), 111-25.

Egan, Geoff. 'Material Culture of Care for the Sick: Some Excavated Evidence from English Medieval Hospitals and Other Sites', in *The Medieval Hospital and Medical Practice*, ed. Barbara S. Bowers (Aldershot: Ashgate, 2007), 66-76.

Frohne, Bianca. 'Individuell organisierte Unterstützungsnetzwerke: Bedarfsfälle und Lösungen am Beispiel Nürnberg im 16. Jahrhundert', in *Dis/ability History der Vormoderne: ein Handbuch/Premodern Dis/ability History: A Companion*, ed. Cordula Nolte, Bianca Frohne, Uta Halle, and Sonja Kerth (Affalterbach: Didymos, 2017), 215-18.

—. *Leben mit 'kranckhait': der gebrechliche Körper in der häuslichen Überlieferung des 15. und 16. Jahrhunderts; Überlegungen zu einer Disability History der Vormoderne* (Affalterbach: Didymos, 2014).

—. '"Mit Wüschen, Wäschen, Wachen und aller anderen gebührenden Pfleg [...]": häusliche Krankenversorgung im 16. Jahrhundert', in *Dis/ability History der Vormoderne: ein Handbuch/Premodern Dis/ability History: A Companion*, ed. Cordula Nolte, Bianca Frohne, Uta Halle, and Sonja Kerth (Affalterbach: Didymos, 2017), 467-70.

Hähner-Rombach, Sylvelyn, ed., in collaboration with Christoph Schweikardt. *Quellen zur Geschichte der Krankenpflege: mit Einführungen und Kommentaren* (Frankfurt am Main: Mabuse-Verlag, 2008).

Harkness, Deborah E. 'A View from the Streets: Women and Medical Work in Elizabethan London', *Bulletin of the History of Medicine*, 82.1 (2008): 52-85.

Heitmann-Möller, Andre and Hartmut Remmers. 'Pflegebett und Agency: eine Untersuchung aus der Perspektive der Akteur-Netzwerk-Theorie von Bruno Latour', in *Pflegedinge: Materialitäten in Pflege und Care*, ed. Lucia Artner, Anamaria Depner, André Heitmann-Möller and Carolin Kollewe (Bielefeld: transcript, 2017), 133-62.

Hölscher, L. 'Handwerkerbriefe aus der Zeit der Reformation', *Zeitschrift der Gesellschaft für niedersächsische Kirchengeschichte*, 7 (1903), 250-74.

Jäggi, Stefan. *Arm sein in Luzern: Untersuchungen und Quellen zum Luzerner Armen- und Fürsorgewesen 1590-1593* (Luzern: Schwabe, 2012).

Jütte, Robert. *Ärzte, Heiler und Patienten: medizinischer Alltag in der frühen Neuzeit* (Munich/Zurich: Artemis & Winkler, 1991).

—. '"Wo kein Weib ist, da seufzet der Kranke" – Familie und Krankheit im 16. Jahrhundert', *Jahrbuch des Instituts für Geschichte der Medizin der Robert-Bosch-Stiftung*, 7 (1988), 7-24.

Kandzha, Iliana. 'Female Saints as Agents of Female Healing: Gendered Practices and Patronage in the Cult of St. Cunigunde', in *Gender, Health, and Healing, 1250-1550*, ed. Sara Ritchey and Sharon Strocchia (Amsterdam: Amsterdam University Press, 2020), 67-90.

[Kempe, Margery.] *The Book of Margery Kempe*, trans. B.A. Windeatt (London: Penguin, 1985), http://d.lib.rochester.edu/teams/publication/staley-the-book-of-margery-kempe (accessed 30 December 2018).

Kollewe, Carolin, André Heitmann-Möller, Anamaria Depner, Daniela Böhringer, Isabel Atzl, and Lucia Artner. 'Pflegedinge – Materialitäten in Pflege und Care; theoretischer Rahmen und interdisziplinärer Ansatz', in *Pflegedinge: Materialitäten in Pflege und Care*, ed. Lucia Artner, Anamaria Depner, André Heitmann-Möller, and Carolin Kollewe (Bielefeld: transcript, 2017), 15-44.

McIntosh, Marjorie K. 'Networks of Care in Elizabethan English Towns: The Example of Hadleigh, Suffolk', in *The Locus of Care: Families, Communities, Institutions, and the Provision of Welfare since Antiquity*, ed. Peregrine Horden and Richard Smith (London/New York: Routledge, 1998), 71-89.

Mummenhoff, Ernst. 'Die öffentliche Gesundheits- und Krankenpflege im alten Nürnberg', in *Festschrift zur Eröffnung des neuen Krankenhauses der Stadt Nürnberg* (Nürnberg: Selbstverlag des Stadtmagistrats, 1898), 1-222.

Munkhoff, Richelle. 'Poor Women and Parish Public Health in Sixteenth-Century London', *Renaissance Studies*, 28.4 (2014): 579-96.

Nolte, Cordula. 'Arbeits(un)fähigkeit und Teilhabe in Alltagswelten des 15. und 16. Jahrhunderts: Erkundungen im Feld einer Dis/ability History der Vormoderne', *Geschichte in Wissenschaft und Unterricht*, 70 (2019), 22-36.

—. '*der leib der hochst schatz* – zu fürstlicher Körperlichkeit, Gesunderhaltung und Lebenssicherung (1450-1550); familien- und alltagsgeschichtliche Perspektiven', in *Fürstin und Fürst: Familienbeziehungen und Handlungsmöglichkeiten von hochadeligen Frauen im Mittelalter*, ed. Jörg Rogge (Ostfildern: Thorbecke, 2004), 45-92.

—. *Frauen und Männer in der Gesellschaft des Mittelalters* (Darmstadt: Wissenschaftliche Buchgesellschaft, 2011).

—. '"She would have disliked her work": häusliche Pflege als Belastung und Verdienst', in *Dis/ability History der Vormoderne: ein Handbuch/Premodern Dis/ability History: A Companion*, ed. Cordula Nolte, Bianca Frohne, Uta Halle, and Sonja Kerth (Affalterbach: Didymos, 2017), 465-67.

Oetheus, Jacob. *Gründtlicher Bericht/Lehr unnd Instruction/von rechtem und nutzlichem brauch der Artzney/den Gesunden/Krancken und Kranckenpflegern*, [...] (Dillingen: Sebald Mayer, 1574), https://reader.digitale-sammlungen.de/de/fs1/object/display/bsb11269358_00005.html (accessed 30 December 2018).

Ott, Katherine. 'Disability Things', in *Disability Histories*, ed. Susan Burch and Michael Rembis (Urbana: University of Illinois Press, 2014), 119-35.

Prühlen, Sünje. '*alse sunst hir gebruchlich is*': *eine Annäherung an das spätmittelalterliche und frühneuzeitliche Alltags- und Familienleben anhand der Selbstzeugnisse der Familien Brandis in Hildesheim und Moller in Hamburg* (Bochum: Winkler, 2005).

[Rem, Lucas.] 'Tagebuch des Lucas Rem aus den Jahren 1494-1541: ein Beitrag zur Handelsgeschichte der Stadt Augsburg', ed. Benedikt Greiff, *Jahresbericht des historischen Kreis-Vereins im Regierungsbezirke von Schwaben und Neuburg für das Jahr 1860*, 26 (1861), 1-110.

Ritchey, Sara. 'Caring by the Hours: The Psalter as a Gendered Healthcare Technology', in *Gender, Health, and Healing, 1250-1550*, ed. Sara Ritchey and Sharon Strocchia (Amsterdam: Amsterdam University Press, 2020), 41-66.

[Sastrow, Bartolomai.] *Bartholomäi Sastrowen Herkommen, Geburt und Lauff seines gantzen Lebens*, [...], ed. Gottlieb Christian Friedrich Mohnike, 3 parts (Greifswald: Universitäts-Buchhandlung, 1823/24), https://reader.digitale-sammlungen.de/de/fs1/object/display/bsb10066512_00260.html (accessed 30 December 2018).

Scheutz, Martin, Andrea Sommerlechner, Herwig Weigl, and Alfred Stefan Weiß, eds. *Quellen zur europäischen Spitalgeschichte in Mittelalter und Früher Neuzeit* (Vienna/Munich: Böhlau, 2010).

Sebastian Fischers Chronik, besonders von Ulmischen Dingen, ed. Karl-Gustav Veesenmeyer, Mitteilungen des Vereins für Kunst und Altertum in Ulm und Oberschwaben 5-8 (Ulm: Nübling, 1896).

Staley, Lynn. *Margery Kempe's Dissenting Fictions* (University Park, PA: Pennsylvania State University Press, 1994).

Stolberg, Michael. 'Kommunikative Praktiken: ärztliche Wissensvermittlung am Krankenbett im 16. Jahrhundert', in *Praktiken der Frühen Neuzeit: Akteure – Handlungen – Artefakte*, ed. Arndt Brendecke (Cologne/Weimar/Vienna: Böhlau, 2015), 111-21.

Strocchia, Sharon T. 'Caring for the "Incurable" in Renaissance Pox Hospitals', in *Hospital Life: Theory and Practice from the Medieval to the Modern*, ed. Laurinda Abreu and Sally Sheard (Oxford: Peter Lang, 2013), 67-92.

Stromayr, Caspar. *Practica copiosa von dem Rechten Grundt Deß Bruch Schnidts* (1559), Faksimile (Munich: Rothacker, 1983).

—. *Practica copiosa von dem Rechten Grundt Deß Bruch Schnidts* (1559), Kommentarband zum Faksimile der Handschrift, ed. and introduced by Werner Friedrich Kümmel, in collaboration with Gundolf Keil and Peter Proff (Munich: Rothacker, 1983).

—. *Practica copiosa von dem Rechten Grundt Deß Bruch Schnidts*, in *Practica copiosa von dem Rechten Grundt Deß Bruch Schnidts (Lindau, 1559-67) & Jakob Ruëff, Practica in arte ophthalmica copiosa (Zürich, um 1550)*, Kommentar zur Faksimile-Ausgabe, ed. Gundolf Keil and Peter Proff (Darmstadt: Facsimilia Art & Edition Ebert KG, 1994).

Van Steensel, Arie. 'Variations in Urban Social Assistance: Some Examples from Late-Medieval England and the Low Countries', in *Assistenza e solidarietà in Europa secc. XIII-XVIII*, ed. Francesco Ammannati (Florence: Firenze University Press, 2013), 135-50.

Vanja, Christina. 'Aufwärterinnen, Narrenmägde und Siechenmütter – Frauen in der Krankenpflege der Frühen Neuzeit', *Medizin, Gesellschaft und Geschichte*, 11 (1992), 9-24.

[Weinsberg, Hermann.] *Liber iuventutis*, in *Die autobiographischen Aufzeichnungen Hermann Weinsbergs: Digitale Gesamtausgabe*, ed. Abteilung für Rheinische Landesgeschichte der Rheinischen Friedrich-Wilhelms-Universität Bonn, www.weinsberg.uni-bonn.de/Edition/Liber_Iuventutis/Liber_Iuventutis.htm (accessed 30 December 2018).

Winckelmann, Otto. *Das Fürsorgewesen der Stadt Strassburg vor und nach der Reformation bis zum Ausgang des sechzehnten Jahrhunderts* (Leipzig: M. Heinsius Nachfolger, 1922; repr. New York: Johnson, 1971).

About the Author

Cordula Nolte is Professor of Medieval History at the University of Bremen. Her main research fields are gender studies, early medieval Christianization, and princely families and courts. Recently she has focused on the history of the body and on dis/ability history. In 2017 she co-edited the first interdisciplinary and international companion on premodern dis/ability.

9 Bathtubs as a Healing Approach in Fifteenth-Century Ottoman Medicine

*Ayman Yasin Atat**

Abstract

The fifteenth-century Ottoman physician Muhammad al-Shirwānī's extensive encyclopedia of pharmaceutical science, *Rawḍat al-ʿiṭr* (Garden of pharmacy/perfumes'), is an important source for understanding Ottoman medicine. The work includes a specific chapter about using bathtubs in urgent cases, along with self-prepared remedies. This essay contextualizes al-Shirwānī's encyclopedia within the traditions of Arabic and Ottoman medicine. It presents the first English translation of al-Shirwānī's chapter on bathtubs and analyses the kinds of ailments that could be treated by this technique, as well as the types of *materia medica* used in therapeutic preparations. Al-Shirwānī's inclusion of an extended chapter devoted specifically to this home-based approach suggests that household medicine was emerging as an authoritative terrain of both Arabic and Ottoman medicine.

Keywords: household medicine, pharmacy, materia medica, balneology

One of the most widespread therapeutic approaches used around the world involves the bathtub as a healing device to treat certain ailments. Using this mode of treatment achieves a number of therapeutic benefits. Bathtubs permit external remedies to achieve a significant amount of contact with the skin surface. Users gain additional benefits from exposure to the warm

* My thanks to Prof. Dr. Bettina Wahrig, head of the Department for the History of Science and Pharmacy at the Technical University Braunschweig, for her guidance in writing this essay; to Mrs. Farah Maghamez for assistance in preparing this essay; and to the Alexander Humboldt Foundation for funding my current project through the Philipp Schwartz Initiative, which is supported by the Federal Foreign Office in Germany.

Ritchey, Sara & Sharon Strocchia (eds), *Gender, Health, and Healing, 1250-1550*. Amsterdam, Amsterdam University Press 2020
DOI: 10.5117/9789463724517_CH09

water in treatment. Moreover, the treatment can be applied at home without the patient's need to leave, thereby eliminating the difficulties associated with out-of-home treatments. This advantage can be especially important in cases of severe pain; indeed, using a bathtub can be considered a form of household medicine.

In the contemporary world, the term 'therapeutic tourism' has emerged, based mainly on the principles of a bathtub approach to therapy.[1] Many specialized clinics have emerged around the world to advance this type of treatment, especially for older people or those suffering from certain movement disabilities, articulated pains, or other conditions.[2] One of the most famous tourist destinations in this regard is Turkey, where many centres can be found in Istanbul and other cities. This is not surprising considering that Ottoman medicine relied heavily on home-based processing using the bathtub. Indeed, visitors to Istanbul can visit a museum that specializes in the culture of Ottoman-era baths and the medical treatment methods used.[3] Furthermore, conferences have been held in Turkey and other countries to study the medical history of the bathtub in various civilizations throughout history.[4]

The bathtub has long been a recommended therapeutic device in Arabic medicine, which was based on humoral theory. Balance between the four humors (blood, phlegm, yellow bile, black bile) was considered essential for the body to remain healthy; any disorders or imbalance would lead to illness. Physicians aimed to recover a correct humoral balance through their treatments.[5] The mid-tenth-century physician al-Qumrī, author

1 According to Connell, 'medical tourism, where patients travel overseas for operations, has grown rapidly in the past decade, especially for cosmetic surgery. High costs and long waiting lists at home, new technology and skills in destination countries alongside reduced transport costs and Internet marketing have all played a role. Several Asian countries are dominant, but most countries have sought to enter the market. Conventional tourism has been a by-product of this growth, despite its tourist packaging, and overall benefits to the travel industry have been considerable'; Connell, 'Medical Tourism', 1093.

2 Many studies discuss medical tourism throughout the world. For an American legal perspective, see Burkett, 'Medical Tourism'; for Poland, Dryglas and Różycki, 'Profile of Tourists'; for Egypt, Helmy, 'Benchmarking the Egyptian Medical Tourism Sector'; for East Asia, Yu and Ko, 'Cross-Cultural Study of Perceptions of Medical Tourism'.

3 The museum is called Bayezid Türk Hamam Kültürü Müzesi, and is located at no. 2, Kimyager Derviş Paşa Sokak, 34134 Fatih, İstanbul.

4 For instance, the Balkan Spa Summit holds an annual meeting in one of the Balkan countries. The first meeting was held in Bulgaria in September 2011, the second in Turkey in October 2012. In addition, there is a biannual International Conference on Swimming Pools and Spas.

5 For a detailed examination of Arabic medicine, see Pormann and Savage-Smith, *Medieval Islamic Medicine*.

of the book titled *al-Tanwīr fī al-Muṣṭalaḥāt al-Ṭubbīīah* (Enlightenment in the medical terms), says that: '*Al-'ibzin* [bathtub] is custom-made for the human being that uses it; it is built in the bathrooms and filled with water to [the point] where, when the patient is in it, his head sits out of the basin'.[6] Since the word *zin* is Persian, it might indicate the existence of a culture of bathtub treatment in Persian civilization as well. This prevalence is confirmed by the fact that physicians like al-Rāzī, al-Majūsī, and Ibn Sīnā from the eastern parts of Islamic civilization in the early eleventh century CE mentioned 'al-'ibzin' in their books.

We note that al-Majūsī (d. 1010) in writing *Kitāb Kāmil al-Ṣinā'a al-Ṭibbiyya* (The entire medical art) relied on the use of the bathtub technique to treat a number of conditions such as fatigue, as well as using it as a prophylactic measure to maintain human health.[7] Ibn Sīnā (d. 1037) also mentioned a prescription based on the use of the bathtub in the treatment of haemorrhoids.[8] The reliance on this therapeutic approach continued in the thirteenth century. In his book titled *Kitāb al-Mukhtarāt fi ṭ-Ṭibb* (The anthology of medicine), Ibn Hubal (d. 1213) mentioned the bathtub in the treatment of a number of ailments like intestinal colic, and as a technique to maintain the health of the elderly.[9] Therefore, it can be said that the bathtub approach in eastern Islamic medicine was commonplace, although used less frequently than other therapeutic methods such as bloodletting or other classical methods that rely on pharmaceutical formulations used orally or topically. In the Byzantine period, however, washing or bathing were frequently only a minor element of the treatment.[10] The Ottoman era then continued what was a common practice in both Arabic and Byzantine medicine; the Ottomans further developed the practice so that it became a cultural aspect of Ottoman medicine in subsequent centuries.

6 Abū al-Qumrī was the leading medical personage of his generation. He was reportedly held in great esteem by the kings of his times. Ibn Sīnā had met this physician when he was very old, and used to attend his medical lessons, which he claimed greatly enhanced his knowledge; Ibn Abī 'Usaibi'a, *'Uyūn al-anbā' fī ṭabaqāt al-aṭibbā'*, 435. In his book *al-Tanwīr fi al-Iṣtilaḥat al-Ṭibbiyyah*, al-Qumrī explained the most important medical terms used in Arabic medicine.

7 al-Majūsī, *Kāmil*, 3: 45.

8 This treatment involved sitting in water in which pennyroyal, myrtle, roses, pomegranates, and oak gall had been boiled; Ibn Sīnā, *al-Qānūn*, 3: 473.

9 Ibn Hubal, *Kitāb*, 1: 198.

10 For further information about bathing culture in the Byzantine period, see Zytka, *Cultural History of Bathing in Late Antiquity and Early Byzantium*. Comparative material on Jewish, Christian, and Islamic bathing practices in the medieval West is developed in the special thematic issue edited by Boisseuil, *Le bain: espaces et pratiques*.

Bathtubs in Early Ottoman Medicine

Bathing culture in Anatolia enjoyed a rich heritage of civilizations that predated the the Turkish conquest. That culture was partially changed by the beliefs and traditions the Turks brought with them from Middle Asia. The Turkish bath had been nurtured by the architectural traditions and bathing rituals of the Seljuks, who brought baths to Anatolia in the eleventh century, and became the most important element of civic architecture and an indispensable part of daily life in the Ottoman period.[11]

To examine the therapeutic culture of the bathtub at the beginnings of the Ottoman Empire in the fifteenth century CE, I will use an important pharmaceutical encyclopedia written by Muhammad ibn Mahmoud al-Shirwānī, who was active *c.*1456 CE. Ottoman pharmacology was one of the most sophisticated branches of medical knowledge and practice that both continued Arabic traditions and adapted them.[12] The encyclopedia itself represents a compendium of medical and pharmaceutical knowledge in the early Ottoman era. Al-Shirwānī devoted an entire chapter to bathtubs as a healing approach and mentioned a number of prescriptions for treating a variety of diseases. Before analysing that chapter, however, it is necessary first to provide a glimpse of the author and his book. Al-Shirwānī was one of the most important Ottoman physicians in the fifteenth century. He was active in the service of many sultans like Murad II and Mohammed I, and was a prolific author of Arabic and Ottoman Turkish medical works. As physician to the Ottoman Sultan, al-Shirwānī was considered the highest medical authority during his service, and his writings were used as references for all practitioners in the field of pharmacy and medicine. Unfortunately, there is almost no additional information regarding his life.

Of all al-Shirwānī's Arabic works, the *Rawḍat al-ʿiṭr* (Garden of pharmacy/perfumes), housed at the Süleymaniye Library in Istanbul, is the most comprehensive. A substantial volume of 239 folios, it is also the most significant of his academic works, employing a careful citation system of the classical authors, such as Ibn Sīnā and Ismail al-Jurjānī. Al-Shirwānī's *Rawḍat al-ʿiṭr* provides rich knowledge about fifteenth-century pharmaceutical practice in the Ottoman realm, including recipes for many remedies and medical

11 For further information about bathing culture in Anatolia, see Özköse, 'Bath Tradition in Anatolia'.

12 Shefer-Mossensohn provides a good synopsis of Ottoman medical theory and practice in 'Medicine in the Ottoman Empire'; a more expansive discussion can be found in Shefer-Mossensohn, *Ottoman Medicine*.

procedures. In fact, this manuscript could be considered an encyclopedia of Ottoman pharmaceutical sciences, shedding much light on the use of simple drugs in Ottoman medical recipes.

Contents of *Rawḍat al-ʿiṭr*

Al-Shirwānī said that the purpose of this book was to provide a reference for all pharmaceutical workers that would give them comprehensive information on medicines and their methods of preparation, as well as prescriptions for all pharmaceutical forms, whether of internal or external use. The introduction began with a statement regarding the ethics of the pharmaceutical profession, and then discussed the identification of simple drugs and how to wash and prepare them before use in the recipes. In addition, he gave the meanings of the names of simple drugs with some of their synonyms listed in accordance with several languages, such as Arabic and Persian, to make them more distinguishable and easily recognized. Moreover, he indicated various alternatives that might be used in the absence of some of these materia medica; he also explained how to distinguish whether simple drugs were counterfeit or blended with other substances. Finally, the introduction ends with a section on the weights used in pharmaceutical preparations.

Al-Shirwānī then divided his book into forty-four chapters. Each chapter included a new pharmaceutical form mentioning a number of the most important prescriptions prevalent in the Ottoman era to treat various conditions and diseases. Readers of the chapter headings may notice that al-Shirwānī started with formulations used internally, like syrups, oxymel, julep, pills, and others. Then he moved to external formulations like lotions and bandages. In chapter 32 he discussed topical douches, which was followed directly with the chapter on using bathtubs in healing (chapter 33). After that discussion, he continued with chapters on other topical formulations. His remaining chapters dealt with other branches of medicine such as ophthalmology, dentistry, and cosmetology, while the final chapter examined patients' diet.

Al-Shirwānī seems to have been the first physician to include an entire, separate chapter on bathtubs as a healing approach in both Arabic and Ottoman medicine.[13] His claim that his book would be an important source for workers in the pharmaceutical field helps us to understand how the use of

13 Although al-Shirwānī stated in the introduction that he cites previous pharmaceutical and medical encyclopedias like Avicenna's *Canon* and al-Shīrāzī's *al-Ḥāwī* (fourteenth century), none of these books devoted a separate chapter to the use of bathtubs. Nor did the famous Arabic

bathtubs in healing became more prominent in Ottoman medical culture. In addition, he provided a number of prescriptions used to treat various ailments, and explained their methods of preparation. Unfortunately, al-Shirwānī did not provide any details regarding the size and physical appearance of bathtubs, the materials of which they were made, or other salient features.

Since the *Rawḍat al-ʿiṭr* was written in Arabic and has never been translated into any other language, I will provide a full translation of the chapter on bathtubs. This translation should facilitate comparative research, so that non-Arabic medical historians can consider its contents in light of other traditions of bathtub use. It can contribute to an analytic lens focused on domestic space and the objects within it. As Cordula Nolte has suggested in her contribution to this volume, using such a lens allows us to better envision the variety of roles played by women householders in the delivery of care.[14] Following the translation, I analyse aspects of this issue for Ottoman medicine, focusing first on the conditions for which bathtubs were used as a kind of home-based healthcare for emergency cases and, second, on the materia medica used in these recipes. In addition, I wish to compare this information with major works in Arabic medicine to understand the development of using the bathtub as a healing technique in the early Ottoman era.[15]

Translation of Chapter 33: 'The al-ʾibzin' ('Bathtubs')

Bathtub: relaxes the leg and knee, and alleviates kidney pain due to kidney stone. Its recipe: chamomile, ribbed melilot, southernwood, and small caltrops (10 dms. each),[16] red rose and fennel peels (7 dms. each), pennyroyal, marjoram, and large dried thyme (3 dms. each), common hollyhock (4 dms.). Boil everything in six *raṭil* of water until reduced by half, pour the mixture in a bathtub, lay the patient in it, and pour the mixture on his leg.[17]

Bathtub: dissolves kidney stones, in addition to alleviating pain in the bladder. Its recipe: chamomile, ribbed melilot, maidenhair fern, and two-rowed barley seeds (10 dms. each), fennel root peel, common hollyhock root, and melon seeds (7 dms. each),

books of formulations by Sābūr ibn Sahl (ninth century) and Ibn al-Tilmīdh (eleventh century) highlight bathtub therapies in separate chapters.

14 Nolte, 'Domestic Care in the Sixteenth Century'.

15 al-Shirwānī, *Rawḍat al-ʿiṭr Istanbul*, Süleymaniye Library Hacı Beşir Ağa 506. This chapter takes up two folios beginning at fol. 209.

16 A *dirham* (dm., pl. dms.) is a unit of weight equivalent to 3.125 grams.

17 A *raṭil* is a unit of weight rather than measure, estimated to be around 406 grams.

sweet violet and white Egyptian lotus leaves (4 dms. each), Egyptian soapwort that has good green colour (3 dms.), small caltrops (6 dms.). Boil everything in 10 *mann* water until reduced by half; then pour the mixture in the bathtub and the patient sits in it.[18]

Bathtub: it works to dissolve kidney stone, and is useful for children who get ischuria due to the existence of stone in the kidney. Its recipe: chamomile, ribbed melilot, red rose, common hollyhock, and small caltrops (10 dms. each), dry peel of melon, two-rowed barley, and maidenhair fern (7 dms. each), green Egyptian soapwort, liquorice root, and fennel peel (5 dms. each), Chinese lantern and fenugreek (4 dms. each), southernwood and sweet violet (3 dms. each), wild carrot and white Egyptian lotus (2 *mithqāl* each).[19] Boil all together in 10 *mann* water until reduced by half, pour it in the bathtub, and the patient sits in it.

Bathtub: it is useful for arthralgia and stones of the kidney and bladder, and it strengthens weak organs. Its recipe: chamomile, ribbed melilot, and southernwood (10 dms. each), dry pennyroyal, large thyme, marjoram, palmarosa, peel of fennel root, common hollyhock, maidenhair fern, and two-rowed barley (5 dms. each), core of safflower (10 dms.). Boil all in 10 *mann* water until reduced by half and pour it while tepid into the bathtub. The patient sits in it and washes the sick organs.

Bathtub: to prevent the abortion of an embryo, so he does not come out before his time while he is in the fifth or sixth month.[20] Its recipe: red rose (10 dms.), white sandalwood (3 dms.), pomegranate flowers (4 dms.), white Egyptian lotus leaves, common myrtle cereal, and gum Arabic (3 dms. each). Boil all in 5 *mann* water until reduced to 2 *mann*, then add to it *Anagyris foetida* (50 dms.), water [distilled] from water skink (30 dms.), and endive water (4 dms.).[21] Mix all ingredients and have the pregnant woman sit in the bathtub.

Bathtub: it is useful for arthralgia, as al-Rāzī said.[22] Water should be boiled in a big boiler several times, then a slaughtered fox or hyena should be thrown into this water to be boiled with dill and salt, and then cooked until it is thoroughly broken down.[23] Then the water should be poured into a bathtub while it is warm and the patient sits in it for two hours; afterwards he rests. At the end of the day, the water should be warmed again and

18 A *mann* is another unit of weight equal to about 816 grams.

19 A *mithqāl* is a unit of weight roughly equivalent to 4.46 grams.

20 Here the original text is gendered male, because in the Arabic language the word embryo (*al-janīn*, الجنين) is masculine. This means that al-Shirwānī did not distinguish the sex of the embryo in this recipe; instead the word could be used for both genders.

21 Skinks are a type of lizard; some species are acquatic.

22 Al-Shirwānī quoted this recipe from al-Rāzī, as he mentions in the text.

23 It is well known that many animal products and organs were used in Arabic and Ottoman medicine. Al-Shirwānī explained that one could slaughter a hyena, fox, zebra, or rabbit, depending on what was available; then the animal was cooked to an extreme and the resulting cooking water poured directly in the bathtub. Alternately, one could add oil and cook until mixed well, then pour this mixture in the bathtub to be used. However, al-Shirwānī did not make any further recommendations about the slaughtering process itself.

the patient sits in it. This should be done twice a day for three days, starting with the first three days of the month, then another three days in the middle of the month, and finally three days at the end of it. The water should be replaced after every three days of use.

Bathtub: it is useful for all gout pain and strengthens the bones; it prevents the corruption of material; and it is used at the end of the last three days of the previous recipe. Its recipe: chamomile, ribbed melilot, and red rose (10 dms. each), sweet violet, roses of common hollyhock, and flower of white Egyptian lotus (5 dms. each), dry leaves of sweet basil handful, white sandalwood (3 dms.). Boil all of the ingredients together in 3 *mann* of water until it becomes 1 *mann*, then it should be poured tepid on the injured organ after the patient sits in the bathtub.

Bathtub: it removes [traces of] smallpox after it has healed but traces of the disease still remain. Its recipe: red rose (7 dms.), sweet violet, leaves of white Egyptian lotus, red sandalwood, seeds of garden lettuce, and seeds of endive (4 dms. each). Boil all of these ingredients in 7 *mann* of water until it is reduced to 3 *mann*, then press and squeeze in a bathtub. After washing, the patient gets in and the mixture is poured on the injured area. If any traces [of smallpox] remain, they will disappear.

Bathtub: it is beneficial for hemiplegia, numbness, and relaxation. Its recipe: leaves of bay laurel, leaves of marjoram, harmal, chamomile, common hollyhock, ribbed melilot, leaves of citron, rue, alfalfa, Roman wormwood, southernwood, chaste tree (equal parts of each), and a half part of *jindibīdister*.[24] Boil all of these ingredients together in a large quantity of water until reduced by half; then add a half part oil. The patient sits in it while the water is warm.

Bathtub: it is prepared from leaves of garden lettuce, white Egyptian lotus, common hollyhock, leaves of common poppy or the common poppy itself, and leaves of common beet cooked all together. It is beneficial for intestinal colic when it occurs, but the body should be rubbed with the following *qīrūṭī* that is made from ointment of sweet violet with pure wax and *Astragalus tragacantha*.[25] After leaving the bathtub, the patient should drink pure water of pomegranate or water of Indian melon or cucumber water with fine white sugar.

Bathtub: to prevent the expulsion of an embryo, so he does not come out before his time while he is in the fifth or sixth month. This recipe is stronger than other bathtub [treatments]. Its recipe: red rose (7 dms.), pomegranate flower, and athel tamarisk (5 dms. each), dry leaves of common myrtle (4 dms.), *shab yamānī*, peel of pomegranate, and oak gall (3 dms. each).[26] Crush all and boil together in 10 *mann* of water until reduced by half, then press and squeeze into a bathtub, and have the pregnant woman sit in it.

24 This term refers to the testis of an otter, which was used frequently as a materia medica in both Arabic and Ottoman medicine.

25 The term *qīrūṭī* refers to an external remedy, which in this case is prepared from an ointment and other simple drugs.

26 *Shab yamānī* is a mineral drug similar to vitriol and verdigris.

Studies on Using the Bathtub in Ottoman Medicine

Two lines of inquiry regarding bathtub therapy merit analysis here: first, the conditions for which bathtubs were used; and second, the materia medica (especially botanical ones) that were used in these recipes. Moreover, it would be useful to compare the results of this analysis with Arabic medicine to understand the interaction between Arabic and Ottoman medical cultures.

Based on the recipes given by al-Shirwānī, the ailments commonly treated with bathub therapy in Ottoman medicine are summarized in Table 9.1. The following conclusions can be drawn from this table. First, we can see that pain relief is the most prevalent aim of treatment. Bathtubs were used therapeutically in connection with arthralgia, cystalgia and nephralgia (with or without stones), and intestinal colic. Second, except for treating smallpox scars, all of the other conditions mentioned required urgent or emergency care. Practitioners did not have the luxury of assessing the precise reasons why a patient was suffering acute pain in the cases of arthralgia, kidney and bladder pains, and intestinal colic; similarly, in the case of preventing an embryo or fetus from being expelled, time was of the essence, since fear and panic on the mother's part could kill the organism. Therefore, the factor of time helps explain why the bathtub method was recommended for certain urgent conditions. In addition, the patient did not need to leave the house to visit a doctor. A home practitioner could apply the treatment directly as soon as the bathtub water was ready.

Table 9.1 Conditions treated by bathtub therapies in al-Shirwānī, *Rawḍat al-'iṭr*, chapter 33

Condition	Category	Number of recipes
Abortion	Gynecology	2
Arthralgia	Arthritis	3
Bladder pain	Urinary system	1
Intestinal colic	Digestive system	1
Kidney stone	Urinary system	2
Nephralgia	Urinary system	2
Numbness	Nervous system	2
Smallpox	Dermatology	1

In the case of smallpox symptoms, which might still be visible in the form of blisters or lesions on various parts of the body, the patient may not have wanted to leave the house. This condition would preferably be treated at home in any case, since doctors were unlikely to make house calls in this situation. The inclusion of this recipe raises important social and medical issues about how Ottoman people dealt with smallpox patients, given its infectious and potentially lethal nature. Were patients forced to stay home? What was the cultural response to smallpox patients? These questions merit further inquiry in light of the many different social structures, political regimes, and medical subsystems encompassed by the Ottoman Empire, even in its early days. Still, we know that both Ibn Sīnā and al-Rāzī thought that people might contract smallpox if they were exposed to hot air containing smallpox matter. Certainly by the early seventeenth century, fear of contagion created anxieties about encountering smallpox patients, making the use of bathtubs inside residential enclosures more understandable in cases of smallpox.[27]

In addition to offering bathtub remedies for diverse ailments, Arabic and Ottoman doctors mentioned other treatments for these same conditions, such as remedies taken by mouth. However, preparations like paste, tablets, and syrups could take several days to make, because some of their ingredients would be placed in the sun to dry and often involved many other steps in preparation. Thus, from a pharmaceutical point of view, the method of preparing recipes in bathtubs was advantageous since, in most situations, it did not require a great deal of time. Rather, these remedies depended on mixing the correct amounts of materia medica and boiling them in water until the desired formula was obtained. Treatment could begin shortly afterwards by laying the patient in the bathtub. Indeed, no special procedures like sifting or refining or drying were required, which made bathtub preparation and application easier, even in the absence of a physician. Therefore, the most important advantages in using bathtubs as a healing approach were the shortened time and ease of preparation. This chapter from al-Shirwānī suggests that household medicine was emerging as an authoritative terrain of both Arabic and Ottoman medicine.

Indeed, a comparison of al-Shirwānī's bathtub remedies with those of his Arabic predecessors demonstrates that the Ottoman physician and pharmacist relied on previous balneological theory and practice, particularly that of Ibn Sīnā. As is well known, Ibn Sīnā is considered one of the most important physicians in Arabic medical history, who exercised

27 In addressing smallpox, it is important to note that Ottoman physicians were famous for the preventive practice of inoculation. See Dinc and Ulman, 'Introduction of Variolation', and Riedel, 'Edward Jenner and the History of Smallpox and Vaccination'. Börekçi, 'Smallpox in the Harem', investigates the anxieties created by an outbreak of smallpox in early seventeenth-century Istanbul and its impact on the Ottoman imperial family.

tremendous influence on the development of Western medieval medicine. Some scholars even consider him to be the most canonical author whose treatment methods became standard in medieval Arabic medicine. By going back to Ibn Sīnā's book *al-Qānūn fī al-Ṭibb* (*The Canon of Medicine*), which includes the same conditions that al-Shirwānī treated using bathtub therapies, we can articulate some of the distinctions between Arabic and Ottoman remedies and ascertain a place for bathtub remedies within these traditions. For example, in his chapter on the treatment of arthritis, Ibn Sīnā says that bathtubs are effective when using 'waters' made with simples.[28] His prescriptions are similar in the treatment of intestinal colic, where Ibn Sīnā stated that using bathtubs could be helpful for patients suffering from this affliction.[29] Although there is agreement in the remedies prescribed by al-Shirwānī and Ibn Sīnā regarding the use of bathtubs for kidney stones and nephralgia, Ibn Sīnā nevertheless had added an important distinction. His instructions prevent patients from staying in the bathtub for a long time, or without a real need for it.[30] However, this agreement is not evident in the case of treatments for smallpox, where Ibn Sīnā makes no reference to the use of bathtubs as a method of healing the disease.

A potential conflict between Arabic and Ottoman medicine arises in the case of abortion. Al-Shirwānī provides two recipes for bathtub therapies to avoid abortion, while Ibn Sīnā mentions that the bathtub is helpful for removing a dead embryo from the uterus. In analysing this seeming contradiction, we should take into consideration first that Ibn Sīnā did not mention whether the bathtub would contain only hot water or also some types of herbs. This issue has great importance, especially for readers of al-Shirwānī. Since symptoms of miscarriage usually begin with bleeding, he prescribes astringent and drier herbs in line with the basic principle of using astringent substances to staunch bleeding in both Arabic and Ottoman medicine. Although the use of astringent substances in internal formulations such as pills and ovules might induce abortion, it seems that al-Shirwānī intended to stop the bleeding by using the bathtub technique. Bathtub therapy would be an extremely quick and useful remedy in this situation. The same would be true if we suppose that Ibn Sīnā intended to use only hot water in the bathtub to facilitate the removal of the dead

28 Ibn Sīnā, *al-Qānūn*, 3: 521.

29 Ibid., 3: 309.

30 According to Ibn Sīnā, using bathtubs for a prolonged period would diminish the power of the kidney. In addition, if bathtubs are used needlessly for purposes of sedation, it makes the kidney ready to accept other substances, leading to its inaction; ibid., 3: 365; 3: 351.

embryo.[31] Unfortunately, this comparison is inconclusive because we cannot know Ibn Sīnā's exact intention when he discussed bathtub therapy here.

With the exception of miscarriage and abortion, it appears that al-Shirwānī was thoroughly influenced by the eastern medical school represented by Ibn Sīnā and later al-Jurjānī.[32] In addition to quoting many of their formulations and other pharmaceutical information, al-Shirwānī also agreed with their medical thinking in using bathtub therapies, generally with only minor differences in details. Therefore, we can conclude that there was a great deal of consistency in Arab and Ottoman medicine with regard to bathtub remedies.

From a medical view, we see that al-Shirwānī depended on bathtubs for healing certain conditions and that his remedies were fairly continuous with those of eastern Islamic physicians. An analysis of the plants used in these formulations provides additional insight, especially when these medicinals are compared with the most important source for materia medica in Arabic medicine, Ibn al-Bayṭār's book, the *Kitāb al-Jāmi' li-Mufradāt al-Adwīya wa al-Aghdhīya* (The compendium of drugs and foods).[33] Table 9.2 abbreviates all the plants mentioned by al-Shirwānī, with their Latin classification and the therapeutic target for which they were used. From this table, we can see that, although al-Shirwānī mentioned many exotic herbs such as sandalwood brought by traders from China or India, readers could recognize that all of them were well-known herbs. Many of them, such as chamomile, were used already in cookery. The prevalence of ordinary herbs used in everyday life presumably indicated their affordability as well, in contrast to remedies containing rare or expensive ingredients used by affluent patients.[34] Al-Shirwānī's use of these familiar herbs in his recipes for bathtubs, as well as their ease of preparation, once again suggests that this therapy was an essential form of household medicine.

31 Many modern studies indicate the benefits of using heated water in the birthing process; see Mackey, 'Use of Water in Labor and Birth'; Church, 'Water Birth'; and Cluett and Burns, 'Immersion in Water in Labour and Birth'.

32 Al-Jurjānī (d. 1136 CE) was the author of the book *al-dhakhīra fī al-Ṭib* (The repertory of medicine). For additional information, see Verma, 'Growth of Greco-Arabian Medicine in Medieval India', 353. Medieval Islamic hospitals functioned as teaching facilities. Five hospitals were built in Baghdad between the ninth and tenth centuries, including the 'Aḍuḍī hospital, which was affiliated with a medical school. This hospital had lecture rooms and a rich medical library. For Arabic medical education in the Middle Ages, see Ragab, *Medieval Islamic Hospital*.

33 Ibn al-Bayṭār's thirteenth-century book is one of the most important reference manuals on simples in Arabic medicine. For more information on this physician, see Sezgin, *'Abdallāh ibn Aḥmad ibn al-Bayṭār*, and Idrisi, 'Gap between the World of Ibn al-Bayṭār and that of Linnaeus'.

34 Shefer-Mossensohn, 'Medicine in the Ottoman Empire', 3.

Table 9.2 Plants used in al-Shirwānī's remedies, *Rawḍat al-'iṭr*, chapter 33

Scientific name	Common name	Medical uses
Acacia arabica	Gum arabic	Abortion
Adiantum capillus veneris	Maidenhair fern (3)	Lower arthralgia, kidney stone
Althaea rosea	Common hollyhock (7)	Lower arthralgia, nephralgia due to stones, kidney stone, intestinal colic
Andropogon schoenanthus	Palmarosa	Lower arthralgia, nephralgia due to stones
Artemisia abrotanum	Southernwood (4)	Lower arthralgia, nephralgia due to stones, kidney stone, numbness
Artemisia pontica	Roman wormwood	Numbness
Beta vulgaris	Common beet	Intestinal colic
Carthamus tinctorius	Safflower	Lower arthralgia, nephralgia due to stones
Cichorium endivia	Endive (2)	Abortion, smallpox
Citrus medica	Citron	Numbness
Cucumis melo	Melon (3)	Nephralgia due to stones, kidney stone, intestinal colic
Daucus carota	Wild carrot	Kidney stone
Foeniculum vulgare	Fennel (4)	Lower arthralgia, nephralgia due to stones, kidney stone
Glycyrrhiza glabra	Liquorice	Kidney stone
Gypsophila struthium	Egyptian soapwort (2)	Kidney stone, nephralgia, pain of bladder
Hordeum distichon	Two-rowed barley (3)	Lower arthralgia, nephralgia due to stones, kidney stone
Lactuca sativa L.	Garden lettuce (2)	Smallpox, intestinal colic
Laurus nobilis	Bay laurel	Numbness
Matricaria recutita	Chamomile (6)	Lower arthralgia, nephralgia due to stones, kidney stone, numbness
Melilotus officinalis	Ribbed melilot (6)	Lower arthralgia, nephralgia due to stones, kidney stone, numbness
Mentha pulegium	Pennyroyal (2)	Lower arthralgia, nephralgia due to stones
Myrtus communis	Common myrtle (2)	Abortion
Nymphaea lotus	White Egyptian lotus (6)	Lower arthralgia, kidney stone, abortion, smallpox, intestinal colic
Ocimum basilicum	Sweet basil	Lower arthralgia
Origanum majorana	Marjoram (3)	Lower arthralgia, nephralgia due to stones, numbness
Oxalis corniculata	Procumbent yellow-sorrel	Abortion
Papaver rhoeas	Common poppy	Intestinal colic
Peganum harmala	Harmal	Numbness
Physalis alkekengi	Chinese lantern	Kidney stone

Scientific name	Common name	Medical uses
Pterocarpus santalinus L.	Sandalwood (2)	Lower arthralgia, Abortion
Punica granatum	Pomegranate (2)	Abortion, intestinal colic
Quercus lusitanica Lam	Gall oak	Abortion
Rosa gallica/ rosaceae	Red rose (4)	Lower arthralgia, nephralgia due to stones, kidney stone, abortion, smallpox
Ruta angustifolia Pers	Rue	Numbness
Thymus glaber	Large thyme (2)	Lower arthralgia, nephralgia due to stones
Tribulus terrestris	Small caltrops (3)	Lower arthralgia, nephralgia due to stones, kidney stone
Trigonella foenum-graecum	Fenugreek	Kidney stone
Viola odorata	Sweet violet (4)	Nephralgia due to stones, kidney stone, lower arthralgia, smallpox, intestinal colic
Vitex agnus castus	Chaste tree	Numbness

Readers of al-Shirwānī's entire chapter would notice that a number of herbs were used repeatedly in the recipes, and that these herbs would have been available in almost every home in both Arabic and Ottoman civilization. This group of herbs includes common hollyhock, chamomile, ribbed melilot, white Egyptian lotus, and sweet violet. Here, I examine the benefits of their use in bathtub recipes, and then compare them with their usage in Arabic medicine. My aim in this comparison is a pharmaceutical and medical one: I wish to determine the reason for using these herbs and to understand the interaction between Ottoman and Arabic medicine in the application of medicinal herbs.

In Arabic medicine, the plant known as common hollyhock (as described by Ibn al-Bayṭār) was used for the same therapeutic purposes mentioned by al-Shirwānī.[35] The only difference is that Ibn al-Bayṭār did not mention using bathtubs to obtain those therapeutic benefits. There is a similar situation with chamomile, where Ibn al-Bayṭār mentions all of the same benefits as al-Shirwānī concerning its analgesic effects, as well as its utility for kidney

35 According to Ibn al-Bayṭār, this plant could be used to prevent inflammation and alleviate pain; moreover, its seeds dissolved kidney stone. The water in which common hollyhock was cooked was beneficial against digestive ulcer, haemoptysis, and diarrhea. If the root was cooked in syrup and then drunk, it would be useful for dysuria, stone, sciatica, and digestive ulcer. If cooked in vinegar and then used to rinse the mouth, it would allay tooth pain; Ibn al-Bayṭār, *Kitāb*, 2: 333.

stone and for strengthening the nervous system.[36] While Ibn al-Bayṭār did not explicitly mention the bathtub as a mode of preparation for these herbs, his reference to a woman sitting in chamomile water bears striking similarities to sitting in the bathtub. Therefore, it appears that al-Shirwānī improved and modernized the usage of both common hollyhock and chamomile by adding the bathtub technique to achieve their full therapeutic benefits.

In the case of ribbed melilot, Ibn al-Bayṭār neither mentioned using it in conjunction with the bathtub technique, nor described its effectiveness in dissolving kidney stone. However, he did discuss its analgesic effect on pains afflicting the joints, kidney, and liver.[37] Thus there is some consensus between Arabic and Ottoman medicine about using ribbed melilot externally to relieve pain. A similar situation can be seen in the case of white Egyptian lotus. Here, Ibn al-Bayṭār did not mention the prevention of abortion in his book, but he did discuss the drying power of this plant.[38] Egyptian lotus might help to stop the bleeding that occurred when the sensation of miscarriage or premature delivery began, so it is understandable that al-Shirwānī took advantage of its astringent properties in his recipe.

The same holds true in the case of sweet violet, although Ibn al-Bayṭār neither mentioned the bathtub technique nor the use of sweet violet in healing the traces of smallpox.[39] However, al-Shirwānī might have added this simple to take advantage of its cold effect on the skin surface. Smallpox is characterized by blisters on the skin that are associated with the sensation

36 Chamomile reportedly alleviated the pain of swollen or inflammed organs, treated fevers, and soothed the abdomen. Since the healing 'virtue' of chamomile was hot, it could act as an emmenagogue, facilitate birthing, and stimulate the urine if a woman sat in the water in which ribbed melilot had been cooked. Its cooking water healed jaundice and liver pain. It strengthened the nervous system and was also good for cold headaches. It could be used in a bandage for the bladder or to alleviate muscle aches in the abdomen; Ibn al-Bayṭār, *Kitāb*, 1: 101.

37 Ibn al-Bayṭār maintained that ribbed melilot was useful for slight inflammation of the uterus, eyes, and the bladder if mixed with egg yolk, fenugreek flour, or flaxseed flour. If combined with water, it would help with malignant sores; if used as a syrup, it would alleviate stomach ache. The juice could be extracted and used as ear drops to alleviate earache. Liquids derived from ribbed melilot also cured headaches and organ pain. Like chamomile, its healing 'virtue' was hot. When used as a bandage with wormwood, it treated inflammation of the liver, intestines, and spleen; Ibn al-Bayṭār, *Kitāb*, 1: 68.

38 According to Ibn al-Bayṭār, its root and seeds have drying power that is useful for intestinal ulcers and metrorrhagia; they also have the power to heal vitiligo; Ibn al-Bayṭār, *Kitāb*, 4: 486.

39 Water made from sweet violets was reportedly beneficial for epilepsy in boys. Since its properties were cold and wet, it benefitted coughs caused by heat. If used in a bandage on the head and forehead, it alleviated the headaches caused by heat. Syrup of sweet violet was useful for odorous urine, bladder pain, and nephralgia, and also had a diuretic effect; Ibn al-Bayṭār, *Kitāb*, 1: 156.

of heat and itching; thus the cooling effects of sweet violet provided topical relief. It seems clear that al-Shirwānī inherited from Arabic medicine the understanding of the effects of particular herbs and thus added them to his formulations.

From a pharmaceutical point of view, we can conclude that al-Shirwānī followed Arabic medicine by using many of the same herbs for specific ailments. However, he modernized and developed traditional recipes by adding herbs that could achieve additional medical benefits based on either their therapeutic effects or on the symptoms of diseases.

Conclusion

The use of the bathtub technique in Ottoman medicine is a continuation of its usage in Arabic medicine, especially among eastern physicians such as al-Majūsī and Ibn Sīnā. The *Rawḍat al-ʿiṭr* book of al-Shirwānī included an extended chapter on the applications of bathtub therapy, in which he mentions various recipes to treat a number of different conditions that included many simple drugs. Hence it is fair to say that Ottoman practitioners developed and modernized the use of bathtubs in therapies that had circulated earlier in the eastern medical tradition. In addition, they clearly took into consideration the availability and familiarity of certain substances, many of which were already used in cookery, when giving instructions on how to prepare these recipes. Like medical systems elsewhere, Ottoman medical practice was entangled in a web of social hierarchies and economic realities that conditioned the range and choice of treatment options.

Several factors likely contributed to al-Shirwani's special treatment of the bathtub method and its rise in Ottoman medicine. On the most obvious medical level, the method was useful and applicable in a variety of situations. From the perspective of gender, bathtub therapies were probably attractive because women of limited means would not need to engage practitioners, least of all male practitioners, and instead could provide healthcare from home.[40] As Sara Verskin discusses in her essay in this volume, in Ottoman Islamic societies where modesty was a concern, the use of the bathtub as a domestic technique enabled patients to negotiate the delivery of care.[41] We

40 Shefer-Mossensohn, 'Sick Sultana in the Ottoman Imperial Palace', discusses the intersection of class and gender in early Ottoman clinical practice, and concludes that elite women may in fact have been more restricted in seeking medical assistance from male physicians.

41 Verskin, 'Gender Segregation and the Possibility of Arabo-Galenic Gynecological Practice'.

might also consider the possibility that Ottoman society regarded illness as a state that required enclosure within the home. Additionally, from an economic standpoint, doctors' fees were often prohibitively expensive, so that home remedies were both desired and necessary.

A study of the ailments treated by al-Shirwānī using bathtub therapy shows that this approach represents a form of domestic care. The basic purpose of using this technique was to shorten the time needed to begin treatment, independent of the doctor's presence. Moreover, the recipes are also easily prepared and applied, which is exactly what patients and practitioners would need in treating domestic cases. As a result, we can say that bathtub therapy clearly was an important mode of treatment within the framework of Ottoman household medicine.

Works Cited

Manuscript

Istanbul, Süleymaniye Library Hacı Beşir Ağa 506, Muhammed ibn Maḥmūd al-Shirwānī, *Rawḍat al-ʿiṭr.*

Printed Works

Boisseuil, Didier, ed. *Le bain: espaces et pratiques*, special issue of *Médiévales*, 43 (2002).

Börekçi, Günhan. 'Smallpox in the Harem: Communicable Diseases and the Ottoman Fear of Dynastic Extinction during the Early Sultanate of Ahmed I (r. 1603-17)', in *Plague and Contagion in the Islamic Mediterranean: New Histories of Disease in Ottoman Society*, ed. Nükhet Varlik (Kalamazoo: Arc Humanities Press, 2017), 135-52.

Burkett, L. 'Medical Tourism: Concerns, Benefits, and the American Legal Perspective', *Journal of Legal Medicine*, 28.2 (2007), 223-45.

Church, L. 'Water Birth: One Birthing Center's Observations', *Journal of Nurse-Midwifery*, 34.4 (1989), 165-70.

Cluett, Elizabeth R. and Ethel Burns. 'Immersion in Water in Labour and Birth', *Sao Paulo Medical Journal*, 131.5 (2013), 364.

Connell, John. 'Medical Tourism: Sea, Sun, Sand and ... Surgery', *Tourism Management*, 27.6 (2006), 1093-1100.

Dinc, G. and Y.I. Ulman. 'The Introduction of Variolation "A La Turca" to the West by Lady Mary Montagu and Turkey's Contribution to This', *Vaccine*, 25.21 (2007), 4261-65.

Dryglas, Diana and Paweł Różycki. 'Profile of Tourists Visiting European Spa Resorts: A Case Study of Poland', *Journal of Policy Research in Tourism, Leisure & Events*, 9.3 (2017), 298-317.

Helmy, E.M. 'Benchmarking the Egyptian Medical Tourism Sector against International Best Practices: An Exploratory Study', *Tourismos*, 6.2 (2011), 293-311.

Ibn Abī 'Uṣaybi'a. *'Uyūn al-anbā' fī ṭabaqāt al-aṭibbā'* (Beirut: Dar Maktabat al-Hayat, 1965).

Ibn al-Bayṭār, *Kitāb al-Jāmi' li-Mufradāt al-Adwīya wa al-Aghdhīya* (Beirut: Dar al Kotob al ilmiyah, 1992).

Ibn Hubal, Muhadhab al-Dīn. *Kitāb al-Mukhtarāt fi ṭ-Ṭibb* (Istanbul: Dā'irat al-M'ārif al-'uthmāniyyah, 1943).

Ibn Sīnā [Avicenna]. *al-Qānūn fi ṭ-Ṭibb* (Beirut: Dar 'iḥyā' al-Turāth al-'arabī, 2006).

Idrisi, Zohor. 'The Gap between the World of Ibn al-Bayṭār and that of Linnaeus', in *Ibn al-Bayṭār al-Mālaqī y la ciencia árabe*, ed. E. García Sánchez (Malaga: Servicio de Publicaciones e Intercambio Científico de la Universidad de Málaga, 2008), 13-34.

Mackey, M.M. 'Use of Water in Labor and Birth', *Clinical Obstetrics and Gynecology*, 44 (2001), 733-49.

al-Majūsī, Ali ibn al-'Abbās. *Kitāb Kāmil al-Ṣinā'a al-Ṭibbiyya = Kitāb al-Malikī* (Cairo: Ministry of Public Education of Egypt, 1968).

Nolte, Cordula. 'Domestic Care in the Sixteenth Century: Expectations, Experiences, and Practices from a Gendered Perspective', in *Gender, Health, and Healing, 1250-1550*, ed. Sara Ritchey and Sharon Strocchia (Amsterdam: Amsterdam University Press, 2020), 215-43.

Özköse, Aysun. 'The Bath Tradition in Anatolia', in *Islamic Urban Heritage* (Istanbul: IRCICA, 2013), 113-23.

Pormann, Peter E. and Emilie Savage-Smith. *Medieval Islamic Medicine* (Edinburgh: Edinburgh University Press, 2010).

al-Qumrī, Abū Manṣūr. *al-Tanwīr fi al-Iṣtilaḥat al-Ṭibbiyyah*, ed. Gāda Ḥasan (Riyadh: Arab Bureau of Education for the Gulf States, 1911).

Ragab, Ahmed. *The Medieval Islamic Hospital: Medicine, Religion, and Charity* (Cambridge: Cambridge University Press, 2015).

Riedel, Stefan. 'Edward Jenner and the History of Smallpox and Vaccination', *Baylor University Medical Center Proceedings*, 18.1 (2005), 21-25.

Sezgin, Fuat. *'Abdallāh ibn Aḥmad ibn al-Bayṭār (d. 646/1248): Texts and Studies* (Frankfurt am Main: Institute for the History of Arabic-Islamic Science at the Johann Wolfgang Goethe University, 1996).

Shefer-Mossensohn, Miri. 'Medicine in the Ottoman Empire', in *Encyclopaedia of the History of Science, Technology, and Medicine in Non-Western Cultures*, ed. Helaine Selin (Dordrecht: Springer, 2014), 1-7.

—. *Ottoman Medicine: Healing and Medical Institutions, 1500-1700* (Albany, NY: State University of New York Press, 2009).

—. 'A Sick Sultana in the Ottoman Imperial Palace: Male Doctors, Female Healers and Female Patients in the Early Modern Period', *Journal of Women of the Middle East and the Islamic World*, 9 (2011), 281-312.

Verma, R.L. 'The Growth of Greco-Arabian Medicine in Medieval India', *Indian Journal of History of Science*, 5 (1970), 347-63.

Verskin, Sara. 'Gender Segregation and the Possibility of Arabo-Galenic Gynecological Practice in the Medieval Islamic World', in *Gender, Health, and Healing, 1250-1550*, ed. Sara Ritchey and Sharon Strocchia (Amsterdam: Amsterdam University Press, 2020), 291-313.

Yu, Ji Yun and Tae Gyou Ko. 'A Cross-cultural Study of Perceptions of Medical Tourism among Chinese, Japanese and Korean Tourists in Korea', *Tourism Management*, 33.1 (2012), 80-88.

Zytka, Michal. *A Cultural History of Bathing in Late Antiquity and Early Byzantium* (New York: Routledge, 2019).

About the Author

Ayman Yasin Atat received his PhD in the History of Medical Science from Aleppo University in 2014 and is currently Philipp Schwartz Fellow in the Department for History of Science and Pharmacy at Technische Universität Braunschweig (Germany). He is an expert on Arabic, Ottoman, and Islamic medicine, and Arabic medical manuscripts.

Part 4

(In)fertility and Reproduction

10 Gender, Old Age, and the Infertile Body in Medieval Medicine

Catherine Rider

Abstract

Medieval medical texts regularly discussed a range of reproductive disorders in men and women. As part of this discussion, they often noted that men and women were infertile in extreme youth and old age. Although medieval medical views of infertility have received scholarly attention, these references to age and infertility have not been analysed. This chapter traces these references in a range of twelfth- to fifteenth-century Latin medical works. It argues that discussions of men and women's fertility in old age were broadly similar, and that age was more important than gender when medical writers thought about age-related infertility. Nonetheless, behind the similarities many medical writers presented age as placing a greater burden on women's fertility than men's.

Keywords: fertility, aging, menopause, reproduction, women's medicine

Age has long been recognized in both medieval and modern medicine as one of the many factors that might delay or prevent the conception of a child. In modern culture the effects of age on fertility are often presented as an issue for women in particular. Since the 1970s, the image of the 'biological clock' and the dangers of 'leaving it too late' have centred on women, while contemporary media stories about older parents have also often focused on women having children in their forties or after the menopause.[1] Medieval medical writers also noted the negative effects of old age on fertility but their approach to gender was rather different. While they generally paid special attention to women, their discussions

1 Jensen, *Infertility*, 148-52; Ylänne, 'Representations of Ageing and Infertility'.

Ritchey, Sara & Sharon Strocchia (eds), *Gender, Health, and Healing, 1250-1550*. Amsterdam, Amsterdam University Press 2020
DOI: 10.5117/9789463724517_CH10

also regularly included men in a way that might seem surprising to a modern reader.

This topic has received relatively little discussion from medievalists. There is a growing body of work on aging and old age in the Middle Ages, but it often says comparatively little about fertility, instead focusing on the question of when one was considered 'old' (variable, but often around the age of 60) and on life for those aged 60 and over, including examinations of retirement, disability, and impairment.[2] Meanwhile, the essays collected in Sue Niebrzydowski's edited volume on middle-aged women focus primarily on issues other than fertility.[3] Studies that consider misogynistic depictions of older women in medieval literature, religious writing, and medicine discuss old women's lack of menstruation and 'barrenness' as well as the ways in which older women were portrayed as sources of sexual knowledge.[4] The essay in this volume by Montserrat Cabré and Fernando Salmón elaborates on many of these themes, showing that, especially after the mid-thirteenth century, medieval and early modern medical texts came to link a lack of menstruation in postmenopausal women to madness, toxicity, and the evil eye.[5] These studies discuss older women's 'barrenness' as part of broader surveys of attitudes to old women rather than focusing on this issue in detail. Therefore, there remains no detailed exploration of the relationship between age and ideas about fertility specifically in the medieval period. This is especially true for men, but more work remains to be done on women also.

This lacuna is surprising in view of significant research in recent decades into fertility, reproduction, and women's medicine in the Middle Ages. This work has greatly increased our knowledge of the transmission and audiences of medical knowledge and texts on these topics, and of what they can tell us about perceptions of women's and (to a lesser extent) men's bodies.[6] It has also underlined the fact that enhancing fertility was an abiding concern in this period, particularly in the fourteenth and fifteenth

2 See, for example, Rosenthal, *Old Age in Late Medieval England*; Shahar, *Growing Old in the Middle Ages*; Youngs, *Life Cycle in Western Europe*, 163-89; Metzler, *Social History of Disability in the Middle Ages*, 92-153.

3 Niebrzydowski, ed., *Middle-Aged Women in the Middle Ages*.

4 Mieszkowski, 'Old Age and Medieval Misogyny'; Pratt, '*De vetula*'; Agrimi and Crisciani, 'Savoir médical et anthropologie religieuse'.

5 Cabré and Salmón, 'Blood, Milk, and Breastbleeding'.

6 Green's extensive body of work has been central here; her book *Making Women's Medicine Masculine* draws together many of her conclusions. On men, see Rider, 'Men and Infertility in Late Medieval Medicine'.

centuries.[7] Fertility enhancement engaged university-educated medical writers as well as collectors and readers of vernacular medical recipes; the recipe collections studied by Sheila Barker and Sharon Strocchia and Julia Gruman Martins in this book, for example, contain substantial material on fertility.[8] Among these studies, however, age has not often figured as a primary consideration. Of the major studies that discuss medieval infertility, only Jean-Claude Bologne's *La naissance interdite* mentions the issue, noting that very few medieval medical writers believed cures for infertility in old age were possible, despite the existence of Bible stories about women such as Sarah who conceived late in life. Medieval medical writers, Bologne suggests, knew their limitations.[9] In part, this gap in an otherwise rich scholarship exists because discussions of age form a comparatively small part of medical writing on impediments to conception. Understandably, research on medieval infertility has tended to examine other causes of reproductive disorders that figure more prominently in the sources, such as humoral imbalances.[10]

By contrast, early modernists have more fully explored the relationship between age and fertility in medicine. Sarah Toulalan has examined the ways in which humoral understandings of the body led medical writers to associate old age with infertility and sexual undesirability. She has shown that, for both men and women, the aging process was believed to lead to a loss of heat and moisture in the body. This deficiency, in turn, affected the quality of both partners' seed as well as the quality of the woman's womb. The loss of heat and moisture was also believed to render older men's and women's bodies physically unattractive and unsuitable for sex.[11] In addition, Toulalan and Sara Read have probed early modern medical thinking about the age at which women experienced the menopause. There was considerable scope for variation here but the general consensus placed the menopause around the age of 50.[12] These two studies suggest that, despite differences in experiences of old age by men and women, with the

7 Green, *Making Women's Medicine Masculine*, documents both the growing volume of medical texts on fertility, and the practical concerns that lay behind them. On the fourteenth and fifteenth centuries, see Park, 'Managing Childbirth and Fertility', 162-63.

8 Barker and Strocchia, 'Household Medicine for a Renaissance Court'; Martins, 'Understanding/Controlling the Female Body'.

9 Bologne, *La naissance interdite*, 59.

10 The chapter on 'Sterility' in Cadden, *Meanings of Sex Difference*, 228-58, does not mention old age; nor does Rider, 'Men and Infertility in Late Medieval Medicine'.

11 Toulalan, 'Elderly years cause a Total dispaire of Conception'.

12 Ibid., 347; Read, *Menstruation and the Female Body*, 180.

menopause marking a clear cessation of fertility in women, in some respects age affected male and female bodies in similar ways – at least in terms of sexuality and fertility – because the humoral model of the body emphasized the importance of heat for reproduction in both sexes. Helen Yallop has gone further, arguing that eighteenth-century medical literature portrayed both older men's and older women's bodies as sexless.[13] Since the same humoral model of the body underpinned medieval and early modern medicine, many of the patterns identified by these scholars probably also applied to medieval medical discussions of aging and fertility. Nevertheless, there are also potential differences between medieval and early modern medical approaches to aging and fertility. For example, when looking at medieval descriptions of the 'ages of man', Sue Niebrzydowski has placed greater emphasis on the differences between male and female aging. Although both men's and women's bodies were believed to grow colder and drier with age, she argues that the loss of beauty and fertility figured more prominently in medieval discussions of women's old age.[14] As we will see, some medieval medical texts also display this pattern of stressing the loss of fertility more for women than for men, and a few linked it to sexual undesirability, even though that is not the only way in which they thought about sex difference.

All of these studies, whether medieval or early modern, suggest that our understanding of the relationship between gender, age, and fertility in the medieval period would benefit from fuller consideration of longer-term continuities and changes, as well as differences between types of source material. They also show that a wide range of medieval and early modern texts mention fertility and old age, from descriptions of the 'ages of man' to poetry. This essay advances this research by examining in greater detail what university-educated medical writers in the later Middle Ages said about the effects of age on fertility for men and women. These works discussed fertility and old age consistently across several centuries, even if their remarks were not always very detailed.

These sources presented age and gender as equally important factors in discussions of fertility. Although medical writers devoted more time to discussing the effects of age on women's fertility than on men's, they often described the effects of age on fertility in similar terms for both sexes. Infertility is therefore a useful case study for thinking about how gender interacted with age in determining attitudes to health and medicine in the Middle Ages.

13 Yallop, 'Representing Aged Masculinity', 201, 205.

14 Niebrzydowski, 'Becoming Bene-Straw', 4.

This essay focuses on a selection of medical works written in Latin between the late eleventh and the fifteenth centuries that discuss the causes of reproductive disorders, their signs, and their cures. Many of these are encyclopedic texts known as *practicas*, which set out the causes and treatment of illnesses, covering the whole body from head to toe. From the twelfth century onwards *practicas* included sections on reproductive disorders in men and women. Over the centuries these sections became longer and more detailed. This elaboration reflected a more general expansion in the length of *practicas*, as well as the increasing volume of medical writing devoted to reproduction, as noted above.[15] *Practicas* discussed impediments to fertility in men and women, including old age, under various headings such as 'impediments to conception', 'difficulty of impregnation', or 'sterility'. They also mentioned the effects of age on women's fertility in their chapters on menstrual problems. When they discussed these topics they drew on a range of earlier texts, including Arabic medical texts translated from the eleventh century onwards and the works of Aristotle translated from Greek in the thirteenth century. The *Canon of Medicine* of Ibn Sīnā (Avicenna), which was translated in the 1180s and used in universities from the mid-thirteenth century, especially influenced *practica* writers' discussions of fertility, prompting many from the mid-thirteenth century onwards to write about the relationship between age and fertility in a way that twelfth-century *practicas* did not.[16] For this reason *practicas* from the late thirteenth to fifteenth centuries will be the focus of much of this study. Nonetheless, as we will see, an earlier translation of another general work on illness and treatment, the *Zād al-musāfir wa-qūt al-hādir* (Provisions for the traveller and nourishment for the settled) of Ibn al-Jazzār, translated as the *Viaticum* by Constantine the African in the late eleventh century, also included important information about the ages at which women began and ceased to menstruate.

In addition to the *practicas*, more specialized treatises discussed the effects of age on fertility. The twelfth-century *Book of the Conditions of Women*, which formed part of the well-known *Trotula* ensemble of texts on women's medicine, discussed the ages at which menstruation started and stopped.[17] In the early fourteenth century, one of a group of treatises that focused specifically on 'sterility', or conception, written at the University of Montpellier, also mentioned youth and old age as causes of female infertility,

15 Demaitre, *Medieval Medicine*, 300.

16 Ibid., 315.

17 *Trotula*, ed. and trans. Green, 66.

although it devoted more space to youth than age.[18] These treatises often gave similar information to that found in the *practicas*, in part because they drew on similar Greek and Arabic sources for much of their material. For example, the *Book of the Conditions of Women* took much of its content (including the information about menstruation) from the *Viaticum*.[19] Later specialized treatises also quoted *practicas*, and so the Montpellier 'sterility' treatise drew on a *practica* written at Montpellier at about the same time, the *Lilium medicine* of Bernard de Gordon.[20]

These Latin treatises employed a technical vocabulary and, as noted above, drew much of their information from earlier written sources. Most were written by physicians who taught medicine at medical schools and universities; often their authors claimed to be writing for their students.[21] Nevertheless, we should not see these texts purely as products of theoretical medicine divorced from more widespread medical understandings or from practice. In the fifteenth century in particular, as Danielle Jacquart has argued, *practica* writers were interested in discussing their own experience and practice.[22] These references to experience included several anecdotes relating to unusual fertility in youth or old age, as we will see. Moreover, by the end of the Middle Ages several of these Latin works were reaching a wider audience. The *Trotula* and several *practicas* were translated into vernacular languages in the fourteenth and fifteenth centuries, and some of the treatments listed in the *Trotula* especially were reproduced in recipe collections, first in manuscript and later in print.[23] These vernacular texts and recipes are beyond the scope of this essay, but their existence suggests that the ideas found in the *Trotula* and the *practicas* had the potential to influence the medical ideas of a wider range of educated readers. In the medieval period, as Monica Green has shown, these educated readers seem to have been mostly (although not exclusively) men, but from the sixteenth century onwards this kind of medical knowledge reached a more mixed audience, including women who wrote recipe collections (such as Caterina Sforza, discussed in this volume by Barker and Strocchia).[24] What

18 *Tractatus de sterilitate*, ed. Cartelle, 74, 84.

19 *Trotula*, ed. and trans. Green, 21; Green, *Making Women's Medicine Masculine*, 49.

20 *Tractatus de sterilitate*, ed. Cartelle, 21.

21 Agrimi and Crisciani, *Edocere medicos*, 157-60.

22 Jacquart, 'Theory, Everyday Practice, and Three Fifteenth-Century Physicians', 140.

23 On this process for fertility, see Rider, 'Men and Infertility in Late Medieval English Medicine', and the references cited there; for the *Trotula* in later print collections, see Jones, 'Generation from Script to Print', 185.

24 On the medieval period see Green, 'Women and the Gendering of Medical Literacy'.

began as elite, Latin medicine for a largely male audience therefore came to incorporate practice and observation and, in the long term, to reach a wider pool of readers.

When they discussed fertility and age, these medical texts gave two kinds of information. On the one hand, they often listed extremes of age – young or old – as causes of infertility in men, women, or (most often) both, among many other causes of infertility. On the other, they included more general discussions of the ages at which women and men were fertile. For women, these discussions focused on the ages at which menstruation began and ended. Writing about men's ages of fertility was less frequent but, as we will see, medical writers who discussed men used a similar language and approach to the one they took when writing about women. This information on age and fertility drew on a wider medical theory of generation which, as Joan Cadden has noted, often (but not invariably) highlighted the symmetries between men's and women's bodies.[25] In particular they reflect the medical theory of generation espoused by many of the medieval medical writers cited here, which held that both men and women contributed 'seed' to the formation of an embryo. This understanding is commonly termed the 'two-seed' theory of conception, and it was often attributed to Galen in the Middle Ages. It was not the only view of generation found in medieval medical and scientific writing. Some writers followed a different view, attributed to Aristotle, that only men contributed a 'seed', which actively formed the embryo, while women contributed 'matter'.[26] Nevertheless the two-seed theory was preferred by many medical writers who influenced the *practicas* and particularly by Ibn Sīnā, as we will see below.

Youth and Old Age among the Causes of 'Sterility'

The first way that many *practica* texts discussed age and fertility was by mentioning old age, often alongside extreme youth, as one among many causes of 'sterility' or 'difficulty of impregnation'. Their comments on this matter were often brief and lacked detail, but they nonetheless reveal some of the ways in which medical writers thought about the effects of age on fertility. Their approach seems to derive from the *Canon of Medicine* of Ibn Sīnā, who listed age as a cause of reproductive disorder in both sexes, first in the section on men's reproductive disorders in Book 3, fen 20, and then

25 Cadden, *Meanings of Sex Difference*, 241.

26 See Jacquart and Thomasset, *Sexuality and Medicine in the Middle Ages*, 61-70.

in the section on women's reproductive disorders in Book 3, fen 21. These passages discussed the effects of age on men and women in similar terms. Ibn Sīnā listed age among a range of other factors in his discussion of men, when talking about the kinds of sperm ('sperma') that cannot generate:

> The sperm of a drunk and a decrepit man [*decrepiti*] and an infant [*infantis*] and a man who has a great deal of sex does not generate. And the sperm of someone who has a damaged penis rarely generates healthy offspring. And when the penis is elongated greatly, the space that the sperm has to move is elongated, so that it comes to the womb with its innate heat already broken; therefore it does not generate, according to many.[27]

In his later section on women and reproduction, Ibn Sīnā again listed age as one of several factors that meant a person's *sperma* would not generate:

> And indeed the sort of sperm from which generation does not happen is the sperm of an infant [*infantis*], and a person suffering from fullness to the point of nausea, and a drunk, and an old person [*senis*], and the sperm of someone [*qui*] who has a great deal of intercourse, and whose body is not healthy. For sperm runs from all the members and a healthy thing is generated from a healthy person, and an unhealthy thing from an unhealthy person, according to what Hippocrates has said. And all these dispositions are found in both sperms together.[28]

The reference to 'both sperms together' is consistent with Ibn Sīnā's more general view that both the man and the woman contributed some form of 'seed' to the formation of an embryo.[29] His adoption of the two-seed position therefore meant that it was easier to present men's and women's seeds as being affected in the same ways by the same factors, including age. For both sexes, age was grouped with a variety of other conditions

27 Ibn Sīnā, *Liber canonis*, bk. 3, fen 20, tract. 1, ch. 13, p. 690: 'Sperma ebrii, et decrepiti, et infantis, et multi coitus non generat. Et sperma habentis membra laesa, raro generat sanum. Et cum prolongatur uirga ualde, prolongatur spacium motus spermatis: quare uenit ad matricem calore eius innato iam fracto, non ergo generat secundum plurimum'.
28 Ibn Sīnā, *Liber canonis*, bk. 3, fen 21, tract. 1, ch. 8, p. 709: 'Et de genere quidem spermatis ex quo non fit generatio, est sperma infantis et patientis nauseativam satietatem, et ebrii, et senis. Et sperma eius qui plurimum utitur coitu, et cuius corpus non est sanum. Sperma enim currit ex omnibus membris: et ex sano, sanum: et ex infirmo, infirmum, secundum quod dixit Hippocrates. Et istae dispositiones omnes inuentae sunt in utriusque spermatibus simul'.
29 McGinnis, *Avicenna*, 241.

which, as Ibn Sīnā explained in the second quotation, rendered the whole body unable to generate healthy sperm. The link between age and fertility here is tied to general health and lifestyle but not closely linked to a particular gender.

Not all later *practica* writers took up Ibn Sīnā's references to age. For example, Guglielmo da Saliceto, one of the first to cite Ibn Sīnā, did not.[30] Conversely, William of Brescia (d. 1326) quoted Ibn Sīnā almost word for word.[31] Others adapted the lists found in the *Canon*, adding or omitting other criteria that might affect the seed. Thus Bernard de Gordon's *Lilium medicine* (1305) offered a discouraging prognosis for certain kinds of infertile men which was similar, but not identical, to Ibn Sīnā's list: 'For boys and the decrepit, drunks, gluttons, and those who have a penis that is too long, and have intercourse too much, do not generate; or only rarely; or their offspring will be horrible'.[32] Bernard's *Lilium* was widely read and quoted, and his list in turn influenced a number of later *practica* writers. John of Gaddesden (*c.*1320) offered the same words as Bernard, as did Michele Savonarola, writing in Ferrara shortly before 1446.[33]

Bernard de Gordon did not mention an equivalent form of age-related infertility in women, but other *practica* authors did. For example, John of Gaddesden noted that women could be made infertile by a range of problems affecting their whole bodies. These included problems with the brain, heart, liver, stomach, or spleen, or 'because her menses are too much retained, or because they flow too much, or because the woman is too thin, or because she is a girl or an old woman [*puella aut vetula*]'.[34] John therefore differentiated between the sexes more stringently than Ibn Sīnā, placing a greater emphasis on women's reproductive organs. Nevertheless, he still maintained the view that both women and men might have problems

30 Gulielmus de Saliceto, *Summa conservationis et curationis*, ch. 176, on difficulty of impregnation.

31 Guilelmus Brixiensis, *Practica*, ch. 125, fol. 137v: 'Ex quo non fit generatio est sperma infantis, et patientis nauseatiuam satietatem, et ebrii, et senis, et utentis multo coytu, et hominis non sani. Sperma enim currit ex omnibus membris corporis, ex sano sanum, exinfirmum [*sic*], et omnes iste dispositiones sunt inuente in utrisque spermatibus simul'.

32 Bernard de Gordon, *Lilium medicine*, pt. 7, ch. 1, fol. 138v: 'Pueri enim et decrepiti, ebrii, crapulati, et qui habent virgam nimis longam, et qui utuntur nimio coitu non generant. aut raro, aut erit feda eorum generatio'.

33 John of Gaddesden, *Rosa anglica*, bk. 2, ch. 17, fol. 96v; Joannes Michaelis Savonarola, *Practica maior*, tract. 32, fol. 238v. On the dating of Savonarola's *practica*, see Jacquart, 'En feuilletant la *Practica maior*', 59.

34 John of Gaddesden, *Rosa anglica*, bk. 2, ch. 17, fol. 95r: 'quia menstrua sunt nimis retenta, aut quia nimis fluunt, aut quia mulier est nimis extenuata, aut puella, aut vetula'.

afflicting their whole body that made conception difficult, and placed age in this category for both sexes.

In many cases, these medical writers did not give reasons why age (or other factors such as excessive drinking) made seed unhealthy; instead, they simply presented the fertile body as one that was healthy, moderate in consuming food and drink and in sexual behaviour, and mature, but not extremely old. However, John of Gaddesden offered a more detailed explanation grounded in the theory of the humors: both children and the elderly lacked heat in their complexions, which in medical theory was deemed essential both for sexual performance and for fertility. This meant that infertility might occur if 'the age is too moist, as are boys and girls; [or] too cold and dry, as in *decrepita* age'.[35] Other *practicas* did not spell out this correlation, but given the predominance of humoral theory it seems likely that similar humoral explanations lie behind the other comments on infertility and old or young age, as they did in the early modern period.

As we can see from the passages quoted here, most of these writers mentioned the effects of age extremes – young or old – on fertility in relatively similar ways for men and women. The young and old of both sexes lacked the necessary physical capabilities to make healthy seed, or had cold and dry humors. Not every writer mentioned both sexes: Bernard de Gordon did not include a parallel discussion of women, whereas the early fourteenth-century *Tractatus de sterilitate* listed 'too young and old' alongside many other causes of infertility in women, but did not mention age in its section on men, even though its anonymous author drew much of his material from Bernard de Gordon and so presumably could have followed him in discussing age for men.[36] Nevertheless, many writers did mention both sexes, and so we see in many of these references a considerable degree of 'symmetry' (to use Joan Cadden's term) between the ways in which age was deemed to have an impact on men's and women's fertility.[37]

However, there were places where this symmetry collapsed. Cadden has noted that, in medieval medical discussions of infertility more generally, when gender symmetry broke down writers tended to focus on the woman as the cause of infertility.[38] Similar patterns held true for discussions of

35 Ibid., bk. 2, ch. 14, fol. 94v: 'scilicet quod etas est nimis humida sicut sunt pueri et puelle, nimis frigida et sicca sicut in etate decrepita'.

36 *Tractatus de sterilitate*, ed. Cartelle, 74.

37 Cadden, *Meanings of Sex Difference*, 241.

38 Ibid., 249.

infertility and age. Both Bernard de Gordon and John of Gaddesden suggested that sleeping with a woman who was either too old or too young might make a man infertile. Here they were not simply stating the obvious that having sex with a woman who was too young or old would not result in conception. Rather, they argued that a woman who was unsuitable because of age or other factors could damage the man's own fertility. Of the two, John of Gaddesden spelled out more clearly how the woman's age, among other factors, could affect the man's generative ability:

> Item there is another cause [of sterility] on the part of the man, because perhaps he has too much sex, or intercourse with a woman who perhaps is not of age, or because she with whom he is having intercourse is an old woman, or because he has intercourse with her in an inept way, or because she is menstruating or scabby [*scabiosa*] or has worms [*tineosa*], or is stinking or of horrible appearance; by reason of these things the man does not take pleasure in sex.[39]

Here the woman's age is emphasized not because she is infertile but because it renders her an unpleasant sexual partner. Although it is not explicit, this passage likely refers to impotence, with the man's lack of desire for the woman making him unable to have an erection. The reference to having intercourse 'in an inept way' suggests that sexual dysfunction is at least part of what is being discussed. I have not been able to trace the source of this information before Bernard de Gordon. Ibn Sīnā had noted that sex with a very young girl could corrupt a man's sperm but said nothing about sex with an old woman or its effects on male pleasure.[40] These passages were not reproduced by later *practica* writers (to my knowledge) but they make clear that, although in many cases the impact of age on men's and women's fertility was discussed in similar terms, a minority of writers placed an additional emphasis on women, in a way that echoed some of the literary stereotypes of disgusting older women.

39 John of Gaddesden, *Rosa anglica*, bk., 2, ch. 17, fol. 94v: 'Item ex parte viri est alia causa: quia forte utitur nimio coitu, vel cum muliere que forte non provenit ad annos, aut quia ipsa est vetula cum qua coit, aut quia cognoscit eam inepto modo, aut quia est menstruosa, aut scabiosa vel tineosa, aut fetida aut horribilis aspectus: ratione quorum vir non delectatur in coitu'; cf. Bernard de Gordon, *Lilium medicine*, pt. 7, ch. 1, fol. 138r.

40 Ibn Sīnā, *Liber canonis*, bk. 3, fen 21, ch. 8, p. 709: 'Et dixerunt quidam quod de causis corruptionis spermatis viri est coire cum illis que nondum sunt magne et hoc currit cursu proprietatum'.

Ages of Menstruation and Fertility

The discussions of infertility quoted above did not generally specify what they meant by too old, or too young. Instead they used general words that might cover a range of ages, such as 'decrepitus', 'senis', or 'infans'. By contrast, the second strand of comments on age and fertility did provide particular ages at which women and, less often, men, were deemed to be fertile. They offer a broadly similar picture to the one discussed above: some degree of gender symmetry but with a greater focus on women. Many of these comments focused on women because they appeared as part of discussions of menstruation, setting out the ages at which women began and ceased to menstruate. Nevertheless, by the fifteenth century, a few medical writers were also discussing the ages at which men's fertility began and ended.

Among educated medical writers, the most widely circulated set of ages for the start and end of menstruation was found in the *Viaticum* of Ibn al-Jazzār, as translated by Constantine the African. By the thirteenth century the *Viaticum* was found on university medical curricula.[41] Beside being influential in its own right, as noted above it was also a major source for another widely circulated work, the *Book of the Conditions of Women*, which became part of the *Trotula* compilation and was translated into many vernacular languages. The *Viaticum* offered broad age ranges for the beginning and end of menstruation, with an especially wide range for the end of menstruation:

> The menses come to women when they reach the age of 14 years; however, if the menses make haste, in the 12th year. Nature may do this. They happen in this way to women just as nocturnal emission [*pollutio*] does to males [...] The lack [of menstruation] is either natural or unnatural, as happens to women after 50 years; to some others in the 40th; others in the 35th, especially to women who are very fat and fleshy.[42]

The *Book of the Conditions of Women* gave similar, but not identical, information, stating, 'This purgation occurs in women around the thirteenth year [...] it lasts until the fiftieth year if she is thin, sometimes until the sixtieth

41 Wack, *Lovesickness in the Middle Ages*, 48.

42 Ibn al-Jazzar, *Viaticum*, trans. Constantinus Africanus (1515), bk. 6, ch. 9, fol. 164v: 'Menstrua mulieribus eueniunt cum etatem xiiii. annorum subeunt. Sed tamen si festinauerint menstrua in xii, hoc faciet natura. Que sic contigunt mulieribus sicut pollutio masculis [...] Eorum ablatio aut est naturalis, aut non naturalis, que mulieribus post l. annos contingit; aliis in xl. aliis in xxxv, maxime multum pinguibus et carnosis'.

or sixty-fifth year if she is moist. In the moderately fat, it lasts until the thirty-fifth year'.[43] Some of these ages at which menstruation might cease look rather high or low compared with modern data about the usual ages of menopause – especially the *Book*'s 35 to 60 or 65 – but it is possible that they were simply designed to encompass a wide range of individual variation, including women who experienced early menopause. Monica Green also notes that the ages given vary considerably between different manuscripts of the *Book* and the same may be true of the *Viaticum*.[44] In singling out fat women ('very' for the *Viaticum*, but only 'moderately' for the *Book*) as likely to cease menstruating early, both sources were in line with wider humoral theory that presented fat bodies as dominated by cold humors, and argued that fat women were likely to suffer a range of reproductive difficulties.[45] Despite this picture of individual variation, however, both the *Viaticum* and the *Book* set clear time limits on women's fertility. Because the focus is on menstruation these limits are specific to women, but it is interesting that the onset of menstruation is linked in the *Viaticum* to a parallel change in men's bodies at puberty. In this way, the *Viaticum* offers a partial similarity between the reproductive development of both sexes.

Many *practicas* included similar comments about ages of menstruation. Bernard de Gordon, for example, noted that '[t]he menses run naturally from the 14th year up to the 45th or 60th, but sometimes earlier and sometimes later according to the [woman's] diverse complexion and other particulars.'[46] However, perhaps tellingly, other fourteenth-century *practica* authors avoided the wide range of ages cited by the *Viaticum* and the *Book*. William of Brescia, in the early fourteenth century, identified 12 to 14 as the starting ages for menstruation and 45 to 50 as the end point.[47] John of Gaddesden followed the *Viaticum* in giving the range 35 to 50: '[The menses] are naturally retained up to the 12th year and after the 50th year; and sometimes they dry up more quickly, such as sometimes in the 35th year, sometimes in the 40th, sometimes in the 45th, depending on the women's different dispositions'.[48]

43 *Trotula*, ed. and trans. Green, 66.

44 Ibid., 191.

45 On this see Toulalan, 'To[o] much eating stifles the child', 74.

46 Bernard de Gordon, *Lilium medicine*, pt. 7, ch. 8, fol. 142v: 'Menstrua currunt naturaliter ab anno xiiii. usque ad xlv vel lx. Aliquando tamen citius et aliquando tardius secundum diversitatem complexionum et aliorum particularium'.

47 Guilelmus Brixiensis, *Practica*, ch. 119, fol. 131r: 'dicitur quod puellis non accidit menstruum ante 12m vel 14m annum [...] et durat usque ad 45m annum vel 50m. annum'.

48 John of Gaddesden, *Rosa anglica*, bk. 2, ch. 17, fol. 100r: 'Naturaliter retinentur usque ad 12m annum et post 50m annum. et aliquando exiccantur citius, scilicet aliquando in 35° anno, aliquando in 40 aliquando in 45° secundum diuersas dipositiones mulierum'.

In bracketing the ages of 45 to 50 as the end point of menstruation, some of these fourteenth-century *practica* writers may in part have been recording their own observation, but they may also have been influenced by a written source that was translated and available later than the *Book* or the *Viaticum*. This source was Aristotle's *History of Animals*, which was translated into Latin in the early thirteenth century by Michael Scot and again by William of Moerbeke later in the century. In these translations, the treatise appeared alongside Aristotle's other works on animals such as *De animalibus*. Here, Aristotle discussed the ages at which both men's and women's fertility ended, and stated that some men could generate children up to the age of 70, and some women up to 50, but that 60 for men and 45 for women were more normal.[49] Fourteenth-century writers such as William of Brescia did not mention Aristotle by name, but their focus on the ages of 45 to 50 suggests that they may have been influenced by his work.

By the fifteenth century, several *practica* writers quoted Aristotle directly, and also followed him in providing ages for the end of men's fertility as well as women's. Thus the Italian physician Antonio Guaineri, writing a treatise on the womb in the 1440s that formed part of a larger *practica*, quoted the ages for male and female fertility given by Aristotle. Guaineri attributed this information to Aristotle's *Parts of Animals* but the information comes, in fact, from the *History of Animals*:

> Age also makes a man sterile, for men after the age of 70 and women after 50 do not conceive, according to Aristotle in *On the Parts of Animals*, 4. In a woman there is no doubt that when the time for menstruation has passed she lacks the essentials for generation; but, in men, although many people say this is true, nonetheless it is not always the case. For I have seen a number of octogenarians who generated children, and one man of more than 90.[50]

49 Aristotle, *De historia animalium*, bk. 5, ch. 14, 144: 'Generat autem homo quidem usque ad septuaginta annos masculus, mulier autem usque ad quinquaginta. Sed hoc quidem rarum; paucis enim facti sunt in hiis etatibus pueri; ut autem in pluribus hiis quidem sexaginta quinque terminus, hiis autem quadraginta quinque'.

50 Antonius Guainerius, *Tractatus de matricibus*, ch. 19, transcribed from the first printed edition by van den Hooff, 'Antonio Guaineri's *De Matricibus*', 63 (I have cited this version because it is easily accessible, but have checked van den Hooff's transcriptions against the early printed text): 'Etas quoque hominem sterilem efficit nam ultra septuagenarium viri et mulieres quinquagenarium, teste Aristotiles in *De partibus animalium* quarto non concipiunt. In muliere illud nec dubium est cum tempore illo transactis floribus careat requisitis ad generationem necessario. In viris vero et si ut plurimum sic sit, non tamen semper, nam octogenarios nonnullos qui genuerunt vidi et quemdam plusquam nonagenarium'.

Writing a commentary on Ibn Sīnā's *Canon* in France a little later, the physician Jacques Despars also followed Aristotle in suggesting that men over 70 rarely had children.[51]

Antonio Guaineri's comments are interesting because, as well as citing Aristotle by name, and discussing both men and women, he included his own observation of men who had children later than Aristotle had described. Guaineri seems to have been especially willing to note his observations of fertility in older age, because he also described cases he had seen of women who conceived quite late in life: 'And I have seen two women who at the age of 45 had never conceived but afterwards had children with their same husband'.[52] Although Guaineri may have been particularly interested in mentioning these cases, his tendency to record his own observations was part of a wider fifteenth-century development in medicine. As noted above, Danielle Jacquart has argued that fifteenth-century *practica* writers were often willing to include more details about their own observations and experience than earlier writers. In the case of infertility and age, two other fifteenth-century writers likewise made brief references to what they claimed were real cases of fertility beyond the normal age limits – either in their own time or in the past. Niccolò Falcucci, a Florentine physician who wrote a voluminous set of *Sermones medicales* around 1400, which shared much information with the *practicas*, quoted the Roman compiler Solinus on the ages at which men's and women's fertility ended, and also added a historical example of fertility in extreme old age: Cato, who had fathered a child at the age of 80. However, he also noted that this was a rare instance and one that Solinus described as a marvel.[53] Michele Savonarola, meanwhile, mentioned another rare case at the other extreme of fertility: 'And Marsilius Paravus saw at Pavia a girl of 9 who was made pregnant, but these cases are rare'.[54]

51 Jacobus de Partibus, *Liber canonis*, bk. 3, fen 20, ch. 8, n.f.: 'Secundo dicit quod decrepitorum sperma non generat. precipue illorum qui septuagesimum transiuerint annum'.

52 Antonius Guainerius, *Tractatus de matricibus*, ch. 19, transcribed in Van den Hooff, 'Antonio Guaineri's *De Matricibus*', 65: 'et ego duas vidi que 45 transacto conceperant nunquam postea cum eisdem maritis prolere habuere'.

53 Falcucci, *Sermones medicales*, sermo 6, tract. 3, ch. 2, fol. 31r: 'Et dixit Avicenna quod de genere spermatis de quo non fit generatio est sperma infantis id est eius qui incipit emittere sperma vel ut dicunt ante 14 annum et sperma senis id est decrepiti ut supra habitum est dixit solinus post 50 annum omni mulierum fecunditas conquiescit et virorum post 60. Cato tamen 80^{0} exacto ex filia solonis clientis sui annum uticensis cathon procreavit hoc autem raro contingit et ideo inter mirabilia descriptum est'.

54 I have not been able to identify this Marsilius. Savonarola, *Practica maior*, tract. 6, ch. 21, fol. 239v: 'Et quedam ut Marsilius parauus vidit puellam Papie annorum noue impregnatam, sed hec sunt raro'.

By the fifteenth century, then, *practica* writers continued to be interested in the same topics as earlier physicians, looking at the ages at which menstruation started and ceased. The age ranges they gave were often comparable with those given by earlier writers, although some omitted the extreme young and old ages found in the *Book of the Conditions of Women*. However, they combined this relatively standard information with a new interest in the limits of men's fertility, prompted in part by Aristotle and in part by a more general interest in discussing examples of unusual fertility, which might include men having children in old age. The result of this method of analysis was that they came to discuss the ages at which men and women were fertile in relatively similar terms. They gave older ages for the end of men's fertility than women's, but they nonetheless believed that both sexes – not only women – experienced a decline and then final end of their fertility, which could be pinned down to a particular age range. They also argued that, for both sexes, these age ranges of fertility were only those experienced by the majority. In rare cases men and women might have children in youth or old age beyond the usual limits.

Conclusion

It is comparatively easy to observe many of the intellectual influences that lay behind these discussions of age and fertility. They can be traced to earlier writers such as Aristotle, Ibn Sīnā, and Ibn al-Jazzār. However, it is much more difficult to assess how closely these medical writers also reflected social practice relating to age and fertility in the world around them, except when they mentioned cases of exceptional fertility that they claimed to have observed. Broadly speaking, we can say that the ages of menopause quoted by most of these medical writers – around 45 to 50 – seem to match modern observations. But is it possible to go further than this? Was there a widespread desire among medieval men and women to have children in what these texts described as old age: over 40 in women, or over 50 in men?

It is certainly possible to think of situations in which medieval men and women might have sought children at these ages: for example, in the event of a late marriage, a second marriage for one partner, or perhaps after the death of a much older child. A few may have had a child in their 40s after some years of childlessness: one example is Constance of Sicily, mother of the Emperor Frederick II, who bore what was likely her only child in 1194 at the age of 40.[55] Other couples may simply have continued to have children into their 40s after beginning at much younger ages. Medieval people, including medical writers, must have been aware of these cases. Their infrequency probably attracted comment and medical writers continued to note similar unusual cases of fertility in old age into the early modern period.[56] But were these cases noted because they were exceptional, in a way somewhat equivalent to the media interest today in women who have children in their 50s and 60s, rather than because many people had children in older age? There are comparatively few records that allow us to calculate the ages at which most medieval men and women had children, and average ages are in any case likely to have varied over time and place, as well as being dependent on wealth and social status. Any conclusions therefore must be tentative. Nevertheless, David Herlihy's demographic work on wealthy fifteenth-century Florentine households suggests that it was not unheard of for women to have children in their 40s, at least among the elite. In his study of the Florentine *catasto* of 1427, Herlihy calculated that 8 per cent of the women aged between 43 and 47 in urban Florence had a child under 2 years old, and just over 18 per cent of women in one of its rural suburbs did.[57] It is likely that among poorer families the numbers would have been lower, given that poorer families tended to have fewer children overall.[58] Thus most women did not continue to have children in their 40s, but in this particular place and time it seems to have been common enough that examples would have been visible. Even if the ages given in the *catasto* were not reported completely accurately, they are likely to reflect a perception of the ages at which some women were still having children.

It seems likely that many medical discussions of fertility and age were not closely focused on the practical task of helping men and women to conceive in later life, even though, as Monica Green has shown, physicians did treat infertility throughout the later Middle Ages.[59] Most *practica* writers listed age as a factor that made people generate rarely, and they did not suggest that it could be cured. This is not to say that there were no possible remedies that could be used in practice. Indeed, *practicas* and recipe collections listed treatments which were simply described as facilitating conception and so could be used for anyone, whatever the 'problem' was deemed to

55 Abulafia, *Frederick II*, 58.

56 Toulalan, 'Elderly years cause a Total dispaire of Conception', 343.

57 Herlihy, *Medieval Households*, 148, table 6.3.

58 Ibid., 147.

59 Green, *Making Women's Medicine Masculine*, 85-91.

be. Humoral cures that increased a person's heat and moisture could also have been used to counter the coldness and dryness of old age. Outside of learned medicine, there were yet other ways of seeking fertility, including consulting unofficial practitioners, going on pilgrimage, performing pious works, or using amulets.[60]

Nevertheless, it was rare for physicians to suggest that treatments could be used specifically to enhance fertility in cases of old age. One exception is Niccolò Bertucci, writing a *practica* in the early fourteenth century. His words offer some indication as to why the topic was mentioned so rarely. Bertucci noted that the age barriers for conception could be remedied with humoral medicine to some degree:

> Hence [women] do not conceive either before this time [the usual ages of menstruation], or after it. And if they do conceive, they miscarry because of any trivial cause, unless a good complexion and regimen and effort should rectify it naturally: hence Hippocrates, in the fifth part of the *Aphorisms*, says 'Any women who are worn out conceive outside nature: they miscarry before they become big. [...]'[61]

In this passage, even Bertucci was cautious about the effectiveness of humoral medicine and diet, ending with the more pessimistic Hippocratic quotation that suggested an older woman was likely to miscarry. Bertucci's caution is suggestive, particularly when viewed alongside the absence of treatments in other *practicas*, when many other causes of infertility were singled out for cures. Perhaps, as Bologne suggested, physicians knew their limits and were wary of overpromising. Instead, the discussions of particular ages at which women, and less often men, were fertile, with their references to unusual fertility in later life, point to a more theoretically driven interest in the limits of natural fertility; in the fifteenth century, this interest combined with a desire to record observations and unusual cases.

Throughout the later Middle Ages, then, learned medical writers argued that old age (like extreme youth) rendered both men's and women's bodies unsuitable for generation because it affected the quality of their seed and their humoral balance. For Bernard de Gordon and John of Gaddesden,

60 Park, 'Managing Childbirth and Fertility', 162-63.

61 Bertucci, *Compendium sive Collectorium*, tract. 9, ch. 1, fol. 178v: 'quare neque ante hoc tempus, neque post concipiunt: Et si concipiant: abortiunt ex omni leui causa, nisi bonitas complexionis, et regiminis, et opus rectificet naturalie: unde Hip. 5. parti. apho. Quecunque preter naturam tenues existentes concipiunt: abortiunt, antequam grossescant'.

men might also be made infertile because very old or young women could not give them sufficient pleasure in intercourse. But in general, medieval medical writers seem to have paid less attention than their early modern counterparts to the sexual undesirability of old bodies.[62] Medical writers also were consistent in citing particular ages perceived as the end dates for women's fertility, to which men were added in the fifteenth century, while acknowledging that a few rare individuals might be fertile much earlier or later. Thus in many respects, discussions of age and fertility considered men's and women's bodies in similar terms, a trend that continued into the early modern period.[63] The reproductive capacity of men and women aged in similar ways and for similar reasons (albeit at different rates); in neither case was there much prospect of treatment.

Nevertheless, behind these similarities there were some subtle differences that often placed greater emphasis on women's infertility in old age. For those writers who gave ages for the end of fertility in both sexes, women lost their fertility earlier than men, and more definitively, at the end of menstruation; medical writers cited exceptional cases of male fertility in extreme old age, but for women the exceptional cases tended to be much younger, like Guaineri's 45-year-old women. Moreover, when Bernard de Gordon and John of Gaddesden stated that a man's fertility could be damaged by an older partner because it reduced his pleasure, they did not mention a similar problem for women who had intercourse with much older or younger men, even though many medical writers recognized that it was necessary for women as well as men to take pleasure in sex if conception was to occur. Finally, as Cabré and Salmón demonstrate, if we look beyond infertility, we find that some medical writers wrote about the negative effects of the end of menstruation on women's bodies in a way that went far beyond what was discussed for men. Thus, in line with what Joan Cadden has observed for discussions of infertility more broadly, medical discussions of infertility and age appeared on the surface to be symmetrical but nonetheless placed a greater burden on the woman as the person responsible for generation. Although age was important, when medical writers thought about fertility, they never rendered gender irrelevant.

Thus even though medical writers may not have spoken directly to common social practice or led physicians to offer cures targeted at age-related reproductive disorders, their discussions of fertility in old age and extreme youth can still shed light on the ways in which gender interacted with other

62 Toulalan, 'Elderly years cause a Total dispaire of Conception', 354-58.

63 Ibid., 359.

factors in determining medical thinking and therapeutic options. Bodies were gendered, and discussions of fertility and age to some extent placed a greater responsibility – and burden – on women, in line with other writing on infertility. Nevertheless, even when the topic was reproduction, gender always interacted with other markers of identity, and in certain circumstances might become subordinate to them. For medieval medical writers, then, the biological clock weighed more heavily on women, but men were often considered too. In this case, a gendered history of healthcare is as much a history of age – in men as well as women – as a history of women's fertility.

Works Cited

Printed Works

Abulafia, David. *Frederick II: A Medieval Emperor* (London: Allen Lane, 1988).

Agrimi, Jole and Chiara Crisciani. *Edocere medicos: medicina scolastica nei secoli XIII-XV* (Naples: Guerini e Associati, 1988).

—. 'Savoir médical et anthropologie religieuse: les représentations et les fonctions de la vetula (XIIIe-XVe siècle)', *Annales: Économies, Société, Civilisations*, 48.5 (1993), 1281-1308.

Antonius Guainerius. *Tractatus de matricibus*, transcribed from the first printed edition by P.C. van den Hooff, 'Antonio Guaineri's *De matricibus, sive De propriis mulierum aegritudinibus*', MA diss, University of Leiden, 2013, https://openaccess.leidenuniv.nl/handle/1887/21559 (accessed 18 October 2019).

Aristotle. *De historia animalium*, trans. Guillelmus de Morbeka, ed. Pieter Beullens and Fernand Bossier (Leiden: Brill, 2000).

Barker, Sheila and Sharon Strocchia. 'Household Medicine for a Renaissance Court: Caterina Sforza's *Ricettario* Reconsidered', in *Gender, Health, and Healing, 1250-1550*, ed. Sara Ritchey and Sharon Strocchia (Amsterdam: Amsterdam University Press, 2020), 139-65.

Bernard de Gordon. *Lilium medicine* (Ferrara: Andrea Gallus, 1486).

Bertucci, Niccolò. *Compendium sive Collectorium artis medicae* (Cologne: Melchiorem Novesianum, 1537).

Bologne, Jean-Claude. *La naissance interdite: stérilité, avortement, contraception au Moyen-Age* (Paris: Olivier Orban, 1988).

Cabré, Montserrat and Fernando Salmón. 'Blood, Milk, and Breastbleeding: The Humoral Economy of Women's Bodies in Medieval Medicine', in *Gender, Health, and Healing, 1250-1550*, ed. Sara Ritchey and Sharon Strocchia (Amsterdam: Amsterdam University Press, 2020), 93-117.

Cadden, Joan. *Meanings of Sex Difference in the Middle Ages: Medicine, Science, and Culture* (Cambridge: Cambridge University Press, 1993).

Demaitre, Luke. *Medieval Medicine: The Art of Healing, from Head to Toe* (Santa Barbara: Praeger, 2013).

Falcucci, Niccolò. *Sermones medicales* (Venice: Bernardinum de Tridino, 1491).

Green, Monica. *Making Women's Medicine Masculine: The Rise of Male Authority in Pre-modern Gynaecology* (Oxford: Oxford University Press, 2008).

—. 'The Possibilities of Literacy and the Limits of Reading: Women and the Gendering of Medical Literacy', in *Women's Healthcare in the Medieval West: Texts and Contexts*, by Monica H. Green (Aldershot: Ashgate, 2000), 1-76.

Guilelmus Brixiensis. *Practica* (Venice: Bonetus Locatellus, 1508).

Gulielmus de Saliceto. *Summa conservationis et curationis* (Venice: Bonetus Locatellus, 1502).

Herlihy, David. *Medieval Households* (Cambridge, MA: Harvard University Press, 1985).

Ibn al-Jazzar. *Viaticum*, trans. Constantinus Africanus, in Ysaac Israeli, *Opera Omnia* (Lyon: Joannes de Platea, 1515).

Ibn Sīnā. *Liber canonis* (Basel: Johann Herwegen, 1556).

Jacobus de Partibus. *Liber canonis Avicenne Principis cum explanatione Jacobi de partibus*, 4 vols. (Lyon: I. Clein, 1498).

Jacquart, Danielle. 'En feuilletant la *Practica maior* de Michel Savonarole: quelques échos d'une pratique', in *Michele Savonarola: Medicina et cultura di corte*, ed. Chiara Crisciani and Gabriella Zuccolin (Florence: Sismel, 2011), 59-81.

—. 'Theory, Everyday Practice, and Three Fifteenth-Century Physicians', *Osiris*, ser. 2, 6 (1990), 140-60.

Jacquart, Danielle and Claude Thomasset. *Sexuality and Medicine in the Middle Ages*, trans. Matthew Adamson (Cambridge: Polity Press, 1988).

Jensen, Robin E. *Infertility: Tracing the History of a Transformative Term* (University Park, PA: Pennsylvania State University Press, 2016).

John of Gaddesden. *Rosa anglica practica medicine* (Venice: Bonetus Locatellus, 1516).

Jones, Peter Murray. 'Generation from Script to Print', in *Reproduction: Antiquity to the Present Day*, ed. Nick Hopwood, Rebecca Flemming, and Lauren Kassell (Cambridge: Cambridge University Press, 2018), 181-94.

McGinnis, John. *Avicenna* (Oxford: Oxford University Press, 2010).

Martins, Julia Gruman. 'Understanding/Controlling the Female Body in Ten Recipes: Print and the Dissemination of Medical Knowledge about Women in the Sixteenth Century', in *Gender, Health, and Healing, 1250-1550*, ed. Sara Ritchey and Sharon Strocchia (Amsterdam: Amsterdam University Press, 2020), 167-88.

Metzler, Irina. *A Social History of Disability in the Middle Ages: Cultural Conditions of Physical Impairment* (London: Routledge, 2013).

Mieszkowski, Gretchen. 'Old Age and Medieval Misogyny: The Old Woman', in *Old Age in the Middle Ages and the Renaissance: Interdisciplinary Approaches to a Neglected Topic*, ed. Albrecht Classen (Berlin: De Gruyter, 2007), 299-319.

Niebrzydowski, Sue. '"Becoming Bene-Straw": The Middle-Aged Woman in the Middle Ages', in *Middle-Aged Women in the Middle Ages*, ed. Sue Niebrzydowski (Cambridge: D.S. Brewer, 2011), 1-14.

—, ed. *Middle-Aged Women in the Middle Ages* (Cambridge: D.S. Brewer, 2011).

Park, Katharine. 'Managing Childbirth and Fertility in Medieval Europe', in *Reproduction: Antiquity to the Present Day*, ed. Nick Hopwood, Rebecca Flemming, and Lauren Kassell (Cambridge: Cambridge University Press, 2018), 153-66.

Pratt, Karen. '*De vetula*: The Figure of the Old Woman in Medieval French Literature', in *Old Age in the Middle Ages and the Renaissance: Interdisciplinary Approaches to a Neglected Topic*, ed. Albrecht Classen (Berlin: De Gruyter, 2007), 321-42.

Read, Sara. *Menstruation and the Female Body in Early Modern England* (Basingstoke: Palgrave Macmillan, 2013).

Rider, Catherine. 'Men and Infertility in Late Medieval Medicine', *Social History of Medicine*, 29 (2016), 245-66.

Rosenthal, Joel T. *Old Age in Late Medieval England* (Philadelphia: University of Pennsylvania Press, 1996).

Savonarola, Joannes Michaelis. *Practica maior* (Venice: Bonetus Locatellus, 1497).

Shahar, Shulamith. *Growing Old in the Middle Ages: 'Winter Clothes us in Shadow and Pain'*, trans. Yael Lotan (London: Routledge, 1997).

Toulalan, Sarah. '"Elderly years cause a Total dispaire of Conception": Old Age, Sex, and Infertility in Early Modern England', *Social History of Medicine*, 29 (2016), 333-59.

—. '"To[o] much eating stifles the child": Fat Bodies and Reproduction in Early Modern England', *Historical Research*, 87 (2014), 65-93.

Tractatus de sterilitate, ed. Enrique Montero Cartelle (Valladolid: Universidad de Valladolid, 1993).

The Trotula: An English Translation of the Medieval Compendium of Women's Medicine, ed. and trans. Monica H. Green (Philadelphia: University of Pennsylvania Press, 2001).

Wack, Mary. *Lovesickness in the Middle Ages: The Viaticum and its Commentaries* (Philadelphia: University of Pennsylvania Press, 1990).

Yallop, Helen. 'Representing Aged Masculinity in Eighteenth-Century England: The "Old Man" of Medical Advice', *Cultural and Social History*, 10.2 (2013), 191-210.

Ylänne, Virpi. 'Representations of Ageing and Infertility in the Twenty-First-Century British Press', in *The Palgrave Handbook of Infertility in History*, ed. Gayle Davis and Tracey Loughran (Basingstoke: Palgrave Macmillan, 2017), 509-35.

Youngs, Deborah. *The Life Cycle in Western Europe c. 1300-c. 1500* (Manchester: Manchester University Press, 2006).

About the Author

Catherine Rider is Associate Professor in Medieval History at the University of Exeter. Her research focuses on the history of medicine, reproduction, magic, and popular religion in the later Middle Ages. She is the author of *Magic and Impotence in the Middle Ages* (2006) and *Magic and Religion in Medieval England* (2012).

11 Gender Segregation and the Possibility of Arabo-Galenic Gynecological Practice in the Medieval Islamic World

Sara Verskin

Abstract

There is a widespread assumption that, in the medieval Islamic world, a cultural emphasis on female modesty and gender separation resulted in male physicians never having the expectation or opportunity to put their gynecological and obstetrical knowledge to practical use. However, a wide range of textual evidence suggests that, in many communities, there was a broad acceptance of intimate interactions between male practitioners and female patients. These interactions included verbal consultations, manual examinations, and physical procedures relating to fertility and childbirth, as well as diseases of the sexual organs. Some male authors of medical texts also convey the expectation that the information in their texts would come to be known and utilized by women themselves, through female medical intermediaries.

Keywords: female patients, gynecology, Islamic medical ethics, midwives, modesty, Sharia

The gynecological section of the only twentieth-century printed edition of al-Rāzī's *al-Manṣūrī fī al-ṭibb* (Rhazes' *Liber medicinalis ad almansorem*) includes a discreetly written editorial footnote. Glossing al-Rāzī's treatment for retained menstruation, the modern editor remarked at the line, 'He gives to the [female] patient':

> It is so in all versions. In these chapters which address women and those diseases of the menses and of the uterus which befall them, the author

Ritchey, Sara & Sharon Strocchia (eds), *Gender, Health, and Healing, 1250-1550*. Amsterdam, Amsterdam University Press 2020
DOI: 10.5117/9789463724517_CH11

> writes as though speaking about a male [practitioner]. Hence 'he gives to the patient', 'he administers', 'he inserts', 'he feeds', etc. We have tried to correct all of the words without pointing out every mistake in the footnotes.[1]

By characterizing the masculine verbs he found in the text as 'mistakes', the editor articulated an assumption commonly found in modern scholarship about the practice of gynecology in the medieval Islamic world. The editor could not imagine that a male physician would have such intimate contact with women. He therefore chose to 'correct' the masculine verbs by substituting feminine and passive verb forms, so that it appears as though the female patient performs these actions on her own, or that a second woman is present to act as a medical intermediary. As he stated in this note, the many 'problematic' references to male practitioners acting on female bodies are too copious to annotate individually.

The notion that in the medieval Islamic world gynecological care could not possibly involve interaction with men is widespread among both Western and Middle Eastern scholars. For example, in his voluminous and groundbreaking study of Islamic medicine, Manfred Ullmann devoted only four paragraphs to gynecology. He reasoned that Muslim physicians did not invest in its study because only female midwives, who received no training in medical theory, had the opportunity to treat gynecological conditions. According to Ullmann, this absence of academic training in medieval gynecology was due to cultural modesty or to 'tradition', a term that he does not clearly define. The end result, according to Ullmann, was a 'backwardness' and lack of 'significant achievement' with respect to gynecology in the Arabo-Galenic medical tradition.[2]

Is it true that male physicians had no interest in or opportunity to practise gynecological medicine, and that therefore book-learned gynecology was an entirely moot endeavour? If so, what should we make of texts such as al-Rāzī's, which instruct physicians to be intimately involved in the care

1 al-Rāzī, *al-Manṣūrī fī al-ṭibb*, 448. The editor notes that the masculine form appears in all manuscript versions of the text.

2 Ullmann, *Die Medizin im Islam*, 250. I use 'Arabo-Galenic' as a shorthand for the system of medicine, explicated in Arabic-language texts, which understood itself to stand on a foundation of Greek-language texts, particularly as they were interpreted by Galen. This system included both non-Muslim physicians writing in Arabic, as well as Muslim physicians who came from or operated in predominantly non-Arab communities but who nonetheless wrote many of their medical works in Arabic. Cabré and Salmón, 'Blood, Milk, and Breastbleeding', this volume, describe several important elements of the gynecological content of this medical system.

of female patients? There seem to be three possibilities for interpreting the historical significance of such texts. One is that medieval gynecological texts were strictly theoretical exercises and had no relation to practice. Second, it is possible that the convention of medieval medical writing cast all medical care in masculine terms, but in reality independent female practitioners or female intermediaries were the ones most likely to supply the intimate care described in the texts; the masculine language of the text is thus an accident of the genre and not a reflection of actual male involvement. Finally, given that female intermediaries often do make an appearance in some but not all gynecological chapters of a medical text, we might argue that the texts hew closer to reality than has previously been assumed, and that in some communities male physicians did in fact interact with female patients and provide gynecological information and care.

This essay makes the case for this last interpretation. I argue that there were indeed opportunities for theoretical gynecology to have an impact on the practical care of women. Sometimes this interaction occurred through the mediation of female medical assistants, who both received theoretical knowledge from male physicians and served as medical informants for them.[3] However, a broad chronological, geographic, and typological view also reveals that medieval Islamicate texts consistently and unambiguously referred to direct male medical interaction with female patients. It is, therefore, a mistake for scholars to assume that modesty concerns always made the male practice of gynecology socially implausible.

Book-Learned Medicine and the Gender Divide

There is little doubt that the primary consumers of Arabo-Galenic writings about gynecology were men. Other than a small number of treatises devoted to the care of pregnant women and newborns, there are few stand-alone

3 Most often medical compendia acknowledge female informants only as reporters of bodily conditions. Only occasionally do physicians acknowledge women contributing knowledge of treatments, often ones with occult elements. For example, the *Paradise of Wisdom* of ʿAlī ibn Sahl Rabbān al-Ṭabarī (d. 923) states, 'The head of the hospital of Jundīshāpūr informed me there is, among a family in the [nearby] village of Ahwaz, a stone which protects the fetus if it is tied to the pregnant woman. Moreover, we have heard that, according to the son of a revered Christian woman in Rayy, if this pregnant woman with the stone inadvertently encounters another pregnant woman, the one who does not have this stone with her will miscarry. Daylamite women inform me that this protective stone is widely available in Jīlān'; al-Ṭabarī, *Firdaws al-ḥikma fī'l-ṭibb*, 39-40. Kandzha, 'Female Saints as Agents of Female Healing', in this volume, shows that professional physicians in medieval Europe also acknowledged such empirical or occult treatments.

gynecological texts in the medieval Arabo-Galenic medical corpus.[4] Instead, gynecology was usually addressed in comprehensive medical encyclopedias. These encyclopedias were organized 'from head to toe' with gynecological matters addressed in sections devoted to the anatomy and physiology of the genitals and their diseases. Sometimes medical encyclopedias also included separate sections devoted to surgery, in which we find descriptions of a variety of operations, including lithotomy, clitorectomy, treatment of an imperforate hymen, excision of cancerous growths, episiotomies during obstructed labour, manipulation of a fetus's position during labour, and the evacuation of a dead fetus or dismemberment of a fetus during obstructed labour. Arabic medical literature also addressed gynecological issues in commentaries on the Hippocratic *Aphorisms*, which included statements about fertility, miscarriage, childbirth, lactation, and menstruation.[5] None of these texts were attributed to female authors and, indeed, we have no direct evidence of women studying these books and scant references to women owning them.[6]

There are only a handful of references to women receiving training in theoretical medicine. Some women in medieval Islamic communities were known to have been taught to read or write, and medieval chroniclers credited them with having mastered the content of particular books; however, to my knowledge, none of the accounts of such learned women mention them engaging with medical literature specifically.[7] The most expansive account of women receiving training from a physician in the Arabo-Galenic tradition can be found in Ibn Abī 'Uṣaybi'a's fourteenth-century

4 For example, al-Qurṭubī's *Kitāb khalq al-janīn wa-tadbīr al-ḥabālā wa'l-mawlūdīn* and al-Baladī's *Tadbīr al-ḥabālā wa'l-aṭfāl wa'l-ṣibyān*.

5 Batten, 'Arabic Commentaries on the Hippocratic Aphorisms'.

6 Ibn Abī 'Uṣaybi'a recounts that al-Rāzī's sister owned his medical papers after his death. She was persuaded to sell them to his disciples, who assembled them to form the *al-Ḥāwī* (*Liber continens*). Ibn Abī 'Uṣaybi'a also describes the sisters of Muwaffaq al-Dīn ibn al-Mūtrān (a physician in the service of Saladin) taking possession of his many medical writings after his death and then losing them or using them as filler in a crafts project; Ibn Abī 'Uṣaybi'a, *'Uyūn al-anbā' fī ṭabaqāt al-aṭibbā'*, 420, 659; English trans. in Ibn Abī 'Uṣaybi'a, *Lives of the Physicians*, trans. Kopf, 542, 828.

7 The conclusion that few women were taught to read is, for the most part, an argument from silence. As for writing, there is an interesting passage in a *ḥisba* manual from early fourteenth-century Egypt which says that a teacher 'must not teach handwriting to a woman or to a slave girl'. Much of the author's advice in the *ḥisba* manual seems to address real-life violations of his prohibitions, so that one could read this passage as indicative that some teachers were in fact instructing women how to write; Ibn al-Ukhuwwa, *Ma'ālim al-qurba fī aḥkām al-ḥisba*, 171. A guide to slave-buying dated a century later also notes that some slave girls could write. See al-'Ayntābī, *al-Qawl al-sadīd fī ikhtiyār al-imā' wa'l-ābīd*, 36.

biographical dictionary of famous physicians. In his description of the multiple generations of the Ibn Zuhr physician dynasty that flourished in Spain, he wrote that the sister and niece of al-Ḥafīd Abū Bakr ibn Zuhr (d. 1233) 'were knowledgeable in the art of medicine and treatment, and they had much experience in matters pertaining to the treatment of women' and served as midwives in the caliph's household.[8] Ibn Abī 'Uṣaybi'a also claimed that the caliph's vizier had both Ibn Zuhr and his niece assassinated, an indication that both occupied positions of power. We know nothing else about these women, not even the assassinated woman's name.[9] With the possible exception of such women, Arabo-Galenic medical books were, as far as we know, the exclusive province of men.[10]

At the same time, many medical texts refer to physicians working alongside or employing women with whom they engaged in a professional exchange, and whose expertise they respected. Additionally, a few treatises include passages that suggest that the author expected that women would become acquainted with the content of his text. These passages all occur in recipes for contraceptives and abortifacients. For example, the tenth-century Tunisian physician Ibn al-Jazzār justified describing these drugs 'so that they will be known and so that women would beware of using them'.[11] His defense implied an assumption that what he wrote would eventually reach women themselves, and that women were ultimately part of his audience or 'readership'. By comparison, Ibn al-Jazzār's Persian contemporary al-Majūsī wrote that sometimes contraception or abortion was medically necessary to preserve the life of a woman, but cautioned the physician against mentioning these medicines 'to prevent their use by women in whom there is no good'; he should describe them only 'to women

8 Ibn Abī 'Uṣaybi'a, *'Uyūn al-anbā' fī ṭabaqāt al-aṭibbā'*, 524; Ibn Abī 'Uṣaybi'a, *Lives of the Physicians*, trans. Kopf, 664.

9 I know of no other references to female relatives of physicians practising obstetrical medicine themselves, but this seems to me to be a likely occurrence. This discussion pertains only to women trained in medical theory. There is little doubt that women in general, as mothers, wives, and preservers of folklore and healing magic provided much of the day-to-day care for sick people and labouring women in particular, both in the Islamic world and in the Western world up until the early modern period; Pormann and Savage-Smith, *Medieval Islamic Medicine*, 103.

10 The feminine noun *ṭabība*, i.e. 'doctoress', is attested to, but nowhere in the pre-Ottoman period does the term appear to refer to a woman trained in Arabo-Galenic medicine or mastering medical texts. Muḥammad b. Ibrāhīm al-Jazarī's (d. 1338) biographical dictionary includes a reference to a Cairene woman named Umm Khayr Khadīja bint al-imām Fakhr al-Dīn al-Nawzarī (d. 1333) who knew how to write and, in her old age, served as a midwife to the sultan's wife. However, her writing seems to be connected to her religious scholarship, rather than to her medical know-how; al-Jazarī, *Ta'rīkh ḥawādith al-zamān*, 3: 701.

11 Trans. from Bos, in Ibn al-Jazzār, *Ibn al-Jazzār on the Sexual Diseases*, 290.

he can trust'.[12] Al-Majūsī's statement implies that women were indirect recipients of his work, rather than his immediate audience. Nevertheless, both Ibn al-Jazzār and al-Majūsī's statements assumed the participation of at least *some* women in their community of knowledge. In this respect, their depiction of their communities is in keeping with what has been shown elsewhere in this volume in regard to others, i.e. that women participated in broader communities of knowledge and practice as bedside caregivers, consumers of recipes, 'ambassadors' of care, and go-betweens.

Islamic Religious Law and the Dictates of Modesty

Since medical books instructed male physicians in the care of female patients, including in reproductive matters, should we accept the notion that there were opportunities for men to treat women? The answer hinges upon identifying what is plausible, and dismissing what is not plausible as merely a literary convention of the writers of medical encyclopedias. To help identify what is plausible, we can turn to depictions of modesty and mixed-gender medical care found in genres that are not known to share this convention.

In a detailed, reproachful treatise, the Cairene jurist Ibn al-Ḥājj al-ʿAbdarī (d. 1336) criticized his own community for what he believed were the many moral degradations of his age. Among the many reprehensible behaviours he condemned were the choices made by his fellow Egyptian Muslims when seeking medical care. Ibn al-Ḥājj was particularly upset with Muslims who summoned non-Muslim physicians to tend members of their household. He laid out many reasons why such conduct was unseemly, one of which focused on women:

> Even if nothing happens except that the infidel describes a Muslim's wife or daughter to someone else [...] it would be too much for Islamic protective jealousy [*al-ghayra al-Islāmiyya*], even if it was not forbidden in the noble Law, God forbid. If someone were to say: 'But the jurists have permitted uncovering nakedness before a physician whether the patient is a man or a woman!' the response is that this is the case when there is a necessity, and there is no necessity that calls for inviting an infidel when there exists a Muslim physician.[13]

12 Trans. from Musallam, *Sex and Society in Islam*, 70.

13 Ibn al-Ḥājj, *al-Madkhal*, 3.4: 318. His reference to the 'noble Law' suggests that, even if the reader were to deny his previous stated arguments showing that choosing non-Muslim physicians

While the central argument in this passage is directed against medical interaction between Muslims and non-Muslims, not against medical interaction between women and men, it is premised on a shared assumption about medical practice crossing gender boundaries. Both Ibn al-Ḥājj and his hypothetical interlocutor assumed that a male physician was expected to see female patients. Moreover, from the interlocutor's statement, we can infer that this environment was one in which it was commonly assumed that, from the point of view of Islamic law (*sharia*), female nudity was perfectly acceptable in medical contexts. Indeed, the religiously zealous Ibn al-Ḥājj did not dispute this point. Instead he claimed that such mixed-gender interactions were only permitted because they were sometimes necessary, meaning there might be no available alternative for a female patient other than to be seen by a male practitioner. By contrast, he argued, there are no medical occasions where the only available practitioner is from both a different gender and a different religion. For this reason, he said, it is sometimes acceptable for women to be attended by male physicians, but not by male non-Muslim physicians.

When compared to discussions in formal legal compendia, this permissive characterization of Islamic legal attitudes towards immodesty in medical contexts is slightly overstated, though it might accurately reflect legal practice in early fourteenth-century Cairo. It is fairly compatible, however, with what appears in formal Islamic legal discussions about medical, and even gynecological, care. Of the four major Sunni schools of Islamic law, only one, the Mālikīs (the dominant legal school in the Maghreb and Islamic Spain), altogether prohibited male physicians from viewing or touching the genitals of a female patient.[14] The other three all permitted a male physician to view and touch a woman's genitals under certain circumstances.[15] The most permissive position was articulated by the highly influential Shāfiʿī jurist al-Nawawī (d. 1278), who explicitly allowed male practitioners to both view and touch women's bodies for purposes of bleeding, cupping, and treating patients, as well as for medical education and for legal and

contravenes the *sharia*, a Muslim man should still disdain such behaviour on the grounds of *ghayra*, appropriate sexual possessiveness.

14 Kan'ān, *al-Mawsūʿa al-Ṭibbiyya al-fiqhiyya*, 748.

15 For examples of Hanafī views see *Fatāwā al-hindiyya*, 5: 330; regarding Hanbalī views see Ibn Qudāma, *al-Mughnī*, 7: 101, and Ibn al-Farrā', *al-Jāmiʿ al-ṣaghīr*, 398. In the *Kashshāf al-qināʿ*, al-Buhūtī (d. 1641) writes: 'A doctor may view and touch whatever it is necessary for him to view and touch, even her genitals and inside her, because this is a matter of obvious need, even if he is a non-Muslim'; al-Buhūtī, *Kashshāf al-qināʿ*, 5: 13.

forensic purposes.[16] Apart from these extremes, most legal discussions about who ought to attend a sick woman articulated an order of preference or precedence rather than offering strict permissions and prohibitions. These texts presume a pressing medical necessity or emergency.[17]

In Islamic jurisprudence, restrictions on male physicians viewing female patients usually do not appear in stand-alone discussions, but appear in the context of discussions about selecting a medical practitioner from an array of imperfect choices. Jurists from the Shāfiʿī legal school in particular took a lively interest in untangling and comparing the various moral hazards posed by medical practitioners who came from outside a female patient's gender, family, or religion. For example, al-Bulqīnī (d. 1403) advanced the following order of preference when choosing practitioners:

> [1] A female Muslim, [2] a prepubescent Muslim boy [*ghayr murāhiq*], [3] a pubescent [*murāhiq*] Muslim boy, [4] a prepubescent infidel boy, [5] a pubescent infidel boy, [6] an infidel woman, [7] a Muslim kinsman, [8] an infidel kinsman, [9] a non-kin Muslim man, then [10] a non-kin infidel man.[18]

Due to certain precedents from early Islamic legal history, childbirth and other scenarios that involved viewing a woman's genitals were placed in a special legal category that was different from other medical situations. This category was particularly hostile to non-Muslim midwives and thus was comparatively more permissive of male practitioners. So, for example, the jurist al-Adhraʿī (d. 1381) argued that it was generally preferable for a Muslim female patient to consult an infidel female practitioner than a Muslim male practitioner from either outside or within the family; however, this principle changed when the patient's genitals had to be examined. In this scenario he gave precedence to any kind of practitioner who could claim to be either a relative or quasi-relative (i.e. slaves, eunuchs, and male minors, including infidel ones). In this case, a relative would be preferable to an infidel woman. Such discussions suggest that mixed-gender medical care was indeed considered to be potentially problematic, but was only one factor to be weighed when seeking treatment. Religion, relationship, age, and gender

16 al-Nawawī, *Minhāj al-ṭālibīn*, 3: 132.

17 ʿAbd Allāh b. Maḥmūd al-Mawṣilī (d. 1284), a Ḥanafī, says that what constitutes medical necessity in this case is the same type of emergency which makes it permissible to drink wine and eat the flesh of pigs (al-Mawṣilī, *al-Ikhtiyār li-taʿlīl al-Mukhtār*, 4: 108). Ibn ʿĀbidīn says the school agrees that a male physician can treat a female patient's genitals only if she is in unbearable pain or might die; Ibn ʿĀbidīn, *Ḥāshiyat Radd al-muḥtār*, 9: 533; cf. *Fatāwā al-Hindiya*, 5: 330.

18 al-Shirwānī, *Ḥawāshī al-Shirwānī*, 9: 40.

were all factors determining the kind of practitioner a woman should seek. Ultimately, jurists like al-Adhraʿī were also of the opinion that outcomes mattered more than demographics. After detailing his order of preference he concluded that one ought to choose 'the most skilled person – even if he is of the opposite gender and religion'.[19] Most Islamic juristic writings thus confirm that, at least in theory, there were some limited times and places in which it was acceptable for male physicians to attend female patients.

We can supplement these rather hypothetical approaches to medicine and sexual propriety with information from a more practical genre of Islamic literature: books of *ḥisba*. These are manuals for market inspectors, who were responsible for ensuring that the market and other public places were safe and hygienic, and who were also charged with preventing fraud and physical and moral pollution. *Ḥisba* manuals from medieval Islamic Spain, Egypt, and Syria portray physicians, pharmacists, surgeons, bonesetters, and other medical personnel having storefronts in the market or in similar settings in which women were present.[20] If theoretical legal discussions tended to depict the medical treatment of women by men as an unfortunate necessity to be considered only in emergencies, by contrast these descriptions of medical practitioners in the marketplace suggest no such compunctions. In his manual for market inspectors, the twelfth-century Syrian author al-Shayzarī mentioned male phlebotomists applying cups to women's thighs to bring down the menses, a practice which was also recommended in the theoretical literature.[21] Similarly, a fourteenth-century Egyptian manual by Ibn al-Ukhuwwa describes male phlebotomists bleeding women. Ibn al-Ukhuwwa offered no modesty concerns in this description, though he did caution against bleeding other classes of people (such as minors without the permission of their parents) and against bleeding women with specific medical contraindications, such as pregnancy.[22] Despite the fact that concerns about the potential for sexual exploitation and lewd or scandalous behaviour feature quite prominently in this genre of literature, neither manual suggests that the market inspector look for lewd behaviour in the context of phlebotomy. Thus a wide variety of texts that are concerned with public morality mention male practitioners providing medical care to female patients, sometimes without any reference to concerns of modesty

19 Ibid.

20 See al-'Aṭṭār, *Minhāj al-dukkān wa-dustūr al-ayān*, 16; Ibn al-Ukhuwwa, *Maʿālim al-qurba fī aḥkām al-ḥisba*, 54-59; Ibn 'Abdūn al-Tujibī, *Séville musulmane au début du XIIe siècle*, §§ 139-40; Chipman, *World of Pharmacy and Pharmacists in Mamluk Cairo*, 70.

21 al-Shayzarī, *Kitāb Nihāyat al-rutba fī ṭalab al-ḥisba*, 96; cf. al-Majūsī, *Kāmil*, 2: 428.

22 Ibn al-Ukhuwwa, *Maʿālim al-qurba fī aḥkām al-ḥisba*, ch. 44.

or impropriety. When issues of propriety are mentioned, antipathy toward male-female medical interaction often appears as only one factor contributing to the drama or complexity of a medical situation.

Gynecology

Having established the social plausibility of male-female medical interactions, we are now in a better position to re-engage with the physicians' own writings about the extent and limits of those interactions. We have attestations of male medical practitioners conversing with, examining, and operating on female patients with a variety of medical concerns, including those pertaining to gynecology and obstetrics. Such references appear across the medieval Middle East wherever there is extant medical literature. It is particularly well attested in writings dating from twelfth- through fourteenth-century Egypt and Syria.

The most common interactions between physicians and female patients were verbal communications, which included discussions of pregnancy and contraception. While such encounters did not require physical contact, and were sometimes conducted via servant intermediaries, they could still be rather intimate. Such intimacy was mentioned, for example, by the ninth-century Syrian Christian physician (who would later convert to Islam), Isḥāq b. ʿAlī al-Ruhāwī. In his medical ethics treatise, al-Ruhāwī invoked the Hippocratic Oath:

> [Hippocrates] said you must not mind the impatience of a woman whom you see distressed and afflicted due to her gestation, and not pity her or give her a remedy to make her fetus fall [...] As to a bad mother, do not show any compassion for her, so that her shame will cause the improvement of many other women. Beware of giving things like these [i.e. abortifacients]; they are prescribed only if you fear the death of the pregnant woman or the fetus. There is no difference whether you administer the drug or you sell it [...] You must adhere to [Hippocrates'] oaths and go along with his beliefs from which the oaths are derived.[23]

23 Trans. in Levey, 'Medical Ethics', 56. The invocation of the Hippocratic Oath in this regard is also present in *ḥisba* manuals from Egypt; for instance, al-Shayzarī, *Kitāb Nihāyat al-rutba fī ṭalab al-ḥisba*, 98; Ibn al-Ukhuwwa, *Maʿālim al-qurba fī aḥkām al-ḥisba*, 167; and Ibn Bassām, *Nihāya al-rutba fī ṭalab al-ḥisba*, 340.

He goes on to caution his male readers not to provide abortifacients to women who seem desperate to end their pregnancies, asserting that 'the physician must warn the drug merchant not to give women drugs which make the fetus fall and menstruation flow without his permission'.[24]

Al-Ruhāwī's exhortations to resist women's entreaties indicate that both physicians and pharmacists could be in close enough communication with women about matters related to pregnancy that they could be emotionally affected by their pleas. We could possibly read this text as simply repeating traditional wisdom, rather than reflecting actual encounters, but the details suggest substantial immediacy. Al-Ruhāwī cautions the physician lest his 'pity' and 'compassion' for a 'distressed', 'afflicted', and 'shamed' pregnant woman move him to violate his professional oath. While al-Ruhāwī certainly urged a pitilessness towards unhappily pregnant women, his hard-heartedness was not borne out of an assumption that it was unusual or inappropriate to talk about reproductive matters with women; rather, he suggested that physicians must steel themselves in the face of such expected, intimate engagements. It is clear that he saw the male practitioner as potentially involved in at least this aspect of obstetric medicine.

To be sure, medical ethics literature depicts charlatans, mountebanks, and disreputable physicians as being on even more familiar terms with women than is proper. Ibn Jumay' (d. 1198), an Egyptian Jewish physician to Saladin, complained that deceptive physicians reach male clientele by 'gaining the favor of their wives through suitable and alluring drugs, like aphrodisiacs, medicaments for conceiving, fattening, and hair-growing and by making common cause with the female bath-attendants, hairdressers and midwives, in order that they should talk about them and praise their wonderful medical skill'.[25] Here the charge against the charlatan was not so much impropriety with women, but rather shameless advertising ultimately aimed at attracting male clientele. The charlatan cultivated a network of relationships with female clientele and with women engaged in forms of bodywork. In this instance, Ibn Jumay' described the charlatan conveying to women information about drugs, rather than learned Galenic theoretical knowledge, and it was not evident that the charlatan has Arabo-Galenic training himself. Nevertheless here too, just as in al-Ruhāwī's description of the medical landscape, there apparently were opportunities for male professionals to be involved in gynecological matters, or at least to share their knowledge with female patients, even if (in Ibn Jumay''s opinion) that information is detestable.

24 Levey, 'Medical Ethics', 62. I use Levey's translation with some significant emendation.

25 Ibn Jumay', *al-Maqāla as-Ṣalāḥ'iya*.

In addition to verbal communications, analysis of the urine and pulse was a perfectly respectable and widely attested form of medical interaction between men and women. Female patients, like their male counterparts, submitted their urine to male physicians for diagnostic purposes that included pregnancy tests and assessments of fetal sex.[26] Taking the pulse was also believed to be useful as a diagnostic tool, although some texts viewed as mere quackery the claim that one could tell whether a woman was pregnant simply by taking her pulse. For example, in his *Da'wat al-aṭibbā'*, the eleventh-century Iraqi physician Ibn Butlān complained that people have absurd and scientifically impossible expectations of physicians. As one example, he mentioned the notion that a physician should be able to distinguish a barren from a fruitful woman by feeling her pulse.[27]

Urinalysis sometimes occurred at a distance via messenger, so that a woman could remain at home while a servant or family member brought the urine to the physician. Pulse-taking, however, required direct interaction. The only reference I have found to measures being taken to preserve modesty or gender segregation during pulse-taking comes from an anecdote in Ibn Abī 'Uṣaybi'a's biographical dictionary of physicians. Ibn Abī 'Uṣaybi'a recounted a story about his older contemporary, the thirteenth-century court physician in Cairo, Rashīd al-Dīn Abū Ḥulayqa. One day Abū Ḥulayqa took the pulse of all the sick women of the court, whom he could not see because they are hidden behind a screen. The sultan himself hid behind the screen with the women and extended to the physician his own arm. The physician recognized by the precise measure of the pulse that it was in fact the king, and not anyone else.[28] The presence of a screen suggests that a physician might touch a female patient without being able to actually see her. However, such measures are not mentioned elsewhere in the biographical dictionary, despite many stories of close interactions with female patients, nor to my knowledge does the screen appear elsewhere in medieval medical texts. It could be that the screen is a mere literary device, meant to show off (as it clearly does) the physician's prowess; or it represents a particular stringency unique to the female members of the royal household.[29]

Thus far we have seen relatively few compunctions about male practitioners conversing with women, or engaging in urinoscopy or phlebotomy,

26 For example, Ibn al-Ruhāwī's *Adab al-ṭabīb*. See Levey, 'Medical Ethics', 74-75.

27 Rosenthal, 'Defense of Medicine in the Medieval Muslim World', 529.

28 Ibn Abī 'Uṣaybi'a, *'Uyūn al-anbā' fī ṭabaqāt al-aṭibbā'*, 592.

29 Shefer-Mossensohn, *Ottoman Medicine*, 130-31, suggests that Ottoman women of the highest rank had more limited access to medical care than those of less exalted social position, owing to modesty demands.

even in matters that pertain to menstruation, pregnancy, and abortion. However, modesty concerns appeared more frequently in matters pertaining to viewing, touching, and operating on the genitals. As a rule, these concerns were depicted as stemming from patients' reluctance to accept help from a physician, rather than from a professional code of ethics or an external source of social pressure. A dramatization of the tensions of such an interaction can be seen in *al-Faraj ba'd al-shidda* (Relief after distress), a compilation of stories combining religious moralism with adventurous high jinks by the tenth-century Iraqi author al-Tanūkhī. A series of such stories depict baffling illnesses, cured in an unusual manner by a brilliant doctor who explains, Sherlock Holmes style, how he reasoned his way to a solution. One story describes a wealthy young woman in the countryside who attempts to conceal pain and discharge in her vagina. She does not let even her own father know of her condition until she is nearing death. Upon learning of her condition, and fearing that his daughter will die, the father calls for a physician, Yazīd, to treat her.

> 'Would you forgive me', Yazīd asked, 'if I make a suggestion? I can issue no prescription unless I am allowed to see the site of the complaint and palpate it with my own hands, and ask the woman questions as to how the disorder may have arisen'. Her condition was now so serious, indeed desperate, that I [her father] consented; but after he had examined her externally and found the site of the pain, his questions went on for so long and had so little to do with her illness that I felt tempted to lay violent hands on him. However, I reminded myself of the good character that he bore, and contained myself with difficulty.

At this point, the physician's palpating of the woman is a matter of some delicacy, such that it requires the father's consent. It is not the touching that mystifies or angers the father, however, but rather the excessive and seemingly pointless questioning.

> At last [Yazīd] said: 'Have someone hold the girl down'. I gave the order. He thrust his hand into her vagina; she screamed, then fainted; blood spurted out, and he withdrew his hand, displaying a creature smaller than a dung-beetle, which he tossed aside. The girl immediately sat up, crying: 'Papa! You must send this man out of my room, for I am well again'.[30]

30 al-Tanūkhī, *al-Faraj ba'd al-shidda*, 4: 215; trans. in Bray, *Writing and Representation in Medieval Islam*, 225.

The story goes on to explain that the source of the trouble was a tick, contracted while tending cattle – a fact that the physician was able to establish through persistent questioning. The insertion of his hand into the girl's vagina seems to carry the valence of a sexual violation, as indicated by the sudden action, the girl's scream, and her fainting. But, in fact, it dramatically restores normal sexual propriety, as the girl is instantly cured and can therefore have the foreign man expelled from her room. In the story, the reassertion of modesty is the privilege of the healthy and a marker of the medical crisis having passed. The ideal physician is therefore not one who avoids female clients or diagnoses them from a distance, but rather one who is so skillful that he can instantaneously restore a woman to health, obviating the need for any further indignities.

Although this story is part of a literary fantasy, the notion that patients might refuse male medical attention for gynecological problems can also be found in books by physicians themselves.[31] The twelfth-century Sevillian physician Ibn Zuhr recounted how in his youth he once came across a woman with a prolapsed uterus who had not sought male medical care. He lamented that, 'it had been that way for a long time. I do not know what happened to her. Had this been recent, the physician would have been able to undo the injury, God permitting'.[32] Just as in the dramatic story of the tick, the physician displayed no doubt in his own competence to provide gynecological care; rather, it was the female patient who hesitated. Interestingly too, Ibn Zuhr noted that, when he encountered the prolapsed uterus, he was still a youth. Perhaps we should understand this detail as supporting the notion that in some communities children really were called upon at times to provide medical assistance, as was suggested by jurists like al-Bulqīnī and al-Adhraʿī.

The most explicit description of the impact of sexual propriety on medical care appears at the beginning of the chapter on removing women's bladder stones in the *Surgery* of al-Zahrāwī (Albucasis, d. 1013), who practised in Cordoba. The operation involved a medical practitioner inserting his finger either into the anus (if the patient was a male or a virgin female), or into the vagina, to feel for the stone; and then, using both the inserted finger and an external hand to press down on the bladder, to manipulate the stone to

31 In Ibn Abī ʿUṣaybiʿa's *ʿUyūn al-anbāʾ fī ṭabaqāt al-aṭibbāʾ*, the story is told of Jibrāʾīl ibn Bukhtīshūʿ ibn Jūrjīs, who cured a woman of paralysis during an examination simply by bending his head down and extending his hand toward her skirt as though he intended to lift it, causing her to jerk away.

32 Ibn Zuhr, *Kitāb al-taysīr*, 308-9.

a location near the groin. The practitioner would then make an incision to surgically cut out the stone. He wrote:

> It is uncommon for a woman to have a stone. But if it should happen to a woman the treatment is indeed difficult and hindered by a number of things. One is that the woman may be a virgin. Another is that you will not find a woman who will expose herself to a [male] doctor if she is chaste or has close male relatives. A third is that you will not find a woman competent in this art, particularly not in surgery. Then a fourth is that the place for cutting open the stone in a woman is a long way from where the stone lies, so the incision has to be deep, which is dangerous. If necessity compels you to this kind of case, you should take with you a competent woman doctor. As these are very uncommon, if you are without one then seek a chaste/eunuch doctor as a colleague or bring a midwife experienced in women's ailments or a woman to whom you may give some instruction in this art.[33]

He then proceeded to explain how the surgeon should instruct the female medical practitioner. Al-Zahrāwī's prologue is interesting because it explicitly addresses the impact of social context on the practice of gynecological medicine. Uncharacteristically, al-Zahrāwī admitted that there were few opportunities for a physician to practise lithotomy, an admission that is absent from most of his other descriptions of performing operations on women. This contrast suggests that, while he viewed those other operations as both socially plausible and medically prevalent, he considered lithotomy as less so. Echoing the sentiments expressed by Ibn Zuhr and others, al-Zahrāwī attributed the rarity of lithotomies specifically to the sensibilities of respectable women, rather than to any reluctance on the part of the physician. He shed additional light on the ways that male gynecological practitioners could handle particularly sensitive operations. Teaming up with women doctors was one possibility, indicating that there were indeed women versed in surgery, even if they were a rarity. More likely alternatives included bringing a sexually non-threatening colleague to accompany him,

33 al-Zahrāwī, *Albucasis on Surgery and Instruments*, bk. 30, ch. 61, 420-21. The translation is a modified version of Spink and Lewis, who translate 'dhawāt al-maḥārim' as 'married' rather than 'having close male relatives'. The Arabic word describing this doctor is *'afīf*, i.e. 'chaste', which is not one of the usual terms for a eunuch, though *'Afīf* seems to have been commonly used as a personal name given to eunuchs. Given the context, I think the interpretation of *'afīf* as eunuch is plausible.

either a male (perhaps a eunuch) known for his chastity, an experienced midwife, or a woman trained for this purpose by the physician himself.

Interestingly, in these statements, al-Zahrāwī does not appear to be recapitulating some other source. While most of the content of this chapter is very similar to a corresponding chapter in the encyclopedia penned by the Byzantine physician Aetius of Amida, all of the passages about a woman's unwillingness to expose herself, as well as the references to chastity, midwives, eunuchs, assistants, and virgins, seem to be original to al-Zahrāwī.[34] By comparison, Ibn Sīnā – writing in the same century but on the other side of the Muslim world – discussed the same operation, but made no mention of a female practitioner or of particular modesty concerns.[35] Al-Zahrāwī's writing about the stone-removal procedure thus reflects an awareness and concern for practicality and social plausibility in his own place and time. His description is not merely a repetition of hypothetical medical wisdom.

Another description of the same procedure, from thirteenth-century Syria, provides a similar account of women's reluctance to undergo surgery for the removal of bladder stones, but articulates concerns and options differently. The author Ibn al-Quff wrote:

> When stones occur in the bladder of women, their treatment is complicated by five factors: one of them is that the woman might be a virgin, and so there is no path for inserting the finger in the vagina so as to find the stone. Second: few women come forward to undergo said treatment, due to the pain of the incision. Third, we do not find a woman who will permit herself such surgical treatment because they are overcome by bashfulness. Fourth: because the location of the stone is further in them and requires a deeper incision, and that is dangerous. Fifth, she may be pregnant and there is a concern that the incision will injure the fetus [...] But, if you want [or: she wants] to attempt to remove it, then seek an expert, intelligent midwife, and order her to do everything that you say [...][36]

Like al-Zahrāwī, Ibn al-Quff placed responsibility for avoiding the procedure on women themselves, and also attributed at least some of their reluctance

34 Spink and Lewis note the correspondence between the two works, but not the discrepancies. Otherwise, they uncharacteristically choose not to comment on the chapter at all, on the grounds that it 'needs no note'; ibid., 420. See Aetius of Amida, *Gynaecology and Obstetrics of the VIth Century*, ch. 99, 105.

35 Ibn Sīnā, *al-Qānūn*, 2: 510 = *kitāb* 3: *fann* 19: *maqāla* 1: *faṣl fī al-tadbīr* [re: *ḥiṣāt al-muthāna*].

36 The verb used here to mean 'want' is ambiguous and can be read as a second-person masculine or third-person feminine form; Ibn al-Quff, *Kitāb al-'Umda fī al-jirāḥa*, 2: 210-11.

to 'bashfulness', or modesty. Both physicians also mentioned the danger of the procedure. Both noted virginity as a complicating factor but, whereas al-Zahrāwī did not explicitly state his reasoning, Ibn al-Quff was clear that the problem was a physical one, rather than a social fear of compromising a woman's integrity. He also suggested several other practical concerns that make such an operation difficult, such as pain, dangers posed to the patient, and dangers posed to a fetus if the patient was pregnant. Although it was conceivable for Ibn al-Quff to imagine a female patient consulting with a male physician on this matter, he nevertheless indicated that the operation itself would be undertaken by a skilled woman, following the guidance (at least nominally) of a male physician. He did not suggest at all that such women are rare.

Midwives as Intermediaries in Arabo-Galenic Medical Texts

If male practitioners could provide some gynecological care, what circumstances necessitated the presence of a female practitioner? What labour did she perform? In medical encyclopedias, descriptions of midwives' roles as intermediaries vary considerably. While there are many references to cooperation between midwives and physicians in the medical compendia, it is just as common for texts not to indicate the presence of a female intermediary at all, even in gynecological situations.[37] When midwives are mentioned, it can be difficult to discern exactly who is performing what work.[38]

Midwives tend to appear in texts when a practitioner needs to touch the cervix or reach into the uterus, either to conduct an operation or to gain diagnostic information. For example, Ibn al-Jazzār, writing in tenth-century Qayrawān, dealt extensively with gynecology, yet he explicitly mentioned the presence of a midwife only twice: once in connection with diagnosing uterine tumours by touch, and once when instructing the midwife to treat

37 The omission of references to female intermediaries where we might expect to find them has been catalogued by Giladi in *Muslim Midwives*. He notes that 'the midwife is altogether – or almost totally – ignored' in the major works by Thābit b. Qurra, al-Ṭabarī, al-Majūsī, Ibn Zuhr, and Ibn al-Nafīs; Giladi, *Muslim Midwives*, 73-74.

38 In part, this ambiguity is due to the frequent use of passive verb forms in these compendia. The matter is further complicated by the fact that it is often grammatically unclear whether the active indicative verbs in Arabic medical manuals are intended to be read as second-person masculine forms or third-person feminine forms, since they look the same on paper. Imperative verb forms make such division of labour somewhat clearer.

hysterical suffocation by rubbing the mouth of the uterus with oils 'from the inside and the outside'.[39]

Unsurprisingly, midwives are frequently mentioned in connection with childbirth. However, authors also mention the male physician's presence in the birthing chamber, particularly when non-invasive techniques are required to manage difficult labour. Consider this passage from Ibn Sīnā's *Qānūn:*

> Know that if the woman has experienced four days of difficult labor, then the fetus is already dead. So busy yourself [masculine] with the life of the mother, and do not busy yourself with the life of the fetus, rather strive [masculine] to expel it. [This] abortion is brought about by means of movements or by means of drugs. The drugs can function either by killing the fetus or by forcefully bringing down menstruation [...][40]

Compare this discussion with another surgical passage about expelling a dead fetus, in which Ibn Sīnā assigned a much larger role to intermediaries. Here, he described the midwife as engaged in the grizzly business of extracting the fetus by means of hooks poked into its body, a technique he attributed to 'the ancients':

> The [pregnant] woman must lay on the bed on her back, with her head tilted downward and her thighs raised. Then women, or a servant, grasp her on either side. If these [people] are not present, then tie [masculine] her chest to the bed with knots so that her body will not be pulled down when it is stretched. Then the midwife opens that which is covering the neck of the uterus, anoints her left hand with oil, brings her fingers together lengthwise, and inserts them into the mouth of the uterus and dilates it with them. More oil is added, and she ascertains whether it is necessary to insert hooks with which the fetus may be drawn out, and the places which are best for inserting the hooks. These places, in a fetus which is presenting head-first, are the eyes, the mouth, the nape [...][41]

He goes on to describe the process for inserting the hooks and piercing, and then how to modify that process when the fetus presented feet first,

39 Ibn al-Jazzār, *Ibn al-Jazzār on the Sexual Diseases*, 275, 277.

40 Ibn Sīnā, *al-Qānūn*, 2: 575 = *kitāb* 3: *fann* 21: *maqāla* 2: *tadbīr al-isqāṭ wa-ikhrāj al-janīn al-mayit.*

41 Ibn Sīnā, *al-Qānūn*, 2: 576 = *kitāb* 3: *fann* 21: *maqāla* 2: *faṣl fī tadbīr li-ba'ḍ al-qudamā' fī ikhrāj al-janīn al-mayit.*

an operation which involved not one hook but two. What is odd about these descriptions is that the first one, featuring a male physician giving his patient expulsive drugs, is quite feasible in terms of medieval medical technique, but the presence of a male practitioner seems surprising. By contrast, the second procedure features a female obstetrical practitioner, which seems more true to life, but used a surgical technique which was difficult to implement.[42] This discrepancy suggests that we should not view the presence of a midwife in a medical text as correlated with the sensitivity of a particular medical problem or the feasibility of a particular form of treatment. Rather, Ibn Sīnā called in his hypothetical midwife when suggesting a particularly invasive operation.

The most detailed description of cooperation and division of labour between a physician and a midwife is found in al-Zahrāwī's chapter on handling difficult childbirth, which indicates that the most invasive interventions were conducted by the midwife. For example, if it was necessary to artificially rupture the membranes of the amniotic sac, it was the midwife who used a scalpel or her nail to do so, although the physician had visual access to the labouring woman and physically touched her.[43] Al-Zahrāwī wrote, 'place [masculine] the woman upon a platform [...] and shake [masculine] the platform'. If the baby emerges feet first, he advises, 'return [masculine] the fetus bit by bit [into the uterus] until you have placed it in a natural position'. If all else fails, the physician should make a compound and 'anoint [masculine] with it the vagina of the woman and her lower abdomen' and later 'press [masculine] gently upon her abdomen'.[44] The chapter thus leaves the reader with an image of both male and female practitioners engaged in gynecological practice, at least during medical emergencies.[45]

In another remarkable depiction of cooperation during an emergency obstetrical operation, al-Zahrāwī explained how to make and use a speculum for opening the womb to extract a (dead?) fetus. He then wrote:

> When you wish to open the womb with this [speculum], make the woman sit on a couch with her legs hanging down, parted; then introduce the two projections [of the speculum] into the orifice of the womb while you hold [masculine] the end of the instrument lower down between her thighs;

42 Savage-Smith, 'Practice of Surgery in Islamic Lands', 315.

43 al-Zahrāwī, *Albucasis on Surgery and Instruments*, 468-71. The translation is Spink's with some additions and emendations to show grammar.

44 Ibid., 471.

45 This can also be seen in Hippocratic and other Greek texts. As Dean-Jones notes, 'there is a division of labor within a single case'; Dean-Jones, 'Autopsia, Historia, and What Women Know', 55.

> then open your hand in the same way as you would with forceps, to the extent to which you wish to open the womb, so as to allow the midwife to see what she desires.[46]

Interestingly, this depiction of the interaction between the physician and midwife does not make clear the hierarchy of roles. One could well read this passage as the male medical practitioner supporting the more expert midwife.

Conclusion

Medieval Arabo-Galenic texts depict a medical landscape in which male physicians provided medical attention to women in all areas, including gynecology and obstetrics. That depiction has been challenged on the grounds that Islamic religious law and social mores would render such interactions highly objectionable, and on the grounds that women would be largely uninterested in men's involvement in feminine matters. A generous depiction of the consequences of such medical segregation is that educated male physicians never became heavily invested in gynecology and obstetrics and thus never tried to wrest control over such matters from midwives, in contrast to the European experience.[47] A more negative articulation of the same conclusion is that the lack of opportunity to interact with women led to physicians taking a 'generally passive role' leading them to 'not perform well in the field of women's diseases, but only [hand] down the ancient traditions'.[48] Such are the consequences of gender segregation.

By contrast, this essay has demonstrated that not only did medieval medical books assert that the barriers between the sexes were porous, but that external evidence supports that assertion. Medical texts describe a situation in which male gynecological knowledge about drugs and surgical techniques were passed along to female practitioners, who in turn collaborated with male physicians or acted as medical informants, examining and operating on female patients for them and possibly steering clientele towards them. But this is not the only, or even the most prevalent, form of cross-gender

46 al-Zahrāwī, *Albucasis on Surgery and Instruments*, 486-89 – Spink's translation with my clarifications in brackets.

47 This interpretation is articulated by Giladi, *Muslim Midwives*, 162.

48 Bos, in Ibn al-Jazzār, *Ibn al-Jazzār on the Sexual Diseases*, 51.

medical interaction depicted in medical texts. Instead, there is a great deal of evidence that direct interactions between female patients and male medical practitioners were commonplace in the communities from which we have extant sources. Female patients communicated verbally with men and were examined, touched, and operated on by them. A culture of modesty thus certainly shaped how medieval learned gynecological medicine was practised, but it did not render that practice impossible.

Works Cited

Printed Works

Aetius of Amida. *The Gynaecology and Obstetrics of the VIth Century*, trans. James Ricci (Philadelphia: Blakiston, 1950).

al-ʿAṭṭār, Abū'l-Munā al-Mūhīn. *Minhāj al-dukkān wa-dustūr al-ayān* (Beirut: Dār al-Manāhil, 1992).

al-ʿAyntābī, Maḥmūd b. Aḥmad. *al-Qawl al-sadīd fī ikhtiyār al-imā' wa'l-ābīd* (Beirut: Mu'assasat al-Risāla, 1996).

al-Baladī, Abū al-ʿAbbās Aḥmad ibn Muḥammad. *Tadbīr al-ḥabālā wa'l-aṭfāl wa'l-ṣibyān* (Beirut: Dār al-Kutub al-ʿIlmīya, 2004).

Batten, Rosalind. 'The Arabic Commentaries on the Hippocratic Aphorisms: Arabic Learned Medical Discourse on Women's Bodies (9th-15th Cent.)', PhD diss., University of Manchester, 2018.

Bray, Julia. *Writing and Representation in Medieval Islam* (London: Routledge, 2006).

al-Buhūtī, Manṣūr b. Yūnus. *Kashshāf al-qināʿ*, 6 vols. (Beirut: Dār al-Fikr, 1982).

Cabré, Montserrat and Fernando Salmón. 'Blood, Milk, and Breastbleeding: The Humoral Economy of Women's Bodies in Late Medieval Medicine', in *Gender, Health, and Healing, 1250-1550*, ed. Sara Ritchey and Sharon Strocchia (Amsterdam: Amsterdam University Press, 2020), 93-117.

Chipman, Leigh. *The World of Pharmacy and Pharmacists in Mamluk Cairo* (Leiden: Brill, 2010).

Dean-Jones, Leslie. 'Autopsia, Historia, and What Women Know: The Authority of Women in Hippocratic Gynecology', in *Knowledge and the Scholarly Medical Traditions*, ed. Donald George Bates (Cambridge: Cambridge University Press, 1995), 41-58.

Fatāwā al-hindiyya, 6 vols. (Būlāq: al-Maṭbaʿa al-Kubrā al-Amīriyya, 1892).

Giladi, Avner. *Muslim Midwives: The Craft of Birthing in the Premodern Middle East* (New York: Cambridge University Press, 2015).

Ibn 'Abdūn al-Tujibī. *Séville musulmane au début du XIIe siècle: le traité d'Ibn 'Abdun sur la vie urbaine et les corps de métiers*, ed. E. Lévi-Provençal (Paris: G.P. Maisonneuve, 1947).

Ibn Abī 'Uṣaybi'a, Aḥmad ibn al-Qāsim. *Lives of the Physicians*, trans. L. Kopf (Bethesda: National Library of Medicine, 1971).

—. *'Uyūn al-anbā' fī ṭabaqāt al-aṭibbā'* (Beirut: Dār Maktabat al-Ḥayāt, 1965).

Ibn 'Ābidīn, Muḥammad Amīn b. 'Umar. *Ḥāshiyat Radd al-muḥtār 'alā al-Durr al-mukhtār*, 14 vols. (Riyadh: 'Ālam al-Kutub, 2003).

Ibn Bassām. *Nihāya al-rutba fī ṭalab al-ḥisba* (Beirut: Dār al-kutub al-'ilmīya, 2003).

Ibn al-Farrā', Abū Ya'lā. *al-Jāmi' al-ṣaghīr* (Riyadh: Dār Aṭlas, 2000).

Ibn al-Ḥājj, Muḥammad b. Muḥammad. *al-Madkhal*, 4 vols. (Beirut: Dār al-Kutub al-'Ilmiyya, 1995).

Ibn al-Jazzār. *Ibn al-Jazzār on the Sexual Diseases and their Treatment: A Critical Edition, English Translation and Introduction of Book 6 of Zād al-musāfir wa-qūt al-ḥāḍir*, ed. and trans. Gerrit Bos (London: Kegan Paul International, 1997).

Ibn Jumay'. *al-Maqāla as-Ṣalāḥ'iya*, in *Treatise to Ṣalāḥ ad-Dīn on the revival of the art of medicine by Ibn Jumay'*, ed. and trans. Hartmut Fähndrich (Marburg: Kommissionsverlag F. Steiner, 1983).

Ibn Qudāma, Muwaffaq al-Dīn 'Abd Allāh ibn Aḥmad. *al-Mughnī*, 10 vols. (Cairo: Maktabat al-Qāhira, 1968).

Ibn al-Quff, Abū al-Faraj ibn Ya'qūb. *Kitāb al-'Umda fī al-jirāḥa*, 2 vols. (Hyderabad: Majlis Dā'irat al-Ma'ārif al-'Uthmānīya, 1937).

Ibn Sīnā. *Qānūn fī al-ṭibb*, 3 vols. (Būlāq: al-Maṭba'a al-Āmira, 1878).

Ibn al-Ukhuwwa. *The Ma'ālim al-qurba fī aḥkām al-ḥisba of Ḍiyā' al-Dīn M. b. M al-Qurashī al-Shafi'ī known as ibn al-Ukhuwwa*, ed. R. Levy (London: Cambridge University Press, 1938).

Ibn Zuhr, 'Abd al-Malik ibn Abī al-'Alā'. *Kitāb al-taysīr fī al-mudāwāh wa'l-tadbīr* (Rabat: Akādīmīyat al-Mamlaka al-Maghribīya, 1991).

al-Jazarī, Muḥammad ibn Ibrāhīm. *Ta'rīkh ḥawādith al-zamān wa-anbā'ihi wa-wafayaāt al-akābir wa'l-a'yān min abnā'ihi*, 3 vols. (Beirut: al-Maktaba al-'Aṣriyya, 1998).

Kan'ān, Aḥmad Muḥammad. *al-Mawsū'a al-ṭibbiyya al-fiqhiyya* (Beirut: Dār al-Nafā'is, 2000).

Kandzha, Iliana. 'Female Saint as Agents of Female Healing: Gendered Practices and Patronage in the Cult of Saint Cunigunde', in *Gender, Health, and Healing, 1250-1550*, ed. Sara Ritchey and Sharon Strocchia (Amsterdam: Amsterdam University Press, 2020), 67-90.

Levey, Martin. 'Medical Ethics of Medieval Islam with Special Reference to Al-Ruhāwī's "Practical Ethics of the Physician"', *Transactions of the American Philosophical Society*, 57.3 (1967), 1-100.

al-Majūsī, ʻAlī ibn al-ʻAbbās. *al-Kāmil al-ṣināʻa fī al-ṭibb*, 2 vols. (Cairo: al-Maṭbaʻah al-Kubrā al-ʻĀmira, 1877).
al-Mawṣilī, ʻAbdallāh b. Maḥmūd. *al-Ikhtiyār li-taʻlīl al-Mukhtār*, 5 vols. (Beirut: Dār al-Risāla al-ʻĀlamiyya, 2009).
Musallam, Basim. *Sex and Society in Islam: Birth Control before the Nineteenth Century* (Cambridge: Cambridge University Press, 1983).
al-Nawawī, Muḥyī al-Dīn Abī Zakarīyā Yaḥyā bin Sharaf. *Minhāj al-ṭālibīn* (Beirut: Dār al-minhāj, 2005).
Pormann, Peter and Emilie Savage-Smith. *Medieval Islamic Medicine* (Washington, DC: Georgetown University Press, 2007).
al-Qurṭubī, ʻArīb ibn Saʻīd. *Kitāb khalq al-janīn wa-tadbīr al-ḥabālā wa'l-mawlūdīn*, in *La livre de la génération du foetus et le traitement des femmes enceintes et des nouveau-nés* (Algiers: Librairie Ferraris, 1956).
al-Rāzī, Muḥammad ibn Zakarīyā. *al-Manṣūrī fī al-ṭibb*, ed. Ḥāzim al-Bakrī al-Ṣiddīqī (Kuwait: Maʻhad al-makhṭūṭāt al-ʻarabīya, 1987).
Rosenthal, Franz. 'The Defense of Medicine in the Medieval Muslim World', *Bulletin of the History of Medicine*, 43 (1969), 519-32.
Savage-Smith, Emilie. 'The Practice of Surgery in Islamic Lands: Myth and Reality', *Social History of Medicine*, 13 (2000), 307-21.
al-Shayzarī, ʻAbd al-Raḥmān ibn Naṣr. *Kitāb nihāyat al-rutba fi ṭalab al-ḥisba lil-Shayzarī* (Cairo: Lajnat al-ta'līf wa'l-tarjama wa'l-nashr, 1946).
Shefer-Mossensohn, Miri. *Ottoman Medicine: Healing and Medical Institutions, 1500-1700* (Albany, NY: State University of New York Press, 2009).
al-Shirwānī, ʻAbd al-Ḥamīd. *Ḥawāshī al-Shirwānī wa-Ibn Qāsim al-ʻAbbādī ʻalā Tuḥfat al-muḥtāj*, 10 vols. (Beirut: Dār al-Kutub al-ʻIlmiyya, 1996).
al-Ṭabarī, ʻAlī ibn Sahl Rabbān. *Firdaws al-ḥikma fī'l-ṭibb* (Berlin: Maṭbaʻat Āftāb, 1928).
al-Tanūkhī, al-Muḥassin ibn ʻAlī. *al-Faraj baʻd al-shidda* (Beirut: Dār Sādir, 1978).
Ullmann, Manfred. *Die Medizin im Islam* (Leiden: Brill, 1970).
al-Zahrāwī, Abū al-Qāsim Khalaf ibn ʻAbbās. *Albucasis on Surgery and Instruments: A Definitive Edition of the Arabic Text with English Translation and Commentary*, ed. M.S. Spink and G.L. Lewis (Berkeley: University of California Press, 1973).

About the Author

Sara Verskin is the author of *Barren Women: Religion and Medicine in the Medieval Middle East* (2020). She holds a PhD in Near Eastern Studies from Princeton University and teaches history at Rhode Island College.

Afterword

Healing Women and Women Healers

Naama Cohen-Hanegbi

Abstract

This essay highlights two main themes explored by *Gender, Health, and Healing, 1250-1550*: women's health and women's roles in healthcare. In reviewing the evidence and main arguments of the studies included in the collection, the essay demonstrates that these two themes are interconnected. A case history of postpartum melancholy reported by the sixteenth-century Portuguese physician Amato Lusitano furnishes a narrative through-line that further exemplifies the value of the information gathered in the book. The afterword proposes several new routes for future research.

Keywords: Amato Lusitano, childbirth, healthcare, melancholy, postpartum

Amato Lusitano (1511-1568), a Portuguese physician and professor of anatomy in Ferrara, documented his consultation with a patient who had fallen into a melancholic state following childbirth.[1] He reports that, on the seventh day after giving birth, the patient began to suffer from fever and stiffness. Her head hurt and she felt severe pain under her left breast near her heart. The patient's fever continued the next day, her stiffness grew, and she could not move. She spoke sparingly. Amato deduced that the patient had not been

1 Amatus Lusitanus, *Curationum medicinalium, centuriae II priores*, 218-33. This massive work contained 700 case histories, both medical and surgical, followed by scholarly discussions ('scholiae'). For biographical information about this notable physician and his work, see Friedenwald, 'Amatus Lusitanus', and Fontoura, 'Neurological Practice in the *Centuriae* of Amatus Lusitanus'. Pomata further situates his contribution within the growing interest in observation and empiricism in this period in 'Sharing Cases'.

Ritchey, Sara & Sharon Strocchia (eds), *Gender, Health, and Healing, 1250-1550*. Amsterdam, Amsterdam University Press 2020
DOI: 10.5117/9789463724517_AFTER

purged properly so he prescribed medicines and bled her. Over the next few days, her situation worsened; she slept poorly and was fearful. Then, her menses became heavy and red, and she became frantic and disturbed, and even spoke immodestly. The women who were assisting the patient attempted to exorcise a demonic spirit, but their efforts failed; consequently, Amato prescribed additional medicines. The physician continued his frequent visits to the patient, whose melancholy eventually subsided, though her sleep became disturbed.

Amato's case of the postpartum patient brings together the two main themes explored by *Gender, Health, and Healing, 1250-1550*: women's health and women's roles in healthcare. The insights and rich new data presented in this collection elucidate the medical context of this case and its underlying social and cultural circumstances. With this exemplum in mind, we might look ahead to the paths for future research inspired by this book.

Women's Health

Among medieval and early modern historians, scholastic explications of humoral theory have traditionally provided a baseline for scholars to identify and classify 'medical' texts and practices. Certainly Amato would be identified in this manner: he supplemented his case notes with a 'scholia' that calculated the critical day of illness when fever followed childbirth; he relied on the ancient authorities of humoral medicine; and he discussed other circumstances of difficult childbirth. But Amato's diagnosis and prescribed course of treatment also point to the elasticity of humoral epistemology that enabled physicians to diagnose patients according to perceived gender differences. Just as Montserrat Cabré and Fernando Salmón document with regard to mania and fascination in their study of the medieval reception of the Hippocratic aphorism 5.40 ('When blood collects at the breasts of a woman, it indicates madness'), so too does humoral imbalance explain the patient's abnormal state for Amato. This notable physician surmises that the parturient's melancholy was caused by insufficient purging and that her symptoms were the result of excessive black bile. Consequently, his medical interventions were directed at resolving this over-abundance. He administered a clyster and then, when the patient's condition worsened, he drew blood and prescribed remedies of 'byzantine syrup' without vinegar, mixtures of fennel and endive, rose oils and melissa, and other herbs in various combinations to reduce the heat of the body.

The attention to the effusion of blood from the patient's body reinforces Cabré and Salmón's argument that medieval academic medicine approached bodies from a humoral perspective, and that physicians engaged more with the function of the organs than with their form. While this notion presented an overriding model of the humoral body regardless of sex, nevertheless the reproductive function engendered the body and determined the ebbs, flows, and directions of its humors. Women's bodies were regularly purged through menses and after childbirth, and their blood turned to milk in breastfeeding. We find this interpretation of the body again in Catherine Rider's investigation into perceptions of fertility in old age. Reviewing references to infertility across a wide range of authors, Rider points out that, despite the basic 'symmetric' understanding that both men and women lost their reproductive potency in old age, medical compendia written in the thirteenth and fourteenth centuries focused more readily on the infertility of women, particularly on the cessation of menses. Although medieval medical authors perceived age to affect the 'seed' of both sexes, clearer biological markers in women inspired a broader discussion within the rubric of amenorrhea. This gendered approach implicitly placed the responsibility for infertility on the female body. Quoting John of Gaddesden, Rider also draws attention to the slippage from medical theory into cultural biases that appears in medical texts. The focus on women's blood is thus set in humoral theory, but is no less bound up with cultural connotations of menstruation.

Read in light of these essays, Amato's analysis of the puerperal patient seems predetermined, even though he does not allude directly to any ancient aphorism or typical diagnosis. Working from a connotation of the humoral body that located gender difference in the function of the uterus, Amato assigned symptoms like fever, chest pains, and headaches to the retention of the menses. Furthermore, although Amato's discourse adheres to strict physical terms (he perceives delirium and fearfulness at night as indications of the abundance of bile), the diagnosis of melancholy links the case to a long-standing association between women, menstruation, and mental instability. Surprisingly, this association is not sufficiently studied with respect to non-literary sources that treat actual cases; as a result, we are not yet able to assess the degree to which such stereotypical imagery fuelled healthcare or other social practices devised for the care of women.

Amato's *scholia*, which accompanies the case history, serves as an example of the kind of source that can illuminate the way that gendered expectations of the body guided healthcare practice. Amato debates whether a physician should begin calculating the critical day of illness from the event of parturition or from the first appearance of fever. The actual argument is perhaps only relevant to medical intricacies, yet it involves broader assumptions about the postnatal period. Amato argues that counting should always begin from parturition, as illness may lie hidden, as it does in rabies. It is therefore necessary to consider the thirty days after childbirth as a time of incubation of some sort. This time frame overlaps with social and religious practices, to which Amato himself refers. He also reveals another distinction between natural and unnatural (or difficult) births of twins, stillbirths, and births with severe pain, with respect to the difference in the period of care they would require. Amato's *scholia* raises questions about the standards by which a particular childbirth would be identified as unnatural and deserving of a longer 'incubation' period. It shows that such standards were invariably as cultural as they were medical.

Women as Healers

Amato's medical case also opens a window onto the array of practitioners making determinations about health and care practices. As the narrative unfolds, we learn that Amato was not actually the patient's main caregiver. Although he observed and conversed with the woman to some extent, he gathered most of the necessary information from the *mulierculae assistentes* that cared for her. In fact, reading backward from the information Amato receives from these women, we learn that they stayed with her at night, changed her clothes, checked her bleeding, monitored her fever, and gave her food. They were also the ones who decided that a priest should be summoned because they feared that she was possessed by an evil spirit. Amato did not criticize this decision. In fact, despite the diminutive occupational marker with which he identified them, his relationship with the women appears to have been a collaborative one.[2] He relies on their care and judgment and seems to see them as important mediators. Furthermore, this nursing role appears in several other cases in the *Centuriae*, mostly of women patients but likely also with regard to men. We are told later in the case that Amato stopped treating a melancholic Jewish youth from Ferrara because the *assistentes* thought exorcism would be more fruitful. It is clear, then, that the women at the bedside maintained some level of authority in providing and even orchestrating care.

2 Similar usage appears in ancient sources. See Flemming, 'Gendering Medical Provision in the Cities of the Roman West', 277.

By pursuing subtle clues like these, this volume demonstrates the vast, largely hidden extent of women's agency and authority in providing healthcare in myriad settings. As caregivers for the sick, beguines and other religious women were engaged in a range of healthcare duties that included the administration of both physical and spiritual remedies. This form of work is usually assumed to have been taught through imitation and via oral modes. In other words, the practical, experiential knowledge embodied in this work is viewed in stark contrast to academic medical knowledge. By expanding the kind of sources traditionally construed as the basis of medical teachings, Sara Ritchey invites us to rethink this disparity. She convincingly argues that prayer books owned by beguines reflect an embedded understanding of the notion of the six 'non-naturals' imperative for the preservation of health according to Galenic medicine. Through prayers, hymns, and images, beguines learned, participated in, and provided affective performances that aimed to generate emotional and spiritual wellbeing in the sick and dying. Since both medieval medicine and devotion attributed salubrious qualities to hope and faith, traditional disciplinary divisions imposed on the work performed by beguines fail to encompass the complexity of their healthcare roles.

Iliana Kandzha makes a similar intervention when she centres relics as healthcare technologies and points to the important role of communal, as opposed to individual, caregiving. Departing from the beaten path in studying miracle collections, Kandzha reveals a fertility cult developing around St. Cunigunde's material remains. This therapeutic use of relics for a specific medical issue maps a network of healing knowledge propagated by persons who possessed some authority and experience. Since this was a cult of a female saint sustained by female devotees, it was a network that blurred the distinction between healthcare providers and their recipients or patients. Replacing the binary image of patient and healer with a more communal sense of healing, in which individuals practised mutual healthcare (perhaps in correspondence with their place in the life cycle), could offer new understandings of how medical knowledge was produced and circulated, as well as documenting women's varied roles within that economy.

By embracing an integrative approach to healthcare, the essays in this volume reveal previously unrecognized swathes of health practitioners, sites of caregiving, and care practices. For example, Eva-Maria Cersovsky surveys gendered perceptions of care through the renditions of a biblical proverb (Sirach 36:27). The religious and secular literary tradition she traces defined wives as being responsible for their husbands' wellbeing, thereby making the wife analogous to a nurse caring for the sick. She shows how this ancient biblical tradition became naturalized over time into an expectation that women were more suited to be compassionate household caregivers. Cersovsky's analysis emphasizes the entrenched nature of these ideals and allows a glimpse into the seams of cultural construction of the traditional role of women as caregivers. Cordula Nolte's essay examining German autobiographical narratives, family records, and images provides the nitty-gritty detail of domestic caregiving and its setting. By recognizing that health was not simply the opposite of illness but rather a condition that demanded ongoing attention and maintenance, Nolte implicates everyday tasks, such as emptying chamber pots and tending beds, as essential components of healthcare. Her essay subtly problematizes the boundaries of care, showing that much of female servants' work can be categorized as bodywork owing to its intimate nature. This is not the case for the work performed by male servants, who are less likely to be described as carrying out such tasks. Here payment becomes a tool of analysis, in which the lists of wages compiled by German householders and civic authorities reveal contemporary valuations of health-related employment. The information Nolte assembles, along with her attention to social status, suggests the need for a comparative history of economic exchange visible in 'bodywork' – one that would include even the unpaid labour of seasonal or ad hoc care provided by neighbours and householders.

Several of the essays in this volume expose the processes of knowledge exchange and empirical testing conducted among female agents of care within domestic settings. For example, Sheila Barker and Sharon Strocchia's study of Caterina Sforza's *ricettario* charts the way that this feminine role could be channelled and managed as part of a larger medical economy. Their study of Sforza's enormous recipe collection shows its author's vast storehouse of empirical knowledge, her authority over others, and her agency in facilitating knowledge transfers across the Italian peninsula. Sforza's expertise both mirrored and complemented the role played by court physicians in caring for household members and visiting dignitaries alike. At the same time, her fame as an erudite maker and broker of medicinal recipes enabled her to form and maintain political ties, indicating the extent to which healthcare was bound up with an array of historical developments.

Other, less renowned women (and men) actively participated in producing medical knowledge on various scales. The essays by Belle Tuten, Julia Gruman Martins, and Ayman Yasin Atat explore the translation and transmission of recipe collections that deal with female maladies to some extent. The geographical span (the Ottoman Empire to England), linguistic range (Arabic, Ottoman Turkish, Latin, Italian, French, and English), and chronological breadth (twelfth to seventeenth centuries) of these three essays suggest the expansiveness of remedy collections as a genre. We learn that these texts were constantly evolving, with translators and copyists amending and expanding them to suit their audience and in line with their own judgment about the efficacy of certain remedies. Thus it is clear that, as a household genre, these recipe collections did not carry the same authorial weight as university treatises. Even when these compendia imported recipes from well-known authorities such as Ibn Sīnā or Bernard de Gordon, they were regarded as malleable knowledge that invited testing and adaptation. Indeed, one wonders about the extent to which Amato's *mulierculae assistentes* may have modified the remedies he prescribed in the course of everyday care. The amalgam of topics included in these collections, ranging from magic tricks to medicinal recipes, reminds us once again that boundaries between healing categories and activities were not innate. In documenting the many emendations made to recipe collections by various historical actors, these essays signal the need to reassess the personal authority of both household caregivers and learned physicians in actual practice. More importantly, they showcase the fact that premodern medical knowledge was anything but static, that ideas, practices, and personnel circulated throughout guilds, university classrooms, courts, domestic spaces, religious houses, and marketplaces.

By prompting us to rethink the boundaries between categories, the study of women's healthcare also reconfigures our understanding of premodern healthcare more broadly. Sara Verskin, for example, clearly establishes that Arab physicians treated women and conducted intrusive, 'immodest' examinations of their reproductive parts. This analysis demands not only a reimagining of medical markets, but also a rethinking of the balance between religious ideals and healthcare needs that conditioned interactions between the sexes in these societies. It also suggests the extent to which women and medical men could exchange knowledge about the female body, even when the evidence for that exchange must be read indirectly. Verskin's observations correspond with similar insights offered by Tuten, Gruman, and Atat, which reveal that both men and women were involved in the transmission and emendation of recipe collections; they also correlate with Amato's testimony of collaboration with the *mulierculae.*

Amato Lusitano and the *mulierculae assistentes* were both healthcare practitioners in sixteenth-century Europe. Thus far, only Amato has enjoyed a place in traditional historical reckonings of the history of healthcare and health knowledge. Yet in their society, they both held recognized healthcare 'roles', to use the conceptual terminology of sociologist Joseph Ben David.

Ben David recognized, in his 1964 *The Scientist's Role in Society*, that 'the persistence of a social activity over long periods of time, regardless of changes in the actors, depends on the emergence of roles to carry on the activity and on the understanding and positive evaluation ("legitimation") of these roles by some social groups'.[3] The formation of a role, he argued, was essential 'for the transmission and diffusion of the knowledge, skills and motivation pertaining to a particular activity and for the crystallization of all this into a distinct tradition'.[4] The essays in this collection show that in the medieval and Renaissance past, such legitimation was not only reserved for male physicians. Female caregivers carried the 'activity' of care over time and it involved 'transmission of knowledge, skill and motivation'.

Ben David's study was concerned with 'pure' science in its positive sense: discovery, innovation, advancement. Its focus was the institutional structures that clustered around legitimized roles and bolstered their innovations and discourse. He devoted, for example, a chapter to the rise of the universities and to the environment these institutions provided for the scientists of the day to elaborate and refine their knowledge. Amato Lusitano, along with most medical authors mentioned in this volume, was part of this relatively new system of formalized authority. To a large extent, they defined how we think of medicine and medical care, even though their theories, as we have seen, were often flexible and culturally imbued. But the *mulierculae assistentes* and their generation and transmission of knowledge has been left out of this progressive narrative of health and healing. Nevertheless, we can use the sociological concept of 'roles' to examine the gendered history of health and healing more broadly. While the role of women in healthcare still largely remains in the shadows of more institutionalized caregiving, Ben David's institutional approach may allow us to consider the structures, whether formal or informal, that upheld the public role of female healers.

The essays in this volume make room for additional roles and their production of knowledge in the medieval and Renaissance medical economy. They chart a divergent path from the historical pursuit of a progressive narrative and the reliance on sources that conform to a strictly disciplinary form of knowledge. This volume is therefore an important step in reconstructing anew the non-institutionalized social structures in which a range of women – the *mulierculae* who treated the melancholic parturient, the beguines, Caterina Sforza, St. Cunigunde – provided important healthcare resources. As noted in the volume's Introduction, the challenge now is to

3 Ben David, *Scientist's Role in Society*, 16-17.

4 Ibid., 17.

conceptualize disparate sources. Alongside the endeavour of assembling information on particular women and groups of women, it is essential to begin reassembling a broader narrative of healthcare that is inclusive of considerations of gender. The essays in this volume eloquently map potential avenues for retelling the history of medicine in a different light. As the essays suggest, these narratives must bridge disciplines, geographies, and faith traditions; they must be more integrative and inclusive. By daring to seek and identify recurring patterns of practices, learning, transmission, compensation, and ideas, we may be able to fill the gaps of an ephemeral, sparsely documented, past.

Works Cited

Printed Works

Amatus Lusitanus. *Curationum medicinalium, centuriae II priores* [...] (Lyon: Apud Gulielmum Rouillium, 1567).

Ben David, Joseph. *The Scientist's Role in Society: A Comparative Study* (Englewood Cliffs, NJ: Prentice Hall, 1971).

Flemming, Rebecca. 'Gendering Medical Provision in the Cities of the Roman West', in *Women and the Roman City in the Latin West*, ed. Emily Hemelrijk and Greg Woolf (Leiden: Brill, 2013).

Fontoura, Paulo. 'Neurological Practice in the *Centuriae* of Amatus Lusitanus', *Brain: A Journal of Neurology*, 132.2 (2009), 296-308.

Friedenwald, Harry. 'Amatus Lusitanus', *Bulletin of the History of Medicine*, 5.7 (1937), 603-53.

Pomata, Gianna. 'Sharing Cases: The *Observationes* in Early Modern Medicine', *Early Science and Medicine*, 15 (2010), 193-236.

About the Author

Naama Cohen-Hanegbi is Senior Lecturer in Medieval History at Tel Aviv University. She is the author of *Caring for the Living Soul: Emotions, Medicine and Penance in the Late Medieval Mediterranean* (2017) and co-editor (with Piroska Nagy) of *Pleasure in the Middle Ages* (2018).

Contributors

Ayman Yasin Atat received his PhD in the History of Medical Science from Aleppo University in 2014 and is currently Philipp Schwartz Fellow in the Department for History of Science and Pharmacy at Technische Universität Braunschweig (Germany). He is an expert on Arabic, Ottoman, and Islamic medicine, and Arabic medical manuscripts.

Sheila Barker directs the Jane Fortune Research Program on Women Artists at the Medici Archive Project (Florence). Her publications include 'Artemisia Gentileschi in a Changing Light' (2017) and 'Cosimo I de' Medici and the Renaissance Sciences: "To Measure and to See"', in *The Brill Companion to Cosimo I de' Medici* (2019).

Montserrat Cabré is Professor of the History of Science at the University of Cantabria, Santander (Spain), and director of the Office for Gender Equality and Social Responsibility. Her research focuses on medicine and sexual difference as well as on women's health practices in the Middle Ages.

Eva-Maria Cersovsky is completing her PhD dissertation on healthcare, charity, and gender in fifteenth- and sixteenth-century Strasbourg at the a.r.t.e.s. Graduate School for the Humanities, Cologne. She co-organized the international workshop, 'Gender(ed) Histories of Health, Healing and the Body, 1250-1550', held at the University of Cologne in January 2018 that forms the basis of this volume.

Naama Cohen-Hanegbi is Senior Lecturer in Medieval History at Tel Aviv University. She is the author of *Caring for the Living Soul: Emotions, Medicine and Penance in the Late Medieval Mediterranean* (2017) and co-editor (with Piroska Nagy) of *Pleasure in the Middle Ages* (2018).

Iliana Kandzha is a PhD candidate at Central European University. Her dissertation examines the medieval cults of the royal virgins St. Henry and St. Cunigunde, with an emphasis on their political and social dimensions. She received her BA in History from the Higher School of Economics in Moscow and an MA in Medieval Studies from Central European University.

Julia Gruman Martins is a PhD candidate at King's College London. Her thesis focuses on the translation of 'secrets of women' in early modern

Europe, especially from Italian into French and English. She holds a joint Master's (honours) degree from the University of Bologna and the University of Paris VII.

Cordula Nolte is Professor of Medieval History at the University of Bremen. Her main research fields are gender studies, early medieval Christianization, and princely families and courts. Recently she has focused on the history of the body and on dis/ability history. In 2017 she co-edited the first interdisciplinary and international companion on premodern dis/ability.

Catherine Rider is Associate Professor in Medieval History at the University of Exeter. Her research focuses on the history of medicine, reproduction, magic, and popular religion in the later Middle Ages. She is the author of *Magic and Impotence in the Middle Ages* (2006) and *Magic and Religion in Medieval England* (2012).

Sara Ritchey is Associate Professor of History at the University of Tennessee, Knoxville, and is author of *Holy Matter: Changing Perceptions of the Material World in Late Medieval Christianity* (2014) and a forthcoming book on late medieval religious women's therapeutic knowledge and healthcare practices (2021).

Fernando Salmón is Professor of the History of Science in the medical school at the University of Cantabria, Santander (Spain). His research focuses on medieval medical scholasticism and he is currently general editor of the *Arnaldi de Villanova Opera medica omnia* (AVOMO).

Sharon Strocchia is Professor of History at Emory University in Atlanta. A social and cultural historian of Renaissance Italy, she has published widely on women, religion, and health-related topics. Her most recent book is *Forgotten Healers: Women and the Pursuit of Health in Late Renaissance Italy* (2019).

Belle S. Tuten is Charles A. Dana Professor of History at Juniata College in Huntingdon, Pennsylvania. Her work concentrates on views of the female breast in medieval medicine and culture.

Sara Verskin is the author of *Barren Women: Religion and Medicine in the Medieval Middle East* (2020). She holds a PhD in Near Eastern Studies from Princeton University and teaches history at Rhode Island College.

Index